THIRD EDITION

Periodontics

J D Manson

M.Ch.D., Ph.D., F.D.S.R.C.S.

Senior Lecturer in Periodontology, Institute of Dental Surgery; Hon. Consultant, Eastman Dental Hospital, London

581 illustrations on
325 figures

HENRY KIMPTON PUBLISHERS
London 1975

106 Hampstead Road, London NW1

First edition 1966
Second edition 1970
Third edition 1975

ISBN 0 85313 788 9

Filmset and printed in Great Britain by
BAS Printers Limited, Wallop, Hampshire

To My Wife

Preface to the Third Edition

Although many important questions about the nature of periodontal disease have yet to be answered our understanding of the subject has grown considerably since the conception of the first edition.

In that time changes in practice and attitudes have taken place, culminating in the development of programmes of preventive periodontics. The needs of the profession have changed therefore and in this edition I have attempted to bring the material up to date so that it can be used by both undergraduate and the interested practitioner. This has involved an almost complete revision of the text, and in this task I have been helped by Mr W. I. R. Davies, Senior Lecturer in Periodontology at the Royal Dental Hospital School of Dental Surgery, who has revised the chapters on occlusion. Along with these changes I have modified the title of the book.

Some mention should be made about terminology. The words 'intrabony' and 'infrabony' are used as in the second edition: more controversial I have used the term 'gingival crevice' rather than 'gingival sulcus' to avoid confusion with the vestibular sulcus.

In rewriting this text I have been helped by many people and I hope that I will be forgiven for not mentioning everyone by name. In the body of the text I have acknowledged my debt to those workers who have allowed me to use or copy their material. I would like to express my gratitude to my colleagues at the Eastman Dental Hospital and especially my friends in the department of periodontology, Dermot Strahan, Ian Waite and Vivian Ward, whose brains I have picked unashamedly.

I would also like to thank Mr W. J. Morgan and the staff of the photographic department, Eastman Dental Hospital, for new photographs.

My especial thanks go to Ian Davies for undertaking the burden of revising the chapters on occlusion, and to Miss Jennifer Middleton for the new drawings.

J.D.M.

Contents

1. Health and Disease

The masticatory apparatus is the first part of the digestive system. Its primary function is the physical breakdown of food so that chemical breakdown is facilitated. Two basic components of this apparatus have evolved, a cutting tool and a locomotor system which brings the cutting parts into effective action. As the diet of all highly evolved animals varies in composition and consistency a sophisticated masticatory mechanism has evolved which can produce the necessary movements and pressures under complete control. This control is effected by neurological feedback systems which also protect the functioning tissues from the stresses involved in this activity.

During evolution many forms of dentition have appeared which vary from the simple and disposable cone-like teeth of the tortoise, which are little more than keratinized thickenings of a moving belt of oral mucosa to the highly sophisticated continuously erupting molar teeth of the guinea-pig. The attachment of tooth to jaw also appears in numerous forms such as the simple fibrous ligament of the shark, and the hinge system of the hake which allows the ingress of food but prevents its escape. In the eel there is an early alveolar process, a bone of attachment on which the single cusp of tooth is perched and which develops with each tooth to be resorbed when its tooth is discarded. The crocodile provides an early example of gomphosis, the system of tooth attachment in Man, where the tooth has a root which is socketed in the alveolar process of the jaw. In Man the tissues which attach the tooth to and support it in its socket, called the periodontal tissues, also contain the proprioceptors of the neuromuscular system which help control the movements of the mandible.

One other important function is served by the periodontal tissues, and that is tissue renewal as tooth substance is worn away by function. All animals in health maintain a functional dentition for life. In the lower animals, fish and reptiles, this is achieved by the continuous development of successional teeth. In a rodent such as the guinea-pig there are a limited number of teeth but these erupt continuously and tissue formation at the apex of the root keeps pace with wear from the functioning surface. As the animal grows the diameter of each tooth increases and as the molar teeth are made up of convoluted layers of enamel, dentine and cementum, the system of tooth formation is highly complex and by comparison makes the system in Man look very primitive indeed.

The two dentitions of Man are meant to span a life-time, and apart from the protective and repair systems inherent in all vital tissue the attachment system is protected from the oral environment by a vital seal, the dento-gingival junction. This is unique in the body. It is the only junction of mineralized and non-mineralized tissue which is exposed to the external environment, and as such is a weak link in the integrity of the oral integument.

Organism – Environment

Every organism exists in a continually changing environment. The temperature, humidity and atmospheric pressure, for example, may change from hour to hour, the amount of sun-light from minute to minute. The quantity of water and of various dietary constituents consumed, and the amount of work performed, varies daily. Health represents the ability of the organisms to function efficiently in such changing and often more extreme conditions.

This tendency for an organism to maintain its integrity within a constantly changing environment is known as homeostasis. Natural selection ensures that those forms disappear which cannot adapt successfully to their environment.

In any attempt to comprehend the behaviour of tissue in health and disease it is necessary to understand the nature of the interaction between tissues and their environment. This can be seen as a state of balance between the internal environment of the organism and its external milieu. Small changes in either system make little demands on the metabolism; small adjustments allow function to proceed normally. Large changes in either the internal or external milieu may upset the balance so that normal function cannot be maintained and tissue changes take place which manifest themselves at a clinical level, *i.e.* as disease.

Individuals vary in their ability to adapt to any given environmental factor. No two individuals are completely alike. There are always differences in general appearance, face, height, behaviour and in the adaptive and regenerative powers of the tissues. Each individual has his own spectrum of adaptability which is termed loosely his 'constitution'. Each tissue possesses a threshold beyond which it fails to adapt to changes in its environment, and suffers changes that interfere with its function. This threshold is not immutable. A multitude of factors alter the ability of the tissues to perform in standardized fashion to a given situation. For example, changes in diet, or in endocrine function such as occur in adolescence, pregnancy or menopause, will alter the way in which the tissues behave, and may lower the threshold of tissue resistance so that an irritant which might normally fail to induce tissue damage may then do so. Factors in immediate contact with a tissue, *i.e.* local factors such as micro-organisms or physical trauma which might be dealt with adequately by the healthy tissues may be able to cause tissue damage when systemic changes occur, and while one local factor may not be sufficient to cause tissue damage its presence might render the tissue incapable of dealing with a second local factor. Thus the overt signs and symptoms of disease are the manifestation of a summation of environmental and host factors. The breakdown of the periodontal tissues must be seen in the same way.

In some individuals tissue breakdown is rapid in the face of apparently little irritation, in others breakdown is negligible although obvious irritation is present. When overt disease is recognized as the end-product of an aggregate of factors this variation becomes more understandable.

A number of defences protect the functioning of tissues:

(i) *the gross anatomy* of the system, as for example the spinal column protecting the spinal cord or proximal tooth contact protecting the interdental gingiva.

(ii) *the integument* provides a vital and mechanical barrier of epithelium which can become increasingly keratinized with function, or increasingly pigmented when exposed to ultra-violet light.

(iii) *surface secretions* such as the lactic acid of vaginal secretions protect against intestinal flora, or saliva with its lysozyme and antibody content.

(iv) *the immunological system* of which the most obvious manifestation is the local inflammatory response.

These systems will be discussed in this text. The essential idea, one which is central to an understanding of the behaviour of tissues, is that of *balance* in the interaction between the organism and its environment. A broadly based system such as occurs in the healthy adult is difficult to upset, a precarious balance such as exists in the diabetic patient can be tipped by a small change in either the internal or external milieu. In the control of periodontal disease it is essential to ask why the tissue in an individual is behaving in a particular way. To answer this question an attempt must be made to identify the many factors involved. This necessitates dealing with the complete individual. To ignore this fact is to invite inevitable failure in understanding the disease process and thus its correction and control.

Periodontal Disease

The mouth provides a unique environment. The oral tissues are exposed to a veritable bombardment of both chemical and physical stimulae, as well as the metabolism of about thirty species of oral bacteria. (The total salivary bacterial count is said to be five thousand million per millilitre of saliva!) Yet for the most part, oral tissues, other than dental tissues, remain healthy.

The tooth-supporting or periodontal tissues appear to be particularly vulnerable. Breakdown of these tissues in the human adult is virtually universal. An understanding of the ecology of the mouth and of the biology of these tissues is essential to prevention of this breakdown and to effective treatment once breakdown has occurred.

Like all other tissues the periodontal tissues are subject to a number of pathological changes; inflammatory, degenerative and neoplastic.

The disease process may be restricted to the gingivae or may involve the deeper periodontal structures, thus inflammation of the gingivae is gingivitis; inflammation of the deeper periodontal tissues is periodontitis. The pathology of the periodontal tissues has been subject to numerous forms of classification based largely on the interpretation of clinical manifestations, and unfortunately not on an understanding of the tissue changes involved. This has given rise to unnecessary complexity and confusion.

Neoplasia of the periodontal tissues are comparatively rare and are not discussed in this text. Degeneration of elements of the periodontal tissues is found under certain situations such as disuse but organ degeneration such as occurs in the myeloid liver is not found.

Inflammation, both acute and chronic, is the principal process involved in pathology of the tooth-supporting tissues. Acute gingivitis is usually associated with specific infection or injury. Acute periodontitis is frequently due to a blow on a tooth, or is a complication of chronic periodontitis. Chronic gingivitis and chronic periodontitis represent the main problems in periodontology, and indeed of dentistry, and form the main subject of this text.

2. The Periodontal Tissues in Health

The Dental Unit

The tooth and its supporting tissues may be regarded as a unit having an edge hard enough to cut food, and a shock-absorbing system which takes up the stresses of mastication. These stresses, which vary considerably in intensity and direction, represent part of the input of a feed-back mechanism which controls the activity of the muscles of mastication. (Fig. 1). The tooth-supporting tissues are invested in oral mucosa, the gingiva.

The surface of the dental unit is smooth and streamlined (Fig. 2). The gingiva forms a tight collar around the neck of the tooth so that contiguous areas of tooth and gum form an almost unbroken surface. In mastication the bolus is crushed and shed across the labial and lingual surfaces of tooth and gum to be returned by cheek and tongue activity to the space between the occlusal surfaces of the teeth. The form of the dental unit is such that the vulnerable junction between hard tooth tissue and soft tissue is protected from injury as food is shed. This junction between tooth and gum is a comparatively delicate and highly specialized mechanism which must be protected from irritation and injury. The marginal ridges and contact points between teeth are so placed that in food-shedding the food is deflected past the interdental papilla (Fig. 3). The convex curvature of the buccal and lingual surfaces of the teeth protect the buccal and lingual margins (Fig. 4).

The tooth-supporting tissues with their investment of oral mucosa constitute the periodontium. Four tissues make up the periodontium: the gingiva; the periodontal ligament; the cementum; and the alveolar process.

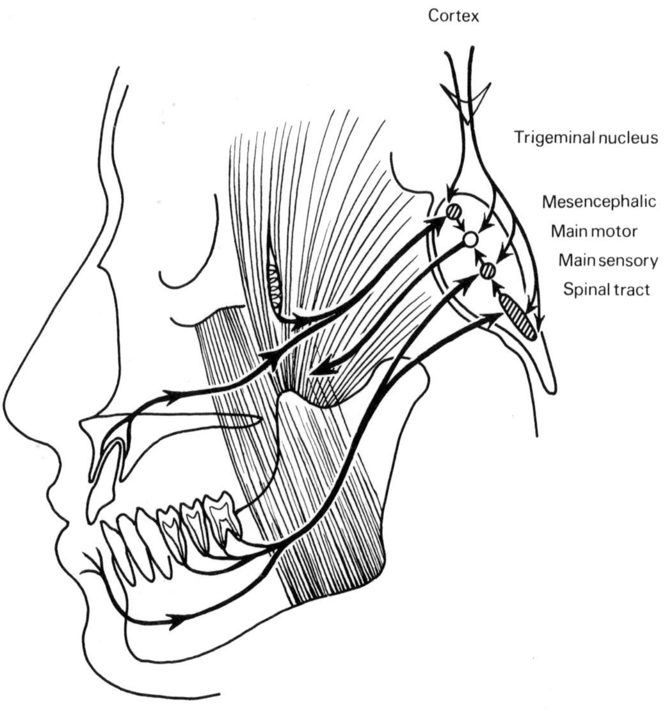

FIG. 1.—Diagram of the masticatory apparatus. The tooth-attachment system forms part of the neuro-muscular mechanism.

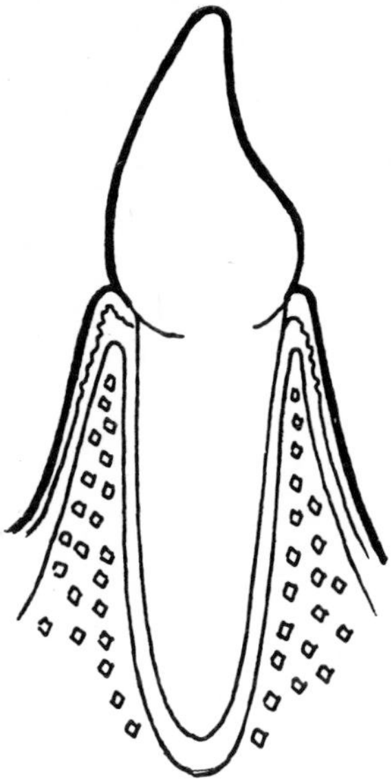

FIG. 2.—The dental unit consists of the tooth and its supporting tissues.

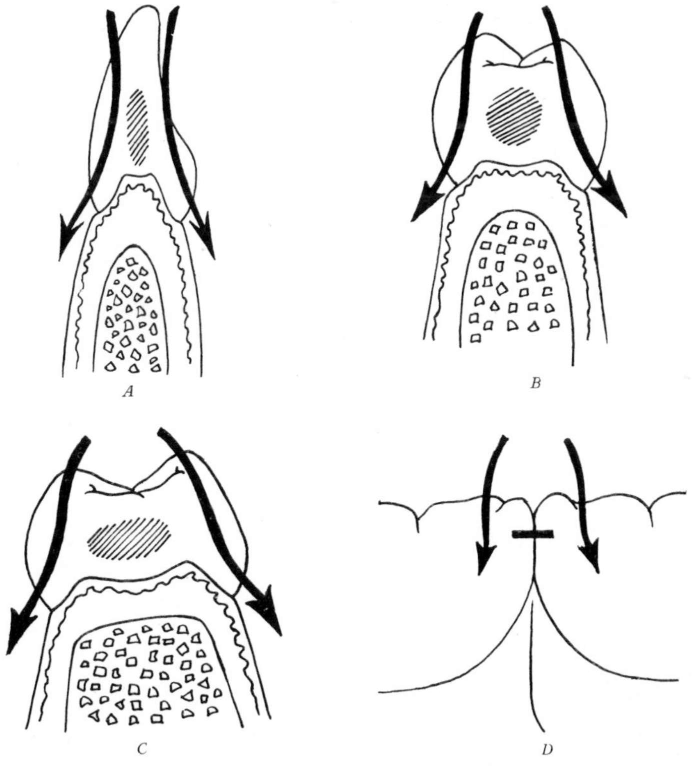

FIG. 3.—Marginal ridges and contact points act in food-shedding to deflect the food past the interdental papilla. The shape of the papilla conforms to that of the contact area between the teeth, while the alveolar bone margin tends to follow the line of the amelo-cemental junction. (*A*) incisor; (*B*) premolar; (*C*) and (*D*) molar.

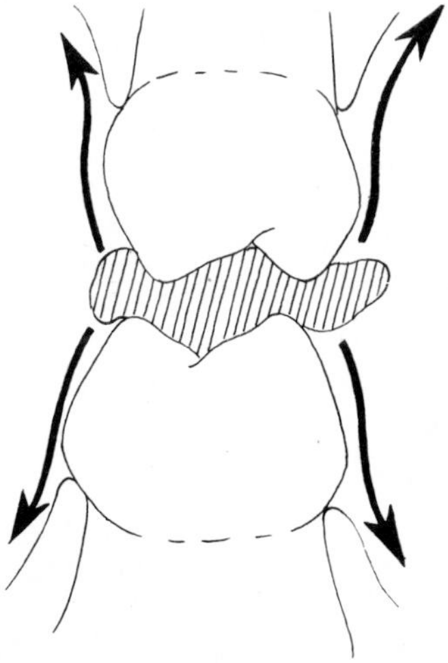

FIG. 4.—The convex curvature of the buccal and lingual tooth surfaces protect the gingival margins in food-shedding.

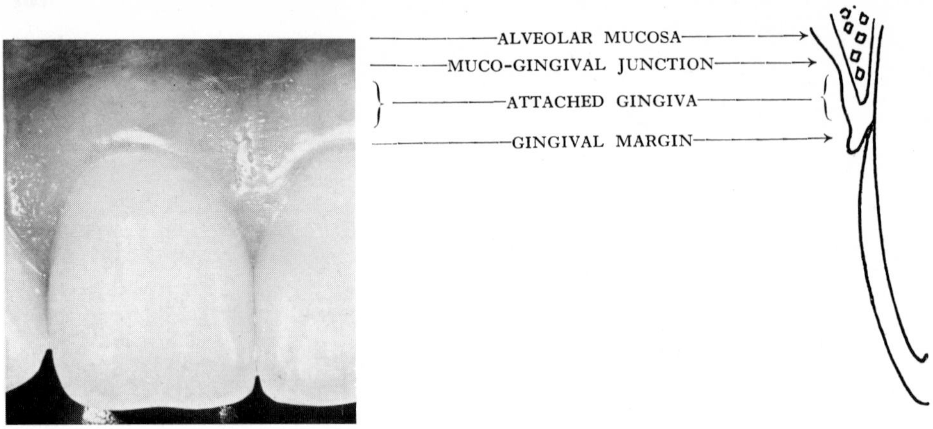

FIG. 5.—Illustration of the terms used in describing the periodontal mucosa.

The Gingiva

The gingiva is that part of the oral mucosa which is bound down to tooth and to the alveolar process, and which extends from the gingival margin to the muco-gingival junction where it joins the more loosely bound alveolar mucosa (Fig. 5). In health the gingiva is pink, firm, knife-edged and scalloped to conform to the contour of the teeth (Fig. 6).

The colour of the gingiva varies in light-skinned individuals, and in dark-skinned people physiological melanin pigmentation may be found as diffuse brown or grey-blue patches (Fig. 7).

The interdental papilla fills the space between the teeth apical to the contact area, and its shape conforms to that of the contact area thus forming the interdental col. The shape of the papilla varies slightly according to the shape and relationship of the teeth; its surface is grooved by an interdental sluiceway (Fig. 8).

The gingiva is divided into two zones, the gingival margin and the attached gingiva.

The Gingival Margin

The gingival margin is a pink, firm and smooth collar of tissue which surrounds the teeth and from which it may be separated by a thin blunt probe. It is 1–2 mm wide and is delineated from the attached gingiva by a shallow groove, the free gingival groove. The gingival margin forms the external wall of the gingival sulcus or crevice which is 0–2 mm in depth. Microscopically the

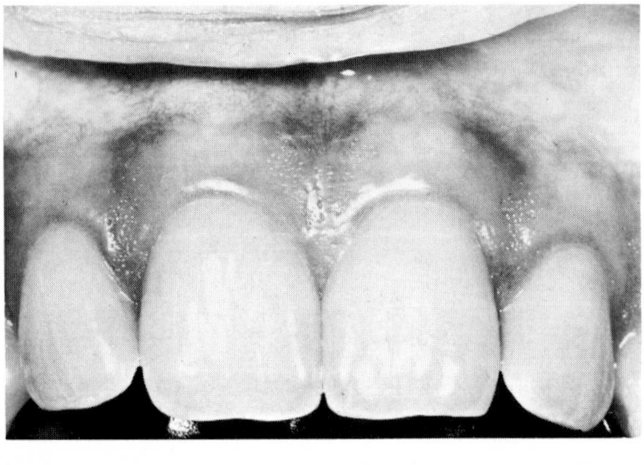

FIG. 6.—Healthy gingivae in a 20-year-old woman.

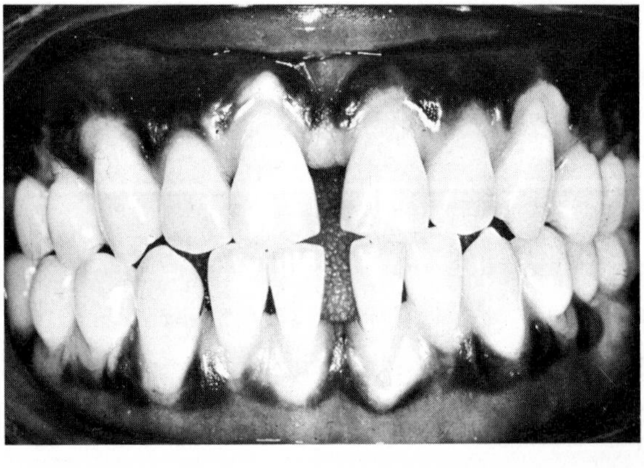

FIG. 7.—Physiological pigmentation in the gingivae of a West Indian.

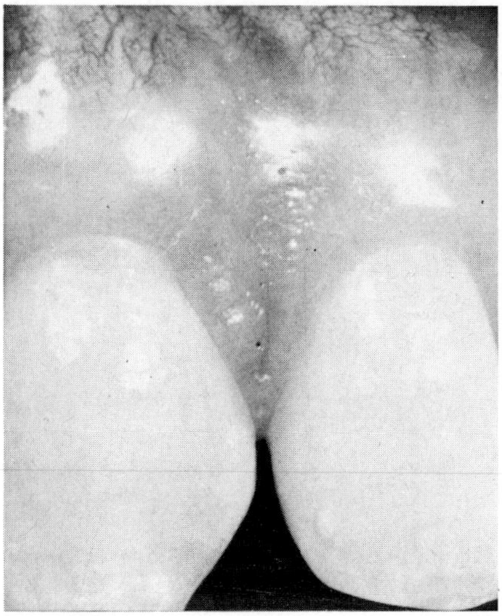

FIG. 8.—The interdental papilla in health fills the space between the teeth and its shape conforms to that of the teeth.

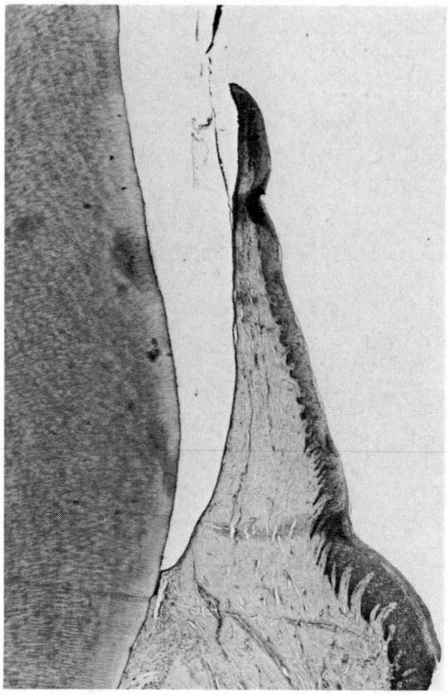

FIG. 9.—Normal gingival cuff in monkey. (By courtesy of Professor B. Cohen.)

gingival margin consists of a core of connective tissue covered by stratified squamous epithelium. The epithelium of the outer exposed surface and crest of the margin demonstrates the characteristic rete peg arrangement and basal cell, prickle cell, granular cell and keratinous layers. The inner surface of the gingival margin is covered by a narrower layer of non-keratinized epithelium, with no rete pegs (Fig. 9).

The difference in morphology of the two sides of the gingival margin appears to reflect the differences in their environment and in particular the presence and absence of mechanical stimulus on the external and internal surfaces respectively.

Attached Gingiva

The attached gingiva is a muco-periosteum tightly bound down to the alveolus between the gingival margin and the mucogingival junction. At this junction which is usually clearly demarcated (Fig. 10), the mucoperiosteum splits and the alveolar mucosa is separated from the alveolar periosteum by loose and vascular areolar connective tissue and muscle. The epithelial surface of the attached gingiva is stratified squamous and may be keratinized. The attached gingiva is firm, pink and unlike the gingival margin is characterized by its stippled or orange peel surface. The stippling is produced by elevations and depressions of the epithelium which may represent an adaptation to function: it does not appear to represent points of special fibrous attachment to the underlying bone. The width of attached gingiva varies considerably. It is usually greatest in the incisor region (3.5–4.5 mm) and narrowest in the first premolar region where it may be under 2.0 mm (Ainamo and Löe, 1966). This zone of firm

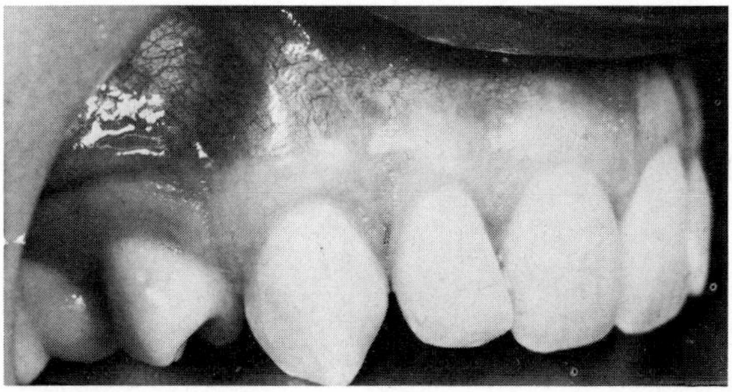

FIG. 10.—There is a clear demarcation between the tightly bound attached gingiva and the highly vascular alveolar mucosa.

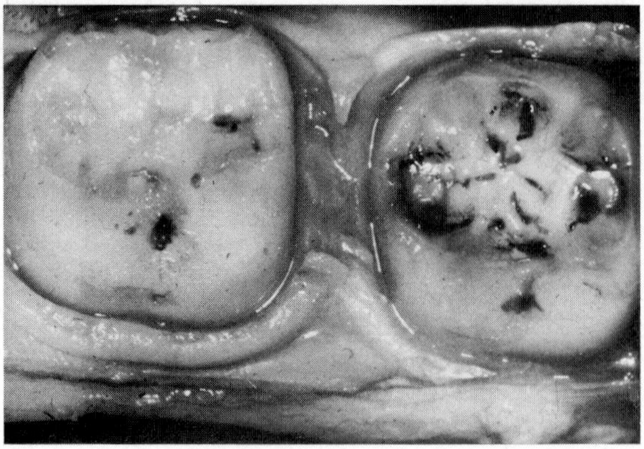

A

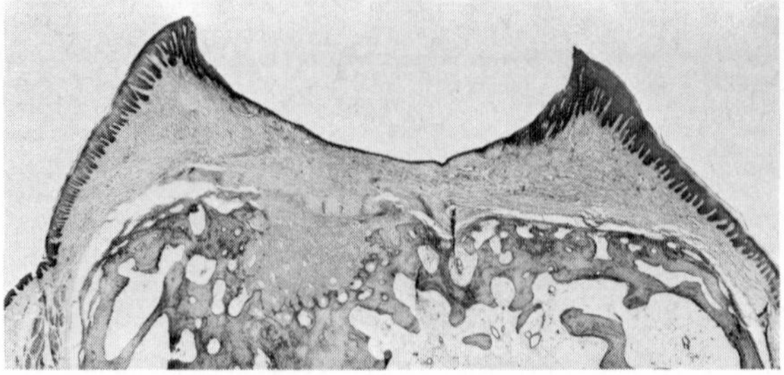

B

FIG. 11.—(*A*) The interdental col seen in a human specimen of mandible which has been decalcified to remove the enamel. (*B*) Section of the interdental col of monkey. (By courtesy of Professor B. Cohen.)

mucoperiosteum appears to separate the vulnerable dento-gingival junction from the mobile tissues of the buccal and lingual fornix.

The gingival epithelium, like all epithelium, undergoes constant renewal. The turnover time for the cells is said to be 10–12 days (palate, tongue, cheek 5–6 days) (Beagrie and Skougaard, 1962).

The Interdental Gingiva

The gingiva between the teeth was first described in detail by Cohen (1959) as a 'col' which joined the buccal and lingual papillae and which conformed to the interproximal shape of the juxtaposed teeth apical to the contact point (Fig. 11). According to Cohen, at eruption and for some months or years after eruption the col is covered by persistent reduced enamel epithelium which is said to be thin and fragile and with limited reproductive and therefore repair capacity, so that in the period before it is replaced the interdental area is particularly susceptible to injury and infection.

However, this idea has been disputed (McHugh, 1971) and it is now generally believed that the col is covered by oral epithelium very soon after tooth eruption. Autoradiographic studies show that epithelial cell turnover in this area is similar to that of epithelium covering other parts of the gingiva, *i.e.* 10–12 days. Col epithelium is certainly thin being made up of only a few layers of cells; this probably reflects the sheltered position of this tissue (by the same token this is also the area of persistent bacterial stagnation).

The Gingival Corium

The connective tissue of the gingiva is a dense network of collagen fibres with some reticulin fibres but few elastic fibres. Next to the epithelium the connective tissue forms papillary projections carrying vessels and nerves between the epithelial rete pegs so that a very large contact area between the two tissues is formed (Fig. 12). Connecting the epithelium and connective tissue is a basal membrane 300–400 Angstroms thick. This consists of two layers, a lamina lucida and lamina densa, and hemidesmosomes of basal epithelial cells

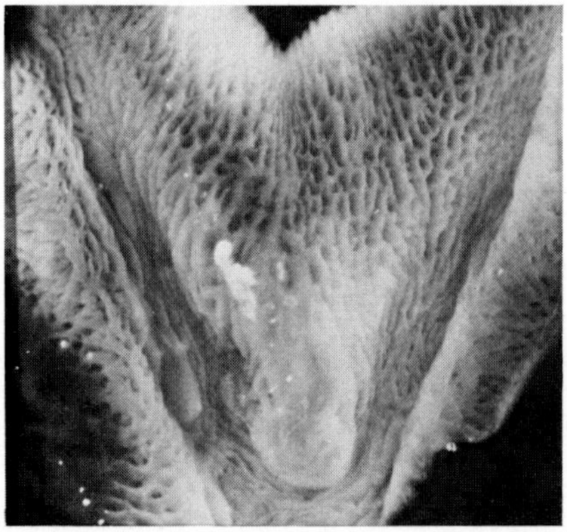

FIG. 12.—Photograph of the undersurface of the epithelium of an interdental papilla of young adult monkey showing boundary architecture between epithelium and connective tissue providing a large surface area and blood supply. (By courtesy of Professor R. D. Emslie.)

extend into the lamina lucida. The basement membrane is permeable to fluid but appears to be impermeable to particulate matter.

The collagen fibre bundles are organized into a number of fibre bundle groups which keep the gingival margin firm and tight around the neck of the tooth. These have been ascribed names according to their general orientation under the microscope. They are usually described as dento-gingival, alveolo-gingival, circular and transseptal fibre groups (see Arnim and Hagerman, 1953).

The dento-gingival fibres fan out from the cementum coronal to the alveolar margin to the crest of the gingiva, to the facial and lingual gingival surfaces, and also extend over the alveolar margin to the periosteum of the attached gingiva (Fig. 13*A*). The alveolo-gingival fibres form a small group of fibres which arise from the alveolar crest and run coronal in the lamina propria of the gingival margin (Fig. 13*B*).

The circular group of fibres encircle the tooth and the transseptal fibres extend from one tooth to another above the alveolar crest (Figs. 13*C* and 13*D*). Glenwright (1970) has described 'longitudinal' fibre bundles which run horizontal completely around the arch along the facial and lingual gingiva both coronal and apical to the alveolar crest (Fig. 13*C*). These arrangements are by no means as simple as the descriptions imply for there is considerable decussation between groups.

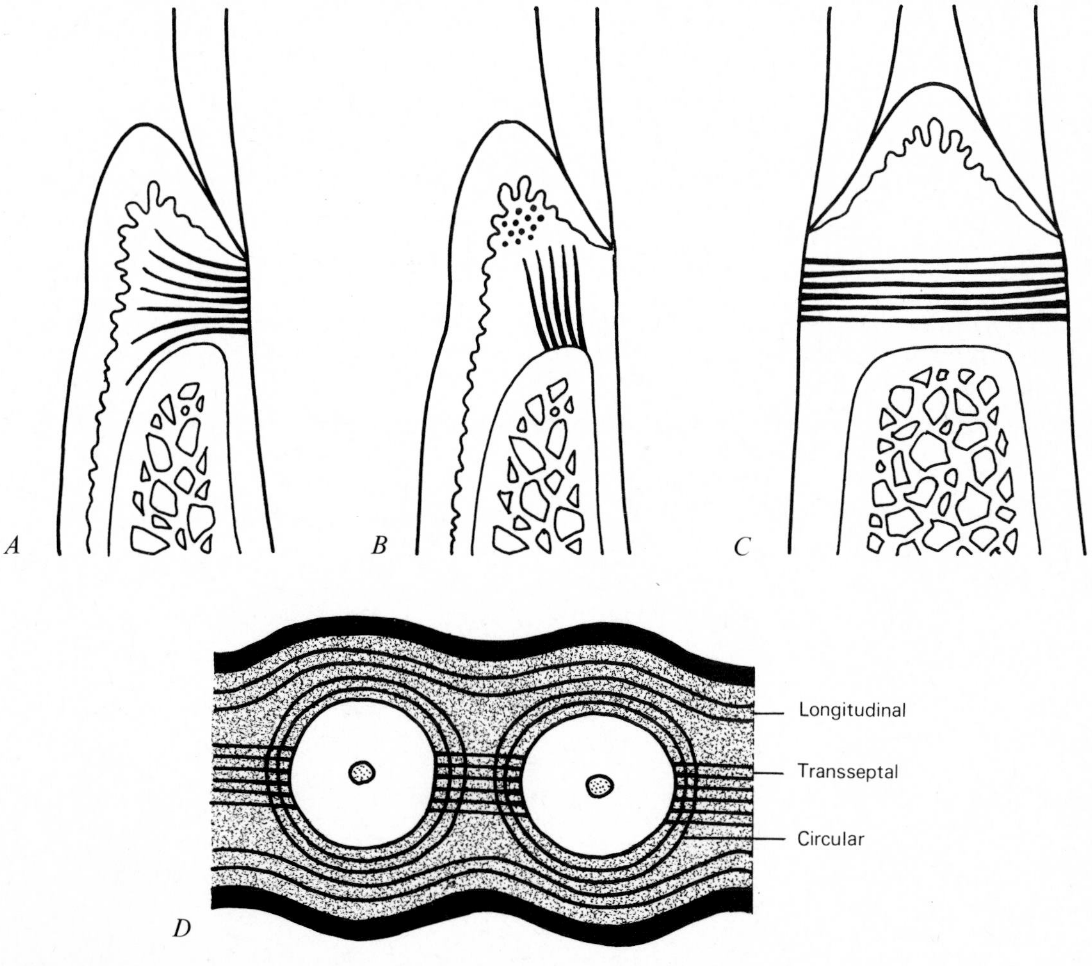

FIG. 13.—Diagrammatic representation of the gingival fibre groups.
(*A*) Dento-gingival fibres. (*B*) Alveolar crest fibres and in cross-section circular fibres. (*C*) Transseptal fibres. (*D*) Cross-section to show transseptal fibres, circular fibres and longitudinal fibres.

Cells of the Gingival Corium

Apart from the principal cells of fibrous tissue, the fibrocyte and fibroblast, several other cells are found as normal inhabitants of the tissue. Many of these cells are associated with chronic inflammation and their presence has given rise to the idea that no gingiva is free of inflammation. Lymphocytes and plasma cells are found most commonly in groups near the base of the crevicular epithelium. Lymphocytes mediate the immune response by storing information about antigens: plasma cells produce antibodies. It was thought that their constant presence represented a response to the oral bacteria and their products. However, these cells are found in the corium of the gut soon after birth (Crabbé, Carbonera and Heremans, 1965) and would appear to represent part of the normal immunological system which is activated as soon as an organism comes into contact with its environment, *i.e.* at birth.

Mast cells are found in oral mucosa and gingiva. They contain histamine, proteolytic enzymes and heparin which appear to play a part in the development of inflammation and in bone resorption. Polymorphonuclear leucocytes are also seen migrating through the intercellular spaces of the sulcular epithelium to be found in great numbers in saliva. All these cells increase in number in inflammation at which time monocytes, polymorphonuclear leucocytes and eosinophils migrate from the blood-stream.

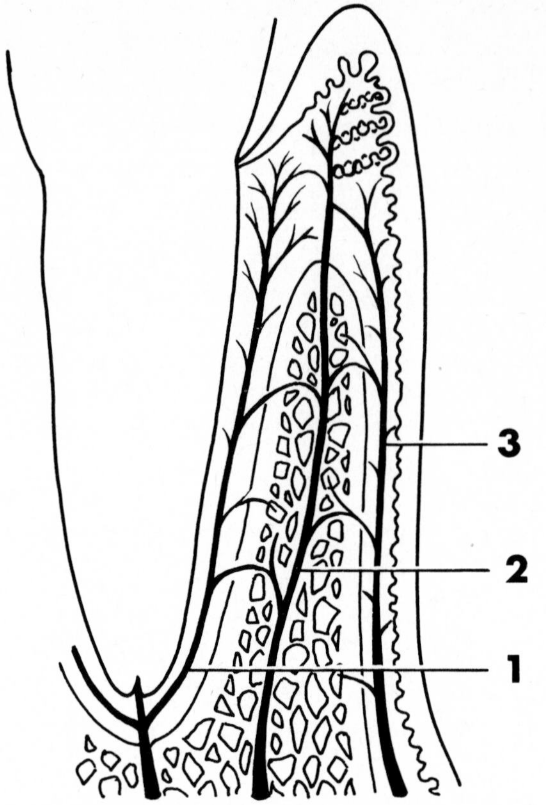

FIG. 14.—Gingival blood supply has three anastomosing sources: (1) Vessels from the periodontal ligament. (2) Vessels from the alveolar process. (3) Supraperiosteal vessels.

Gingival Blood Supply

The gingiva has a rich blood supply which stems from three sources (Kindlova, 1965) (Fig. 14).

1. Supra-periosteal vessels pass over the buccal and lingual surfaces of the alveolus to the gingiva. Some branches of these vessels pass through the bone to the periodontal ligament.
2. Vessels pass from the crest of the alveolar process.
3. Vessels extend from the periodontal ligament.

There is anastomosis of the capillaries from these sources. These capillaries form loops in the papillae of connective tissue between the epithelial rete pegs (Karring and Löe, 1967). Capillaries also lie parallel to the tooth surface below the crevicular epithelium. A network of lymph vessels has been identified; these drain into regional lymph nodes. A variety of nerve structures have also been identified, including specialized nerve endings such as Meissner corpuscles and Krause corpuscles.

The Dento-gingival Junction

The nature of the relationship between the tooth and the gingiva has been debated for over half a century and many ideas have been put forward.

In 1921 Gottlieb described an 'epithelial attachment'. He believed that this is formed by the union of the stratum intermedium of the reduced enamel epithelium and oral epithelium when the tooth erupts. The reduced enamel epithelium, the remnant of the ameloblast layer, is organically attached to its product, the enamel, and the epithelial attachment is similarly attached (Fig. 15). The ideal depth of the gingival crevice is therefore zero. In eruption the tooth moves in an occlusal direction with the united epithelium moving down the tooth surface towards the

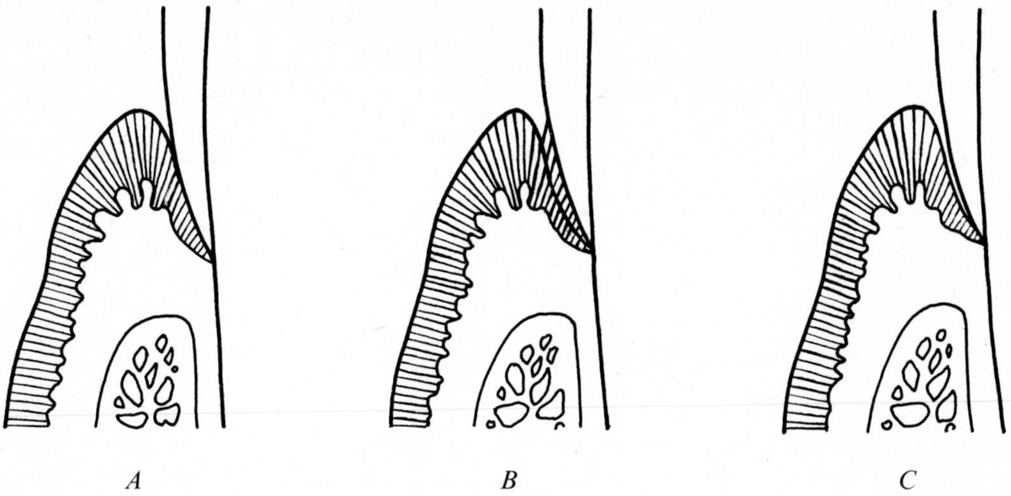

FIG. 15.—Diagrams to illustrate some theories about the nature of the dento-gingival attachment.
(*A*) Gottlieb: organic epithelial attachment to enamel and shallow gingival crevice. (*B*) Weski: split in epithelial attachment produces gingival crevice. (*C*) Waerhaug: crevicular epithelium lines, tight gingival cuff. No attachment to enamel and deep gingival crevice.

amelo-cemental junction. Gottlieb further postulated that the occlusal movement of teeth continued for life together with a continuing but very slow apical migration of the epithelial attachment (passive eruption). Weski (1922) and others contested this interpretation of the histological appearance and stated that the gingival crevice is formed by a split in the epithelial attachment rather than an epithelium separation from the tooth (Fig. 15*B*). Becks (1929) also contended that the reduced enamel epithelium degenerates and takes no part in the formation of the epithelial attachment.

In 1952 Waerhaug disputed Gottlieb's theories, and maintained that there is no organic epithelial attachment to the enamel. He stated that the gingival margin forms a cuff which is tightly apposed to the tooth surface but from which it can be separated down to the amelocemental junction by a very thin probe, *e.g.* a mylar strip (Fig. 15*C*). Thus in children the gingival crevice around the partially erupted tooth may be 10 mm deep while around the fully erupted tooth it is 1–2 mm deep.

The dispute stemmed essentially from the limitations of the light microscope. Clinically one can certainly probe a deep gingival crevice in children, which reduces with tooth eruption, but the microscopic appearance of a decalcified section of the dento-gingival junction often indicates that the soft tissue–hard tissue relationship is more intimate than mere apposition. The split in the epithelium described by Weski occurs very frequently and points to considerable tension on the epithelium during histological preparation. Also specially prepared non-decalcified sections of the dento-gingival junction demonstrate an intimate relationship between the surfaces of the enamel and the epithelium of the gingival crevice (Weinreb, 1960). This and other evidence persuaded Orban (1956) to produce a compromise between these views, and he put forward the idea of an 'attached epithelial cuff'.

More recently the electron microscope has allowed detailed examination of non-decalcified material showing the intimate relationship of the enamel and the gingiva. The nature of related cellular activity has been investigated by autoradiography, and tissue culture work has provided information about the characteristics of epithelial cells.

Using the electron microscope Schroeder and Listgarten (1971) presented a very detailed picture of the dento-gingival junction which is different from that put forward by either Gottlieb or Waerhaug. Schroeder and Listgarten have retained the term 'epithelial attachment' while giving it a completely different meaning.

These investigators describe the gingival epithelium as consisting of three components, 1. oral epithelium, 2. sulcular (or crevicular) epithelium, 3. junctional epithelium (Fig. 16). The oral epithelium extends from the muco-gingival junction to the gingival margin. The sulcular epithelium forms the wall of the gingival sulcus or crevice and extends from its junction with the gingival margin apically to the base of the crevice where it joins the junctional epithelium. The latter extends from the base of the crevice down the surface of the tooth to which it is attached by its basement lamina. The junctional epithelium extends 2–3 mm on the enamel coronal to the enamel-cementum junction except where there is gingival recession when it is located on cementum.

Electron microscopic examination reveals a basement lamina at the junction of epithelium and the underlying connective tissue. It is a product of the epithelial cell and is composed of two layers, a lamina densa (350–600 Å wide) and a lamina lucida (300–500 Å wide). Hemidesmosomes are epithelial cell surface structures which join adjacent epithelial cells to form desmosomes – the 'spines' of the spinous layer of epithelium (Fig. 17). At the basement lamina hemidesmosomes join epithelial cells to the connective tissue and the junctional epithelium to the tooth surface.

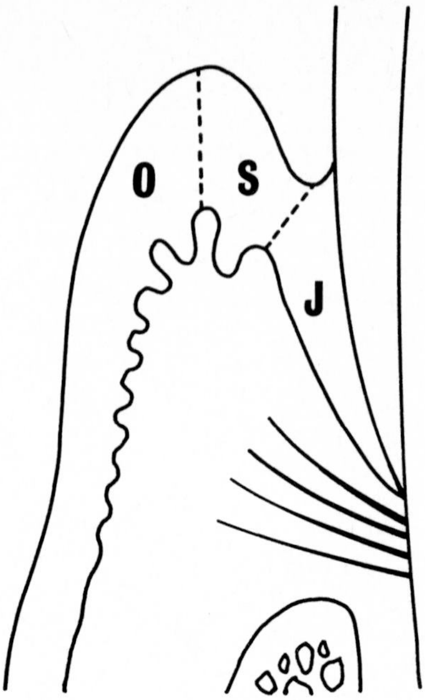

FIG. 16.—Dento-gingival junction according to Schroeder and Listgarten. J—junctional epithelium attached by basement lamina and hemi-desmosomes to enamel. S—sulcular epithelium. O—oral epithelium.

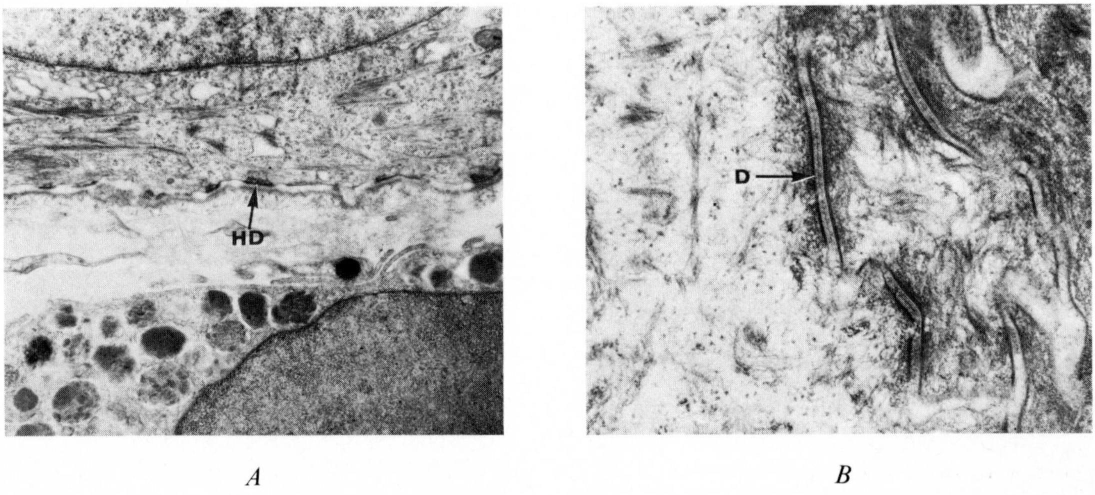

FIG. 17.—Electronmicrographs of oral mucosa showing (*A*) Hemidesmosome (HD) between epithelium and connective tissue. (*B*) Desmosome (D) connecting epithelial cells. (By courtesy of Dr N. El-Labban.)

This basement lamina plus the related hemidesmosomes is the 'epithelial attachment'. It is thought that the apical portion of the junctional epithelium is derived initially from reduced enamel epithelium, while its coronal aspect and sulcular epithelium derives from oral epithelium; subsequent renewal of the junctional epithelium is achieved by a flow of cells from the oral epithelium (Fig. 18). If the gingival epithelium is completely removed by surgery new oral, sulcular and junctional epithelia are all reformed from oral epithelium and a new basement lamina with hemidesomosomes attach the junctional epithelium to the tooth surface whether on enamel, dentine or cementum.

Crevice Depth

According to Listgarten (1972) the intercellular spaces of junctional epithelium are larger than those of oral epithelium, and frequently contain large numbers of leucocytes. The junctional epithelium is therefore very fragile and does not provide a firm barrier against probing. Thus while the histological crevice may be 0.5 mm deep the clinical crevice as measured by probing is deeper as the probe may disrupt cells and actually penetrate the junctional epithelium (Fig. 19).

The depth of penetration of an instrument into the gingival crevice must depend on the pressure applied, probe thickness and the integrity of the tissue as determined by the degree of inflammatory infiltration of the junctional epithelium and adjacent connective tissue. Thus the epithelial attachment to the tooth is stronger than the bond between the cells of the junctional epithelium. If this is indeed the case the variety of observations made by earlier workers would appear to be reconciled. Gottlieb's attachment, Weski's split and Waerhaug's crevice represent factors of the method of examination of the dento-gingival junction. However in referring to the gingival crevice it is essential to distinguish between the clinical crevice and the histological crevice.

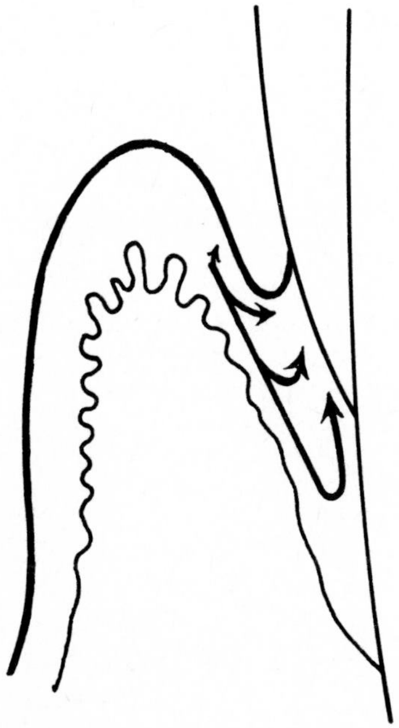

FIG. 18.—Epithelial cells produced in the broad germinal layer migrate to the surface to be shed from the constricted (sulcular) area of junctional epithelium. (After Dr M. Listgarten.)

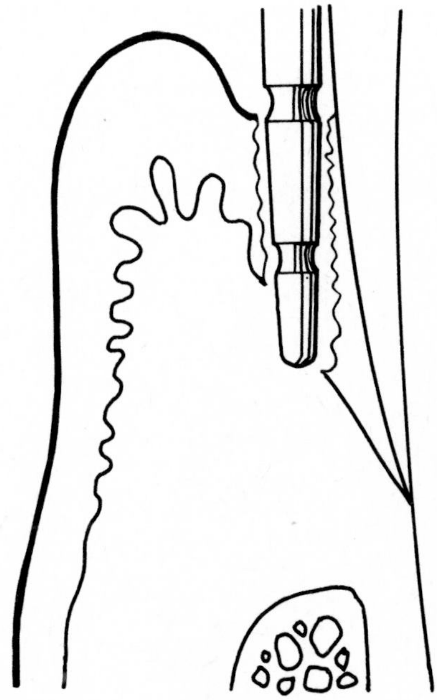

FIG. 19.—Diagram to show difference in depth between the shallow histological crevice and the clinical crevice when blunt pocket measuring instrument disrupts fragile junctional epithelium. (After Dr M. Listgarten.)

There is constant renewal of the gingival epithelium including the junctional epithelium, but whereas desquamation from oral and crevicular epithelium takes place from a surface similar in area to the area of the germinal or basal layer, the desquamation of junctional epithelium appears to be concentrated in the small area at the apical end of the gingival crevice (Fig. 18).

The junctional epithelium is also relatively permeable. It has been shown that proteins (Tolo, 1971) and enzymes (McDougall, 1971) which cannot penetrate keratinized gingival epithelium can diffuse through junctional epithelium. A growing body of evidence points to a two-way movement of elements through the junctional epithelium; leaving the tissues are leucocytes and gingival fluid while a variety of substances largely from the flora of the oral cavity enter the tissue (see Chapter 3).

Gingival Fluid

When foreign particles are introduced into the gingival crevice they are quickly washed away. The passage of fluid from the crevice was first demonstrated by Brill and Bjorn (1959). When the dye fluorescein is administered by mouth or intravenous injection it soon appears in the gingival crevice and even in bacterial deposits or calculus if present. Diffusion in the opposite direction, *i.e.* into the tissue, is demonstrated by the fact that carbon particles are absorbed from the crevice into the underlying corium (Brill, 1959). The outward flow of fluid is stimulated by the insertion of filter paper strips into the crevice and by chewing, and it is greatly increased when inflammation is present. It is debatable whether this fluid flow is physiological, *i.e.* a defence fluid, or is a product of inflammation. The flow of fluid occurs before the clinical manifestations of gingivitis appear, but it contains polymorphonuclear leucocytes (Löe, 1961). Electrophoretic analysis has shown at least seven plasma proteins are present and the concentration of various inorganic ions is similar to that of serum: in this respect it resembles an inflammatory exudate. Also it may have antimicrobial properties (Cowley, 1966).

Löe and Holm-Pederson (1965) state that in completely healthy gingiva no fluid can be collected on filter paper strips. In their experiment filter paper is placed over the mouth of the crevice while other workers collect fluid by placing the strip in the crevice and probably thereby stimulate the flow of liquid. It seems quite irrelevant to debate whether the presence of fluid is a sign of disease if it can be regarded as an immediate response to gingival irritation and part of the dento-gingival junction defence system. Indeed if health is defined in dynamic terms rather than static terms, *i.e.* as the ability of the tissues to react adequately to a changing environment, then the prompt production of gingival fluid on irritation would seem to be a proper and therefore healthy response.

THE PERIODONTAL LIGAMENT

The periodontal ligament attaches the tooth to its socket, supports the tooth under a variety of functional stresses, and may even cope adequately with powerful forces such as those operating in tooth-grinding or clenching. It can within limits adapt itself to changes in this stress system. The periodontal ligament is composed mainly of bundles of collagen fibres which are attached to cementum on one side and the alveolar process on the other (Fig. 20). The fibre bundles are arranged in a complex manner and are usually described as being in groups (Fig. 20*B*).

1. Alveolar crest fibres which run diagonally from the neck of the tooth to the alveolar crest.
2. Horizontal fibres running perpendicularly between tooth and the margin of the socket.
3. Oblique fibres running from the bone in a slightly apical direction to the tooth. These form about two-thirds of all bundles.
4. Apical fibres which radiate from around the tooth apex to the base.
5. Interradicular fibres, *i.e.* transseptal fibres in the furcations of multirooted teeth.

Thus the main orientation of the fibre bundles is such that an axial force on a tooth is most effectively absorbed. Masticatory forces have a considerable lateral component which produces slight tipping of the tooth about its fulcrum near the midpoint of the root (Fig. 21).

In histological section bundles of collagen fibres follow a wavy course from cementum to alveolar bone. The fibres are not elastic but because they are not normally fully extended they allow a limited physiological tooth movement within the socket. The fibres cannot be traced all the way

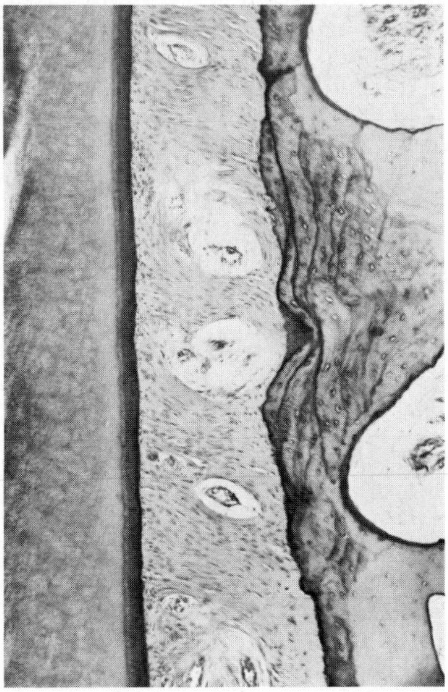

A

B

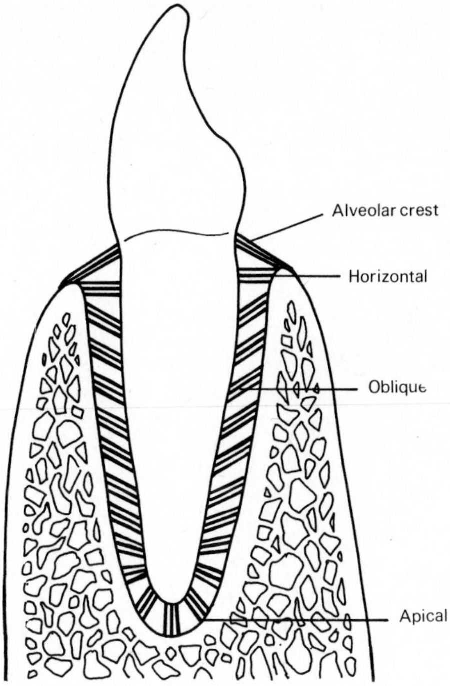

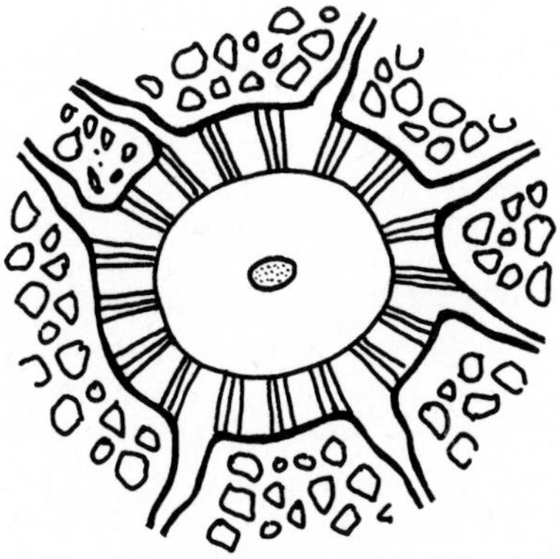

C

FIG. 20.—(*A*) Principle periodontal fibre bundles (human). Cementum – left; bone – right. (*B*) Diagram to show general arrangement of periodontal ligament fibre bundles. (*C*) Cross-section diagram of tooth and socket to show radial arrangement of periodontal fibre bundles.

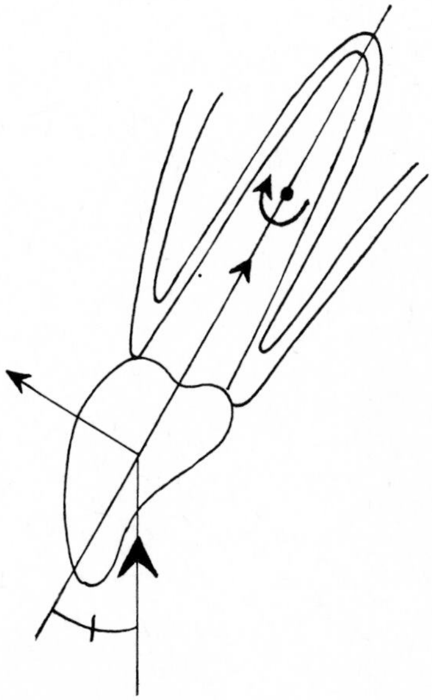

FIG. 21.—The axial and lateral components of a functional force producing a slight rotation of the tooth about its fulcrum.

from the cementum to their insertion into the alveolar bone as Sharpey's fibres. At about the mid-section of the ligament the fibres appear to interweave in an 'intermediate plexus' and it was thought that here splicing of the fibres takes place which permits a rearrangement of fibres during eruption and in response to changes in function. This may be the case with teeth of continuous eruption; however, there does not appear to be any extra cellular activity in the intermediate region which would mediate this fibre rearrangement and it seems likely that the intermediate plexus merely represents the crossing over of fibres travelling in different directions as seen in two-dimensional histological section. Spindle-shaped fibroblasts are aligned along the length of the collagen fibres, and between fibre bundles vessels and nerves run in loose connective tissue.

The periodontal ligament has a rich anastomosing blood supply which penetrates the cribriform plates at many points (Fig. 22). Thus there is an intimate connection between the blood supply to the trabecular spaces and the periodontal space. Trigeminal nerve bundles pass into the ligament from the periapical region and the alveolar bone following the course of the blood vessels. The nerves appear to terminate as free nerve endings or spindle-like structures. No other form of specialized proprioceptive receptors appear to be present.

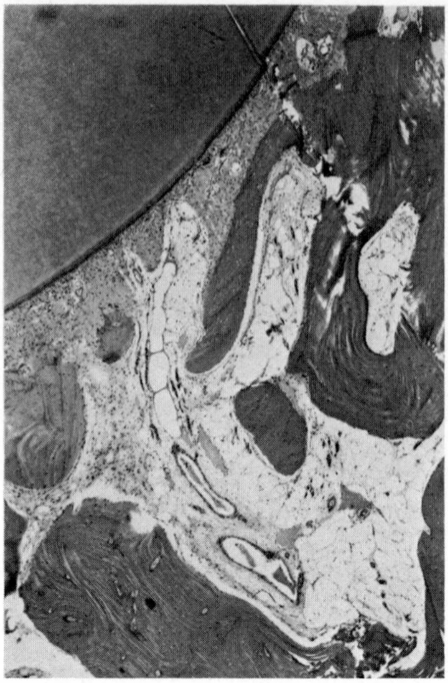

Fig. 22.—Horizontal section showing a large thin-walled vessel linking the periodontal ligament and trabecular space.

Other cellular elements found in the periodontal ligament include macrophages and the epithelial rests of Malassez which are remnants of the Hertwig root sheath.

The structure of the ligament is affected by age and function. In normal function it is 0.25–0.1 mm thick. It has an hourglass shape, being narrowest at the level of the tooth fulcrum and widest at the alveolar margin and at the apex. When functional stresses are increased the ligament widens, fibre bundles become thicker and Sharpey's fibres increase in number and size. When stresses decrease, as when opposing teeth are absent, the ligament becomes narrower and the fibre bundles become thinner as the number of fibres reduces. The orientation of the bundles changes so that they become more parallel with the tooth surface. Because of this variation the width of the periodontal space cannot be used as a critical diagnostic tool. Nevertheless, marked enlargement of the space usually indicates a significant change in function. If subject to increased functional stress over an extended period the increase in width may be sufficient to be observed on the dental radiograph (Fig. 23).

There is a constant activity of connective tissue cells and turnover of collagen in the periodontal ligament. Radioactive proline can be seen to be taken up as collagen is synthesized (Carneiro and Fava de Moraes, 1965). At the same time collagen is being broken down and collagenese has been demonstrated in the tissue (Fullmer *et al.*, 1969). Thus the mechanisms for constant adaptation exist.

A special fibre, called the oxytalan fibre has been demonstrated lying at right angles to the principal collagen fibres (Fullmer and Lillie, 1958). Oxytalan fibres are said to be inserted into the bone and cementum. They may be elastic fibres but this is disputed. Groups of epithelial cells, epithelial rests (the debris of Malassez), are also found in histological section close to the cementum. They represent a mesh of epithelial cells, the remnant of Hertwig's sheath, which surrounds the root. Their function is unknown.

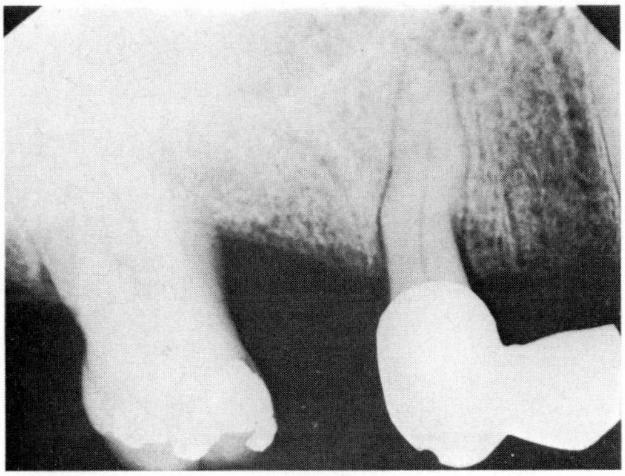

FIG. 23.—Widened periodontal space and funnelling of socket around tooth used as abutment.

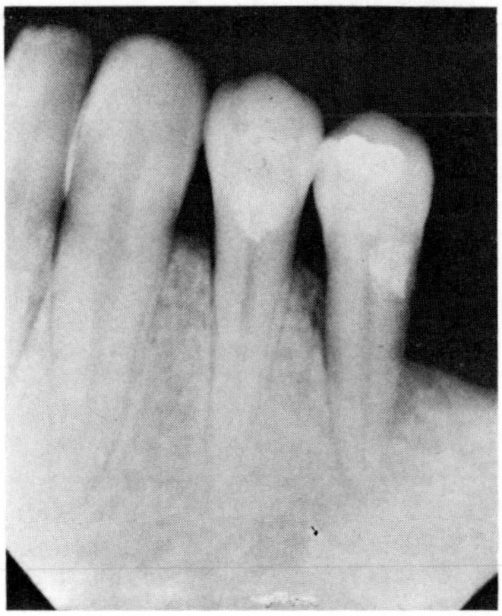

Periodontal Ligament Ground-Substance

The above structures, especially the principal fibres, are seen clearly in the light microscope and their obvious presence has dominated thinking about the function of the periodontal ligament. However, all these structures as well as nerve endings are embedded in a relatively amorphous mucopolysaccharide matrix, the ground substance. The importance of this matrix in tooth support is slowly being clarified and it seems possible that this together with the principal fibres provide a variety of mechanisms to absorb the many forms of stress to which the periodontium is exposed (Parfitt, 1967). These mechanisms are described in the Chapters on Occlusion.

Cementum

Cementum, like bone and dentine, contains hydroxypatite crystals deposited parallel to the collagen fibrils of the organic matrix. The inorganic content of cementum is similar to that of bone – about 40%. Cementum is found in an acellular and cellular form; the former does not contain cementocytes and appears as a thin and relatively homogeneous layer laid down by cementoblasts at the beginning of root formation. It is frequently restricted to the cervical portion of the root. In the formation of cellular cementum the cementoblast becomes embedded in the calcified matrix to become the cementocyte just as the osteoblast becomes the osteocyte. Canaliculi radiate from the cementocyte lacunae.

The collagen fibrils of cementum (and bone) are of two types. The principal fibres are periodontal fibres which can be traced from the periodontal ligament through the layer of cementoid (precementum) to be embedded as Sharpey's fibres in the calcified matrix. These are formed by fibroblasts of the periodontal ligament and gradually become embedded as more cementum is laid down.

The other fibrils form a dense meshwork in the cementoid and cementum matrix. In acellular cementum Sharpey's fibres are closely packed and for the most part completely calcified. In cellular cementum the Sharpey's fibres are more widely spaced; many are completely calcified while others retain an uncalcified core.

The cementum surface is formed into conical projections about single fibrils or bundles. Cementum spurs and tubercles are found as in bone where there is a direct insertion of a tendon or ligament.

From a structural point of view cellular cementum is very like bone, but unlike bone there is no evidence of cementum remodelling, *i.e.* a process of resorption and deposition which alters the form of the tissue without necessarily changing its volume. A single layer of well ordered cementoblasts line the cementum surface and cementum deposition continues throughout life (Zander and Hurzeler, 1958) but it is very slow so that even on the old adult tooth only a few incremental layers are evident. The greatest thickness of cementum is found at the apex and in the furcation area. With any occlusal movement of the tooth further deposition of the cementum in these regions takes place. Apical deposition takes place continuously together with deposition of bone at the alveolar margin as compensation for loss of tooth substance by attrition so that the vertical dimension of the face is maintained.

Cementum hyperplasia is occasionally found usually involving the apical third of the root. This may be associated with excessive occlusal stress or more commonly with pulp disease. Root resorption is also found as a consequence of excessive occlusal stress or chronic pulpitis and it seems possible that the difference in cementum response is associated with variation in the degree and kind of irritation. Areas of cementum resorption are frequently seen in tooth sections and while some of these do appear to be the result of excessive forces on the tooth the cause is not evident in most cases.

The relationship between enamel and cementum varies. In about 60% of teeth cementum overlaps enamel; in about 30% they abut, while in the rest there is a small gap between the cementum and enamel.

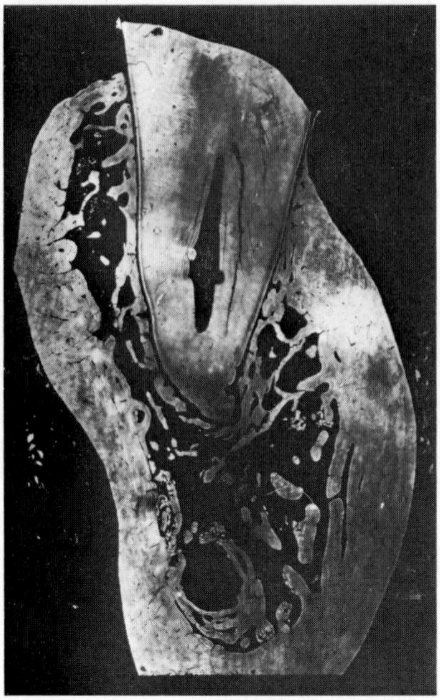

FIG. 24.—Microradiograph of undecalcified section of human mandible showing general morphology.

The Alveolar Process

The alveolar process is that part of the jaw which supports the teeth. It consists of trabecular bone within facial and lingual cortical plates (Fig. 24). The tooth socket, or cribriform plate, is a thin plate of bone perforated in many places so that a large number of vascular and neural connections are made between the periodontal ligament and surrounding trabecular spaces (Fig. 25). Fibres of the periodontal ligament are embedded as Sharpey's fibres in the socket wall. The Sharpey's fibres consist of bundles of parallel collagen fibrils. Some of these bundles (as in cementum) are completely calcified, others retain an uncalcified core.

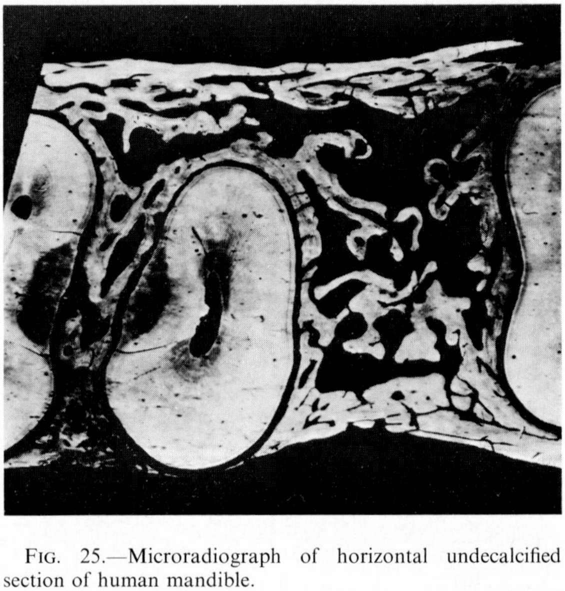

FIG. 25.—Microradiograph of horizontal undecalcified section of human mandible.

Note (*a*) irregularity of trabecular pattern; (*b*) variation of form of connection between periodontal space and trabecular spaces; (*c*) absence of cortical plate where root is placed to one side.

Alveolar Morphology

There is considerable variation in the morphology of the alveolar processes. Size, shape, thickness of cortical plates and interdental septa vary between individuals, between the maxilla and the mandible and in different parts of the same jaw.

The contour of the alveolar crest usually conforms to that of the root contours and the amelocemental junction, and any variation in tooth

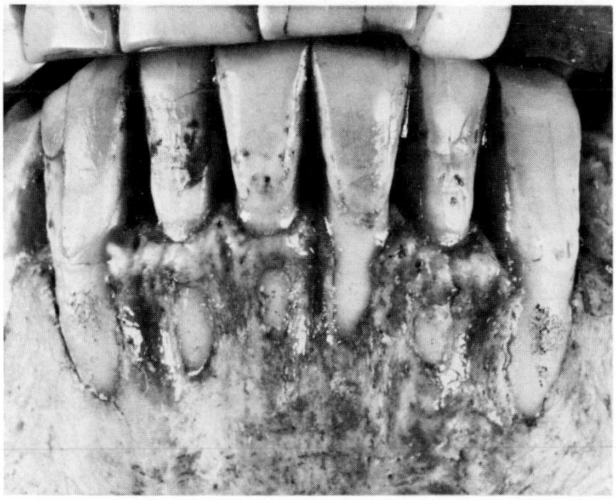

FIG. 26.—Dried skull of a young adult showing developmental faults in the alveolar bone.

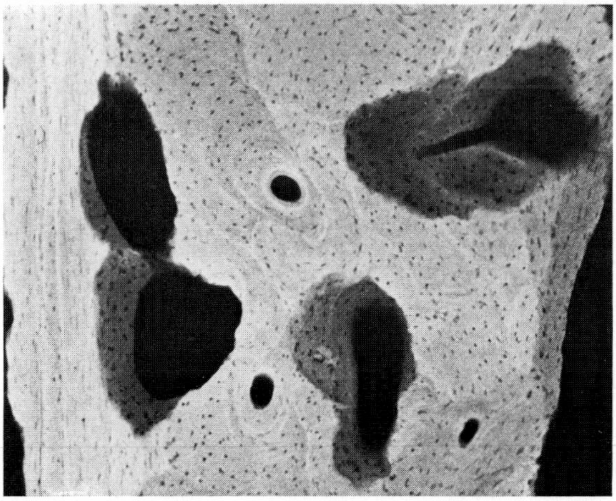

FIG. 27.—Microradiograph of undecalcified section of mandible from young individual showing considerable activity. Deposition is indicated by dark areas: resorption by crenated surfaces.

shape or alignment means some variation in bone contour. However, there seems to be a limit to the degree to which the bone conforms to variations in tooth position and morphology, and where a tooth or individual root is displaced out of the arch the facial or lingual plate may become very thin or even perforated so that fenestrations (circumscribed holes) or dehiscences (splits) are found (Fig. 26). With even moderate malalignment the bone margin may be apically placed so that the gingiva is not supported by bone. Where there is crowding and the roots of neighbouring teeth are close together (or even touching) the interdental bone is absent.

The shape of trabecular spaces and the connections with the periodontal spaces vary considerably (Fig. 25) and it seems reasonable to assume that spread of inflammation via vascular pathways is associated with bone morphology. These variations are very important therefore from a clinical point of view; they affect the course of the pathological process and therefore the treatment.

Bone Activity

As a tissue there is no difference between alveolar bone and any other bone. It undergoes constant remodelling, and like all bone it has two basic functions – to act as a mechanical framework, and as a reservoir of inorganic ions (Fig. 27). Cancellous bone is more reactive than cortical bone and has a faster turnover. In health the remodelling process maintains the total volume of bone at about the same level, but the pattern of tissue may change in response to changes in function. Remodelling activity is slightly greater in alveolar bone than in the body of the mandible and this difference probably reflects changes in functional stress, mesial drift, and occlusal movements which compensate for attrition (continuous eruption). Mesial drift is indicated by resorption of mesial surfaces of sockets and deposition on distal surfaces (Fig. 28).

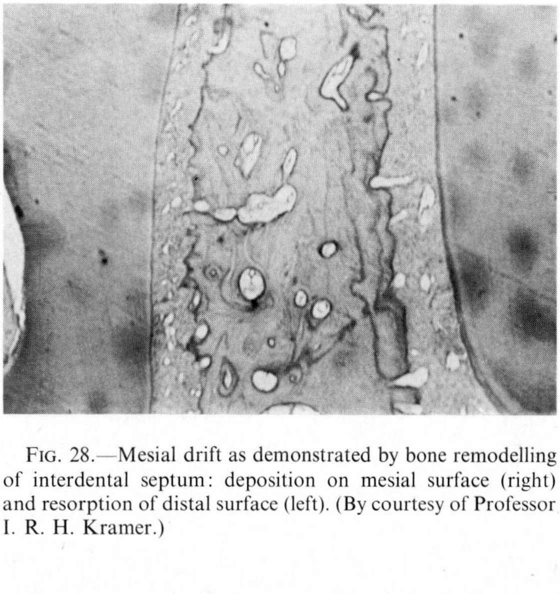

FIG. 28.—Mesial drift as demonstrated by bone remodelling of interdental septum: deposition on mesial surface (right) and resorption of distal surface (left). (By courtesy of Professor I. R. H. Kramer.)

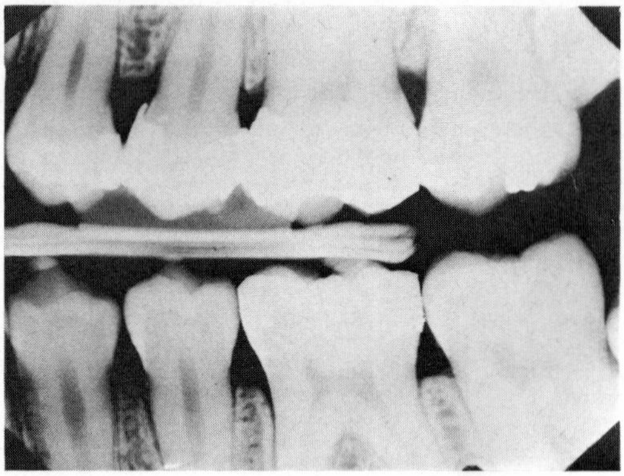

FIG. 29.—Healthy alveolar bone margin in a 17-year-old girl, showing the variation in appearance of the bone margin. Note the relative radiodensity of the flat-topped bone between the molars compared with that of the more convex crest between pre-molars.

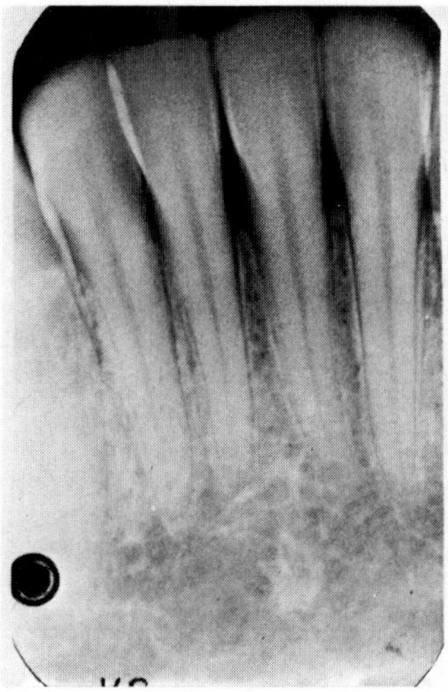

FIG. 30.—Healthy alveolar bone in a 19-year-old girl, showing the delineation of the bone by the radio-opaque line, the lamina dura.

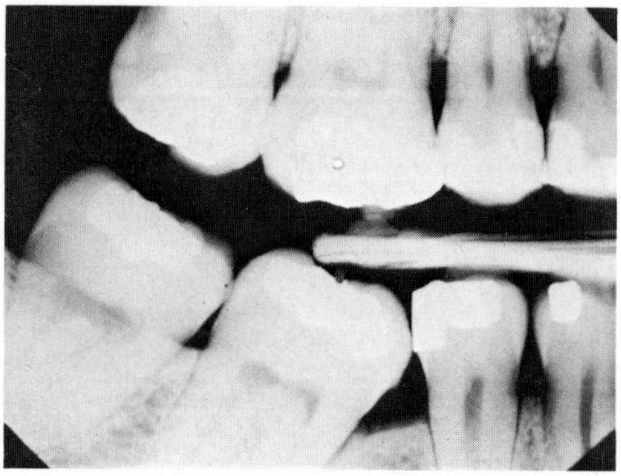

FIG. 31.—The angulated bone margin in relation to a tilted lower molar in an 18-year-old girl.

Radiographic Appearance of The Healthy Periodontium

Familiarity with the normal radiographic appearance of the periodontal tissues is essential for the diagnosis and treatment of periodontal disease. The radiograph registers the radiodensity of all the tissues in the path of the X-ray. The radiographic image represents the product of the radiodensity of several layers of tissue so that only the most radiodense tissue in the path of the beam may be discernible. Thus the interdental bone is registered on the radiograph while the buccal and lingual plates of bone are almost completely obscured by the tooth (Fig. 29).

The socket walls and crests of the interdental septa usually register as linear radio-opacities, the white line of the lamina dura delineating the tooth socket (Fig. 30).

The contour of the alveolar crest depends upon the shape and relationship of neighbouring teeth. For example, the crest mesial to a second premolar is usually a different shape from that distal to this tooth, and where a tooth is tilted the bone crest appears to run towards the tooth in a slightly apical direction (Fig. 31). The radiodensity of the bone margin is determined not only by the actual density of the bone, but by the labio-lingual shape of the margin; a broad flat-topped interdental crest will produce a well defined white line on the radiograph while a convex or pointed crest registers more faintly (Fig. 29). The appearance of the lamina dura also varies with the shape and position of the tooth root in relation to the X-ray beam. Indeed, in radiographs of healthy teeth this feature may be partially or completely absent (Fig. 32). Similarly the width of the periodontal space as seen on the radiograph may be altered by the angulation of the beam and the shape and position of the root. Minor variations in these features in the absence of other signs of disease should not be allowed to dictate diagnosis and treatment.

A completely standardized procedure must be used in taking radiographs when establishing a periodontal diagnosis. Variation in beam angulation, in exposure time and developing time may render interpretation difficult and comparison of radiographs impossible, and thus contribute to a misdiagnosis (Fig. 33).

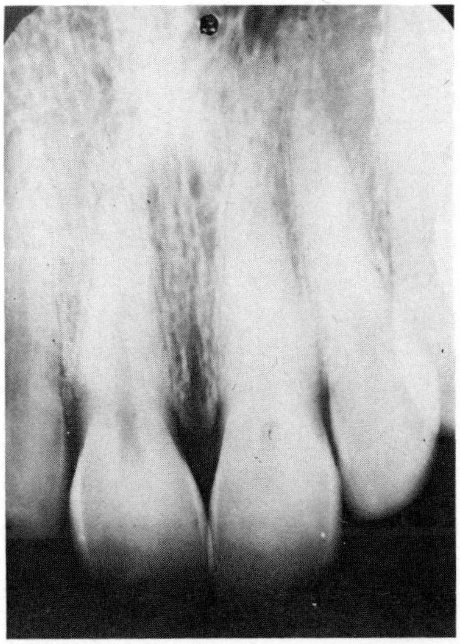

FIG. 32.—Healthy incisors, showing lack of clarity of lamina dura and periodontal space.

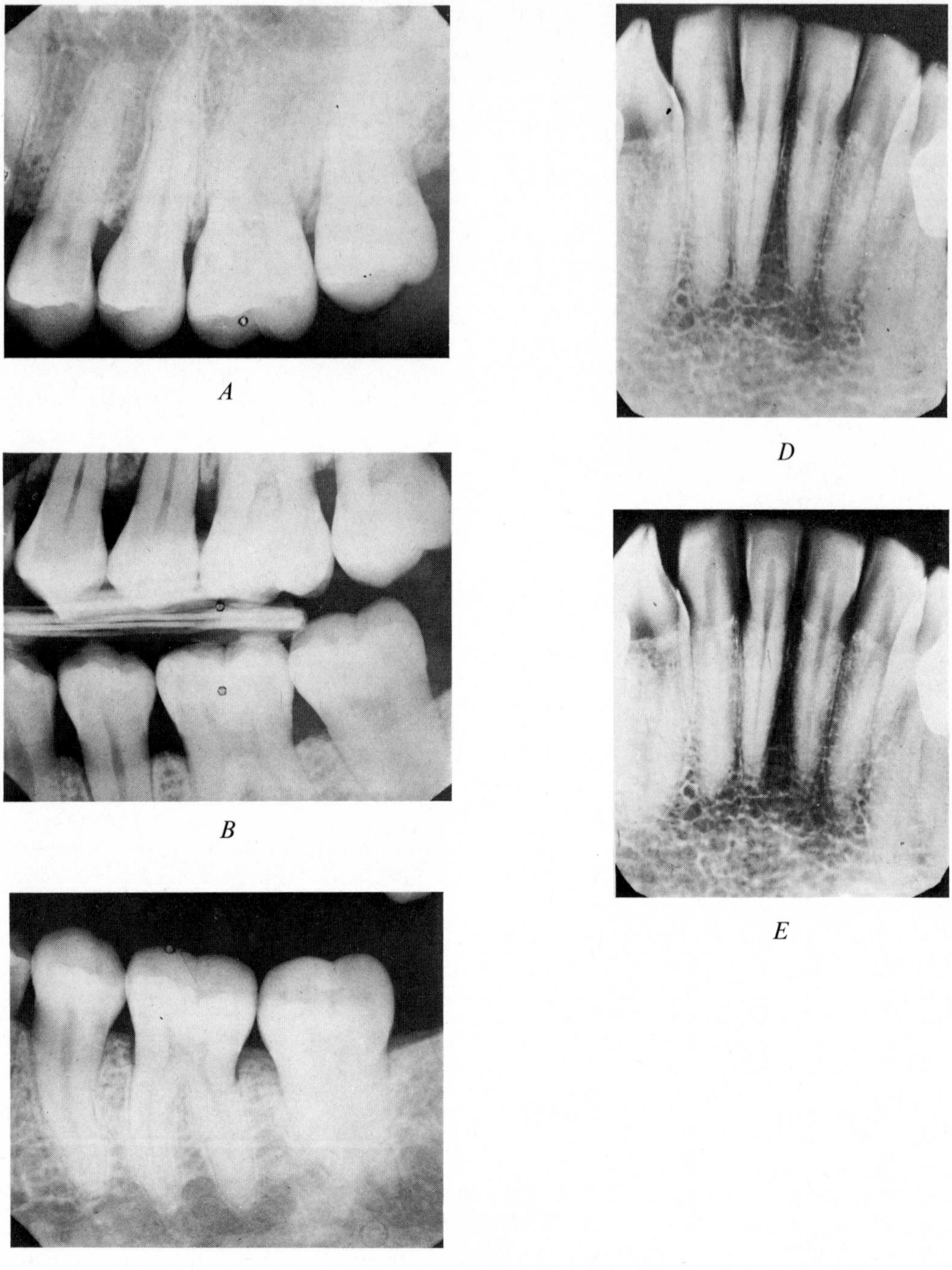

FIG. 33.—Radiographs demonstrating the variation in appearance caused by beam angulation and in exposure time. (*A*), (*B*) and (*C*) show that the bitewing radiograph gives the most reliable evidence of the relationship of the bone margin to the amelo-cemental junction.

A healthy interdental septum (*D*) is almost completely obscured by over-exposure (*E*).

REFERENCES

AINAMO, J. and LÖE, H. (1966). Anatomical characteristics of gingiva. I. A clinical and microscopical study of the free and attached gingiva. *J. Periodont.*, **37**, 5.

ARNIM, S. S. and HAGERMAN, D. A. (1953). Connective tissue fibers of the marginal gingiva. *J. Amer. dent. Ass.*, **47**, 271.

BEAGRIE, G. S. and SKOUGAARD, M. R. (1962). Observations on the life cycle of the gingival epithelial cells of mice as revealed by autoradiography. *Acta odont. scand.*, **20**, 15.

BECKS, H. V. (1929). Normal and pathologic pocket formation. *J. Amer. dent. Ass.*, **16**, 2167.

BRILL, N. (1959). Removal of particles and bacteria from gingival pockets by tissue fluids. *Acta odont. scand.*, **17**, 431.

BRILL, N. and BJORN, H. (1959). Passage of tissue fluid into human gingival pockets. *Acta odont. scand.*, **17**, 11.

CARNEIRO, J. and FAVA DE MORAES, F. C. (1965). Radioautographic visualization of collagen metabolism in the periodontal tissues of the mouse. *Arch. oral Biol.*, **10**, 833.

COHEN, B. (1959). Morphological factors in the pathogenesis of periodontal disease. *Brit. dent. J.*, **107**, 31.

COWLEY, G. C. (1966). Fluorescence studies of crevicular fluid. *J. dent. Res.*, **45**, 655.

CRABBÉ, P. A., CARBONERA, A. O. and HEREMANS, J. F. (1965). The normal human intestinal mucosa as a major source of plasma cells containing YA. Immunoglobulin. *Lab. Invest.*, **14**, 235.

FULLMER, H. M. and LILLIE, R. D. (1958). The oxytalan fiber: a previously undescribed connective tissue fiber. *J. Histochem. Cytochem.*, **6**, 425.

FULLMER, H. M. *et al.* (1969). The origin of collagenase in periodontal tissue in Man. *J. dent. Res.*, **48**, 636.

GLENWRIGHT, H. D. (1970). Observations on circular and longitudinal gingivae collagen fibres in the rhesus monkey. *Dent. Practit.*, **20**, 337.

GOTTLIEB, B. (1921). Der epithelansatz am Zahne. *Dtsch. Mschr. Zahnheilk.*, **39**, 142.

KARRING, T. and LÖE, H. (1967). Blood supply to the periodontium. *J. periodont. Res.*, **2**, 74.

KINDLOVA, M. (1965). Changes in the vascular bed of the marginal periodontium in periodontitis. *J. dent. Res.*, **44**, 455.

LISTGARTEN, M. A. (1972). Normal development, structure, physiology and repair of the gingival epithelium. *Oral Sci. Rev.*, **1**, 3.

LÖE, H. (1961). Physiological aspects of the gingival pocket – an experimental study. *Acta odont. scand.*, **19**, 387.

LÖE, H. and HOLM-PEDERSEN, P. (1965). Absence and presence of fluid from normal and inflamed gingiva. *Periodontics*, **3**, 171.

MCDOUGALL, W. A. (1971). Penetration pathways of a topically applied foreign protein into rat gingiva. *J. periodont. Res.*, **6**, 89.

MCHUGH, W. D. (1971). The interdental gingivae. *J. periodont. Res.*, **6**, 227.

ORBAN, B. *et al.* (1956). Epithelial atachment and the attached epithelial cuff. *J. Periodont.*, **27**, 167.

PARFITT, G. J. (1967). The physical analysis of the tooth-supporting structures. *In* The Mechanisms of Tooth Support, p. 154. John Wright, Bristol.

SCHROEDER, H. E. and LISTGARTEN, M. A. (1971). Fine Structure of Developing Epithelial Attachment of Human Teeth. Karger, Basel.

TOLO, K. J. (1971). A study of permeability of gingival pocket epithelium to albumin in guinea pigs and Norwegian pigs. *Arch. oral Biol.*, **16**, 881.

WAERHAUG, J. (1952). Gingival pocket; anatomy, pathology, deepening and elimination. *Odont. Tidskr.*, **60**, Suppl. 1.

WEINREB, M. M. (1960). Epithelial attachment. *J. Periodont.*, **31**, 186.

WESKI, O. (1922). Die chronischen marginalen Entzundungen des Alveolar – fortsatzes mit besonderer Berucksichtigung der Alveolar pyorrhoe. *Kerteljahxschr. Zahnheilk.*, **38**, 1.

ZANDER, H. A. and HURZELER, B. (1958). Continuous cementum apposition. *J. dent. Res.*, **37**, 1035.

3. The Oral Environment

The clinical crown of the tooth, the gingiva and oral mucosa are bathed in saliva and exposed to the rich oral flora. These two elements form the major components of the environment for the tissues, with the addition of a large number of occasional factors associated with the diet, the mechanisms of eating and oral habits. The interaction of saliva and the oral flora, with the intermittent influence of the diet, produces a variety of deposits on the teeth, acquired pellicle, bacterial plaque, materia alba, dental calculus and stains.

SALIVA

The chemical and physiological characteristics of saliva are fully described in the appropriate textbooks (Jenkins, 1966), but several aspects need to be recalled because of their significance in periodontal health and disease.

Saliva flows constantly day and night. This flow is markedly increased by oral and olfactory stimulus as well as by pain and psychological factors. Salivary secretion is reduced in old age, with disease of salivary glands, by radiation and several pharmacological agents.

Apart from its role in digestion, saliva provides a protective coating for the oral tissues. When its flow is reduced as in xerostomia the mucosa becomes rough and dry, the tongue red and smooth, heavy bacterial deposits form and if irritated, the tissues bleed easily, caries appears to increase and periodontal destruction becomes more severe.

The protective function of saliva is served in a variety of ways:

1. The flow of saliva removes food and bacterial debris which can be swallowed or expectorated.
2. Glycoproteins and mucoids coat the mucous membrane preventing dehydration, acting as a lubricating agent and as a barrier to chemical irritants.
3. Because of its bicarbonate and phosphate content it can act to buffer acids from food or micro-organisms.
4. The mineral content is in constant interaction with tooth enamel.
5. It contains a range of antibacterial factors:
   (a) Lysozymes which lyse certain micro-organisms, *e.g.* some staphylococci and Gram-negative organisms, by breaking up cell walls.
   (b) Antibody, mainly Gamma-globulins, primarily as IgA, which enter into antibacterial mechanisms.
   (c) A variety of enzymes effective against many bacteria including streptococci and lactobacilli.

Saliva also contains a large number of leucocytes, mainly polymorpho-nuclear leucocytes, which migrate through the epithelium of the gingival crevice. The rate of migration increases with gingival inflammation and the 'orogranulocytic migration rate' has been used as an index of the severity of inflammation (Klinkhamer and Zimmerman, 1969).

Micro-organisms are normally present in saliva (Gibbons, Kapsimalis and Socransky, 1964) but in much lower numbers than in the gingival crevice or in bacterial plaque. Streptococcus salivarius is the predominant organism in free saliva. Saliva plays an essential role in the formation of deposits on the teeth, in particular bacterial plaque and calculus.

The Oral Flora

Within a few hours after birth the mouth becomes populated by aerobic or facultative micro-organisms, mainly streptococci with smaller numbers of staphylococci, lactobacilli, and even Candida. Anaerobic organisms have appeared by the time of tooth eruption.

Micro-organisms flourish generally in the mouth but are found in largest concentrations on the dorsum of the tongue, the gingival crevice and tooth crevices. The number and types of organisms vary from time to time and is influenced by many factors including the presence or absence of teeth and the state of oral hygiene. The number of micro-organisms colonizing the clean and healthy gingival crevice while much greater than that of saliva is still relatively low compared to the flora of the dorsum of the tongue. There is a large variety of bacteria consisting mainly of anaerobes, including Gram-positive cocci with smaller numbers of Gram-negative cocci and Gram-positive bacilli. There are also some Gram-negative bacilli, fusobacteria, spirochaetes and filamentous forms (Socransky, 1970). If food stagnation is allowed to occur bacterial growth is promoted by this rich medium and the number of micro-organisms increases considerably.

Whether the base of the healthy gingival crevice is sterile has been the subject of much dispute. It is difficult to examine the contents of the bottom of the crevice without having some contamination from the gingival margin, but careful studies indicate that most healthy crevices give no growth on culture. If we accept the distinction between the clinical and histological crevice described by Listgarten (1972) then the base of the clinical crevice is actually within vital tissue and is therefore sterile. It seems likely that from time to time a number of micro-organisms find their way into the depths of the crevice, *i.e.* into tissue, to be eliminated by the effective self-cleansing mechanism of the crevicular tissues. These organisms like all those that inhabit the body are in a state of balance with the host tissues as well as between themselves. Disease can result from an upset in the host-parasite relationship or a change in the balance between micro-organisms. One of the most common of the latter changes is seen when antibiotic therapy depresses certain oral organisms and allows Candida to flourish and produce a Candidiasis.

TOOTH DEPOSITS

The Acquired Pellicle

This is a thin layer of salivary proteins, mainly glycoproteins, which is formed within minutes on tooth surfaces or other firm surfaces in the mouth, *e.g.* dentures, after they have been polished. It is about 0.5 mm thick, acellular and initially bacteria-free. It is a smooth, colourless, translucent film which adheres firmly to the underlying tooth surface. Although it is said that the formation of dental plaque can proceed directly on tooth surface it does appear to commence on the acquired pellicle.

Dental Plaque

Dental plaque is a soft non-calcified bacterial deposit which accumulates on the surfaces of teeth and other firm objects in the mouth such as restorations, dentures and dental calculus. It adheres tenaciously to these surfaces and can only be detached by mechanical cleaning, *e.g.* toothbrushing. It cannot be removed by rinsing or water sprays and it is this characteristic which distinguishes it from soft easily removed deposits known as materia alba. In small amounts it is not visible and its presence can be revealed only by staining with special disclosing dyes (Fig. 34).

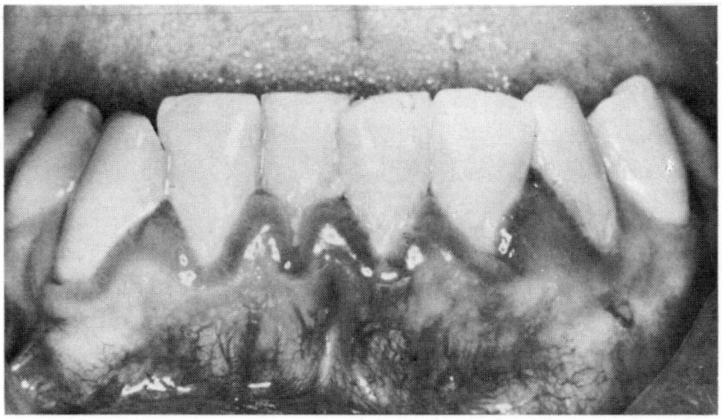

A

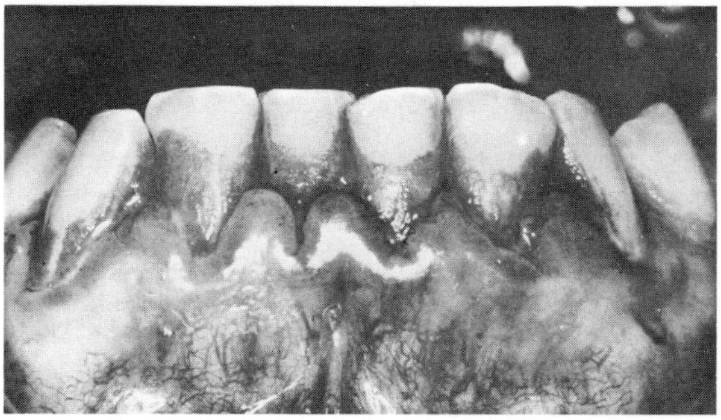

B

FIG. 34.—(*A*) Appearance before using disclosing agent. (*B*) After staining plaque with disclosing tablet (4% erythrocine).

In thicker layers it is seen as yellowish or grey deposits on the teeth. It is important to understand that the presence of food is not necessary to the formation of plaque (Egelberg, 1965). As stated the formation of plaque on a clean tooth surface usually starts with the rapid deposition of salivary proteins to form a relatively bacteria-free acquired pellicle. There appears to be an electrostatic affinity of the hydroxyapatite of enamel for glycoprotein. The pellicle is then colonized by salivary bacteria. Isolated colonies mainly of Gram-positive cocci and rods deposit rapidly (Fig. 35*B*), usually in sheltered areas such as the gingival margin. The time taken for aggregates of colonies to appear seems to be related to the health of the neighbouring gingiva. In the presence of gingival inflammation and increased crevicular fluid flow aggregates may appear within thirty minutes of tooth cleaning. Gram-negative cocci and rods appear and the colonies fuse. Fusobacteria and filamentous forms appear as the plaque deposit thickens and favours the proliferation of anaerobic organisms; they are well represented by the fifth day (Figs. 35*C* and 36). Shed epithelial cells and leucocytes become involved so that a dense mass of bacteria in an inter-cellular matrix is formed. The percentage of filamentous forms increases and the percentage of streptococci decreases as the plaque matures. Bacteria constitute 70% of the mature plaque: the matrix is mainly protein containing mucopolysaccharide groups derived from both saliva and bacteria. It is basophilic, metachromatic with toluidine blue and positive to the periodic-acid-Schiff reaction. The chemical composition varies from one individual to another and in different parts of the same mouth; its composition

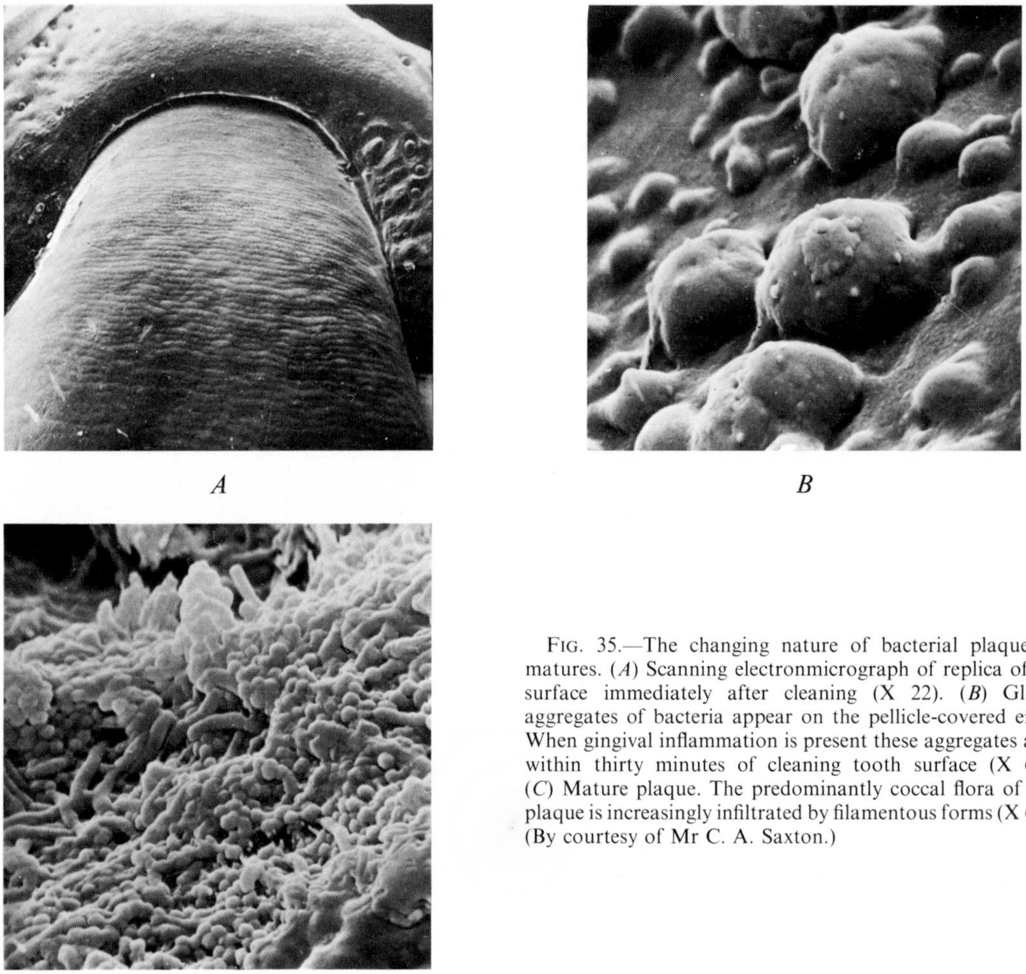

A

B

C

FIG. 35.—The changing nature of bacterial plaque as it matures. (*A*) Scanning electronmicrograph of replica of tooth surface immediately after cleaning (X 22). (*B*) Globular aggregates of bacteria appear on the pellicle-covered enamel. When gingival inflammation is present these aggregates appear within thirty minutes of cleaning tooth surface (X 6,400). (*C*) Mature plaque. The predominantly coccal flora of young plaque is increasingly infiltrated by filamentous forms (X 6,400). (By courtesy of Mr C. A. Saxton.)

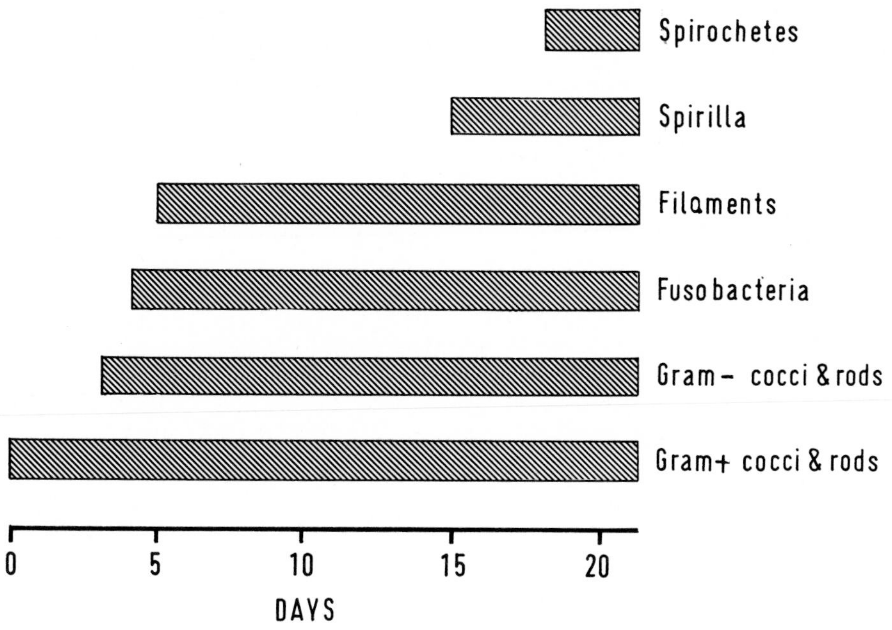

FIG. 36.—The changing flora of plaque as it matures during a three-week period without oral hygiene. (By courtesy of Dr H. Löe.)

appears to be influenced by diet.

Plaque forms most heavily in those areas which are sheltered from the friction of mastication and tongue movements. Occlusal surfaces of teeth in function support less plaque. The gingival crevice is the site of heaviest plaque deposition. In the gingival crevice the concentration of bacteria may be 10^8 micro-organisms/mg net weight of plaque.

Mature plaque consists of tufts of filamentous and thread forms with colonies of cocci between, held together by an adhesive interbacterial matrix (Gibbons, 1970). It seems to form more rapidly during sleep perhaps because of decreased salivary flow and the absence of the mechanical action of eating. It also forms more rapidly on a soft diet than on hard chewy diets.

Dental plaque has been established as the primary cause of gingival inflammation; the relationship between plaque, plaque products and gingival disease is discussed in the chapter on the aetiology of gingivitis.

Materia Alba

Deposits formed by bacteria and epithelial cells which can be washed away by rinsing or water-sprays are called materia alba. They are clearly visible as a white or yellow soft deposit, usually on teeth near the gingival margin. Materia alba may contain food products but needs to be distinguished from undegraded food debris. It may play a part in gingival disease but its presence is usually transient except where oral hygiene is very poor.

Dental Calculus

Pathological calcifications occur in several sites in the body, the kidney, gall-bladder and duct, salivary ducts and in the mouth. In the mouth calculus forms on tooth surfaces and on other hard surfaces, *e.g.* restorations and prostheses, which are not exposed to friction.

Dental calculus or tartar is classified according to its position on the tooth in relation to the gingival margin, as supragingival or subgingival calculus (Fig. 37).

Supragingival calculus is found coronal to the gingival margin. It is deposited first on tooth surfaces opposite salivary ducts, *i.e.* lingual surfaces of lower incisors and facial surfaces of upper molars, but may be deposited on any surface

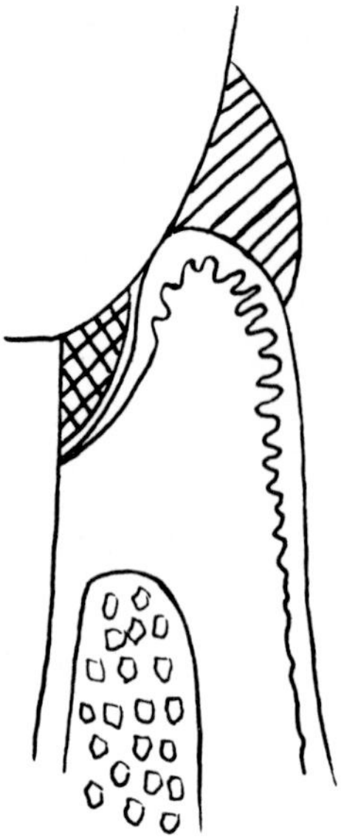

FIG. 37.—The relationship of supragingival and subgingival calculus to the gingival margin.

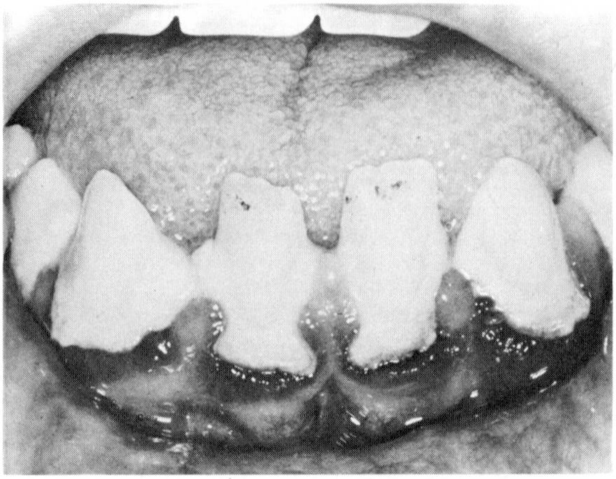

A

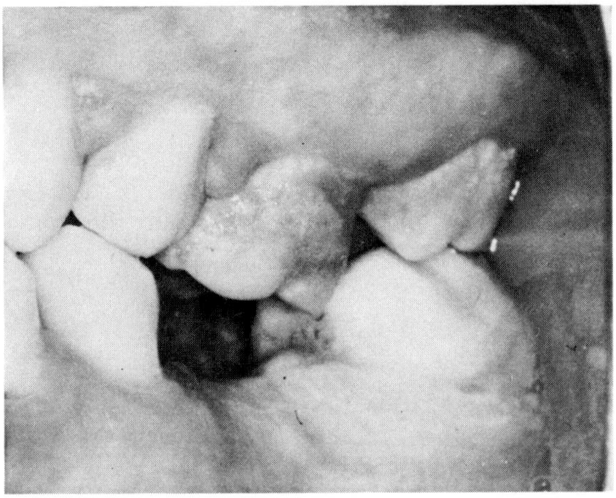

B

FIG. 38.—(*A*) Gross deposits of supragingival calculus in the neglected mouth of a 26-year-old woman. (*B*) Supragingival calculus on a non-functional upper molar.

including dentures if oral hygiene is poor (Fig. 38). Occasionally it is found on the occlusal surfaces of unopposed teeth. It is light yellow in colour when recently deposited, is fairly soft but becomes harder and more brittle with time.

Subgingival calculus is deposited on tooth surfaces below the gingival margin. It is dark brown or green, very hard and strongly attached to the root surface (Fig. 39).

Supragingival calculus is also known as salivary calculus while subgingival calculus is also called seruminal calculus because of the assumption that its origin is not from saliva but from blood serum.

Supragingival calculus is rarely found on deciduous teeth and is not common on the permanent teeth in young children. However by the age of 9 it becomes increasingly common (Everett, Tuchler and Lu, 1963) and in the adult is found in virtually all mouths.

Subgingival calculus is not found so commonly except in the presence of gingival pathology; it is very common in adults.

Composition

The composition of calculus varies slightly according to its site in the mouth, age of deposit and geographical location of the individual.

It consists of about 80% inorganic matter, some water, an organic component made up of desquamated epithelial cells, Gram-positive filamentous micro-organisms such as leptotricia, some Gram-negative filamentous forms and cocci, leucocytes and an amorphous ground-substance. This organic matrix is largely protein with 12–20% carbohydrate. The surface of calculus is covered by bacterial plaque but the centre of thick calculus may be sterile.

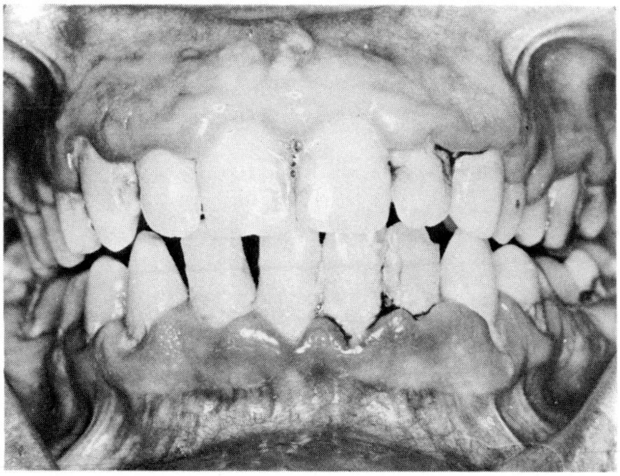

A

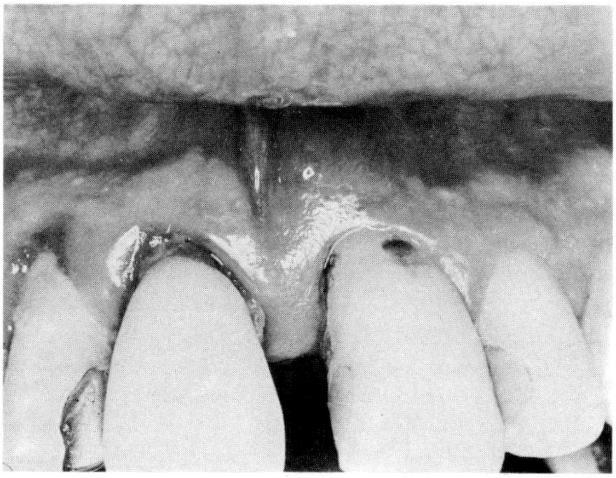

B

FIG. 39.—Generalized subgingival calculus. (*A*) Very poor oral hygiene showing thick plaque deposit, and subgingival calculus at 23 and 12. (*B*) Subgingival calculus showing under gingival margin, with little plaque deposition.

The inorganic component consists mainly of calcium phosphate as hydroxyapatite and other crystalline forms of calcium phosphate such as brushite, whitlockite and octacalcium phosphate. There is also a small amount of calcium carbonate and magnesium phosphate as well as fluoride.

The composition of subgingival calculus is similar to that of supragingival calculus. It has more whitlockite, less brushite and octacalcium phosphate. The Ca/P ratio is higher and the sodium content is also greater in subgingival calculus. Salivary proteins are not found in subgingival calculus, a fact which supports the idea of a non-salivary origin for this substance.

Deposition

Early theories of the formation of calculus describe the precipitation of inorganic salts from a supersaturated saliva into the passive organic matrix provided by the plaque. Now it is thought that the plaque plays a more active role in providing nucleation sites where calcium, phosphorus and other ions can accumulate to form crystals of hydroxyapatite. Some change in the chemical composition is thought to take place which encourages the growth of filamentous bacteria. At the same time some plaque constituent (as yet undefined) changes to act as a seeding agent which results in the crystallization of calcium phosphate from the supersaturated saliva. In early plaque concentrations of calcium and phosphorus are high but no apatite crystals are present. Electron microscope studies suggest that apatite is deposited in or on filamentous organisms; these filamentous organisms can form intracellular crystals of apatite, therefore the seeding substance may be formed by these organisms. However as calculus is formed in germ-free animals it is likely that more than one substance can act as a seed. Once calcification has begun it can continue by crystal growth. With increasing thickness the internal population of filamentous organisms falls until, as stated, the centre of thick calculus may be sterile.

Other theories of calculus formation which centre on the release of calcium and phosphorus ions are briefly as follows:

1. The CO_2 tension is relatively low in the mouth, therefore CO_2 is lost from saliva which can be regarded as an unstable supersaturated solution of calcium phosphate, with consequent deposition of insoluble calcium phosphate.
2. During periods of reduced salivary flow, such as sleep, ammonia is formed from salivary urea producing a rise in pH which favours precipitation of calcium phosphate.
3. Concentrations of both acid and alkaline phosphatase in the plaque is higher than in saliva. The phosphatase releases the phosphorus ion from the organic phosphates resulting in precipitation. The idea is supported by the fact that oral actinomyces in

plaque can produce phosphatases.

4. Proteins may hold calcium in high concentrations in saliva and when saliva comes into contact with teeth the protein comes out of solution leading to reduced stability of salivary calcium and phosphorus.

It is thought that the origin of subgingival calculus is not saliva. Saliva does not seem to have access to the subgingival area in which the calculus is formed, and subgingival calculus never forms on the experimental mylar strips on which supragingival calculus is collected. Also the composition of subgingival calculus is similar in different locations and does not vary with the distance from the salivary ducts as does supragingival calculus. It is very rare in children. It is never found except in association with gingival inflammation and it is thought that inflammatory exudate into the pathologically deepened crevice (the pocket) forms the source of its mineral content. The old name 'seruminal' calculus may well be correct.

Both forms of calculus are attached to the acquired pellicle, or to irregularities in the tooth surface or via organisms which penetrate cementum and are embedded in calculus. Calculus acts as a tissue irritant by virtue of its bacterial content and the plaque on its surface.

Tooth Stains

A number of tooth stains are found. They are very tenacious and may be the result of the pigmentation of acquired pellicle by chromogenic bacteria, food and chemicals.

Tobacco produces a brown stain, wine a brown-green stain. A green stain is found commonly in children's teeth. Its origin is uncertain; it may be a remnant of enamel cuticle or a product of fluorescent bacteria or fungi. Metal salts produce a variety of stains, silver and iron black, copper green.

These stains produce an aesthetic problem but there is no evidence that they cause gingival irritation.

REFERENCES

EGELBERG, J. (1965). Local effect of diet on plaque formation and development of gingivitis in dogs. III. Effect of frequency of meals and tube feeding. *Odont. Revy*, **16**, 50.

EVERETT, F. G., TUCHLER, H. and LU, K. H. (1963). Occurrence of calculus in grade school children in Portland, Oregon. *J. Periodont.*, **34**, 54.

GIBBONS, R. J., KAPSIMALIS, B. and SOCRANSKY, S. S. (1964). The source of salivary bacteria. *Arch. oral Biol.*, **9**, 101.

GIBBONS, R. J. (1970). *In* Dental Plaque (ed. W. D. McHugh). Livingstone, Edinburgh.

JENKINS, G. N. (1966). The Physiology of the Mouth. Blackwell, Oxford.

KLINKHAMER, J. M. and ZIMMERMAN, S. (1969). The function and reliability of the orogranulocytic migratory rate as a measure of oral health. *J. dent. Res.*, **48**, 709.

LISTGARTEN, M. A. (1972). Normal development, structure, physiology and repair of gingival epithelium. *Oral sci. Rev.*, **1**, 3.

SOCRANSKY, S. S. (1970). Relationship of bacteria to the etiology of periodontal disease. *J. dent. Res.*, **49**, 203.

4. The Aetiology of Chronic Periodontal Disease

Two fundamental ideas are now generally accepted:

1. That gingival inflammation is produced by accumulations of bacterial plaque in proximity to the gingival margin. It follows that all factors which encourage such accumulations or prevent their removal tend to promote gingival inflammation.
2. That chronic periodontitis is the sequel to persistent gingival inflammation. This does not mean that destruction of the periodontal tissues inevitably follows gingival inflammation but that the latter is the essential precursor of the former.

BACTERIAL PLAQUE

In 1683 Anthony Van Leeuwenhoek wrote in a letter to Francis Aston, Secretary of the Royal Society, ''Tis my wont of a morning to rub my teeth with salt, and then swill my mouth out with water; and often, after eating, to clean my back teeth with a toothpick, as well as rubbing them hard with a cloth: wherefore my teeth, back and front, remain as clean and white as falleth to the lot of few men of my years, and my gums (no matter how hard the salt be that I rub them with) never start bleeding. Yet notwithstanding, my teeth are not so cleaned thereby, but what there sticketh or groweth between some of my front ones and my grinders (whenever I inspected them with a magnifying mirror), a little white matter, which is as thick as if 'twere batter. On examining this I judged (albeit I could discern nought a-moving in it) that there yet were living animalcules therein. I have therefore mixed it, at divers times, with clean rain water (in which there were no animalcules) and also with spittle, that I took out of my mouth after ridding it of air-bubbles (lest the bubbles should make any motion in the spittle): and I then most always saw, with great wonder, that in the said matter there were very many very little living animalcules, very prettily a-moving.'

Historically it has been accepted that there is a relationship between the state of oral hygiene and periodontal disease, but perhaps because of the chronic nature of the periodontal lesion it was believed to be produced by the physical irritation of calculus on the gingiva. This notion still persists, despite the weight of evidence pointing as Van Leeuwenhoek evidently suspected, to a relationship between the oral flora and the production of disease.

Observation shows that where there is gingival inflammation or periodontal pocketing the number of organisms increases. The types of organism and their relative proportions do not alter a great deal except for a significant increase in spirochaetes (Rosebury, 1947). However, such observations merely indicate a co-existence of bacteria and periodontal disease, they do not prove a cause and effect relationship. The evidence for the bacterial aetiology of periodontal disease derives from several observations.

1. The direct correlation between oral hygiene scores which indicate the amount of bacterial debris, and the severity of gingival inflammation as measured by gingival indices (Arno *et al.*, 1958; Ash, Gitlin and Smith, 1964). However this data could be interpreted as indicating that inflamed gingiva provide a better environment for bacteria.
2. The correlation between the state of oral hygiene and the amount of periodontal destruction as indicated radiographically by the amount of alveolar bone loss (Schei *et al.*, 1959). This study also shows a direct correlation between age and the degree of bone loss from which one might assume that both the oral hygiene state and degree of bone loss are merely functions of age, *i.e.* co-existent factors.
3. The experimental production of gingivitis by the withdrawal of all forms of oral hygiene, Löe, Theilade and Jensen (1965) showed that when a group of 12 dental students stopped cleaning their teeth and allowed plaque to accumulate gingival inflammation appeared. When oral hygiene measures were recommenced and plaque removed the inflammation disappeared (Fig.

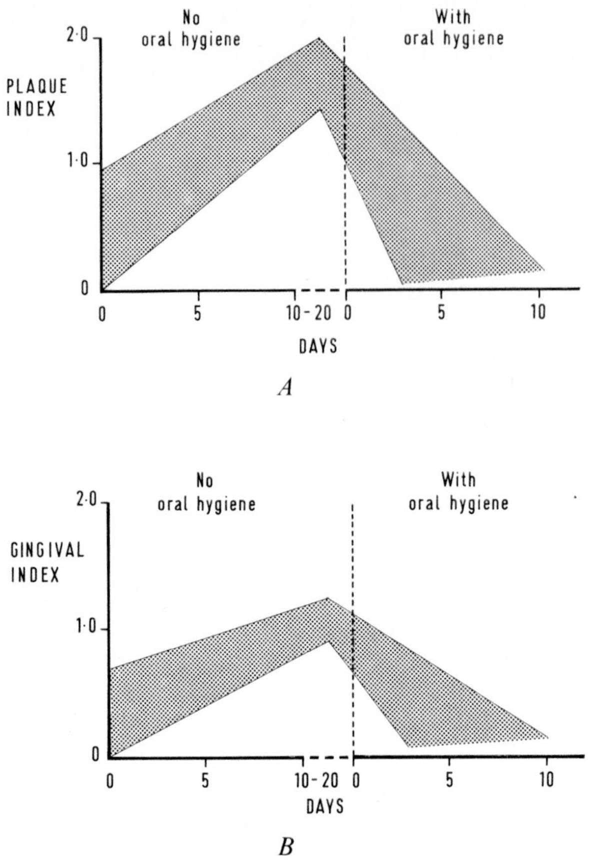

FIG. 40.—The development of gingival inflammation with plaque accumulation during withdrawal of oral hygiene measures followed by resolution of inflammation as plaque control is resumed. (*A*) Plaque index against time. (*B*) Gingival index against time. (By courtesy of Dr H. Löe.)

40). This experiment was repeated in beagle dogs with similar results (Saxe *et al.*, 1967).

It has been argued that these experiments could be interpreted to mean that the withdrawal of physical stimulus produces inflammation but such a conclusion is contradicted by subsequent studies (*vide infra*).

4. The finding that inflammation produced by withdrawal of oral hygiene measures can be resolved by the application of non-specific antiseptics such as chlorhexidine to the tooth and gingiva in human and dog subjects.
5. A related piece of evidence is the observation that acute ulcerative gingivitis is highly susceptible to the action of topical or systemic antibiotics (Schuessler, Fairchild and Stransky, 1945).
6. Injection of oral bacteria into guinea pigs produces inflammation and abscess formation (Socransky and Gibbons, 1965).
7. In germ-free animals mechanical abuse of the gingiva by silk ligatures placed between the teeth does not appear to produce either gingival inflammation or alveolar bone loss. However when micro-organisms are present the same procedure produces both gingival inflammation and bone loss (Rovin, Costich and Gordon, 1966). The results of germ-free animal studies must be viewed with some reserve as Baer and Lieberman (1959) have shown alveolar bone loss in germ-free mice, which appears to vary considerably with the species studied.
8. When gingiva is traumatized by mechanical irritants such as rough or overhanging fillings little gingival inflammation is present unless the filling has a covering of bacterial plaque (Waerhaug, 1956a; 1956b).
9. Enzymes extracted from cultures of human gingival sulcus bacteria can destroy elements

of gingival tissue. These bacteria have been shown to produce collagenase, proteases, hyaluronidase and many other enzymes.

Although individual observations are open to criticism the total weight of evidence would seem to be overwhelming (Socransky, 1970). Materia alba may also act on the tissues in the same way as dental plaque. However its presence, except in very dirty mouths, is usually transient.

Dental calculus may be regarded as calcified plaque. At one time it was thought that its physical presence produced mechanical irritation of the gingiva. Such a belief has never been substantiated and the calcified deposits which form on the teeth of germ-free animals do not appear to produce gingival inflammation. The surface of calculus is covered with a layer of plaque and it is this which produces the gingival irritation and inflammation. Despite all this research no specific organism or group of organisms has yet been identified as causal. Also the exact mechanism whereby bacterial plaque induces gingival inflammation has not been elucidated. However a likely train of events has been worked out mainly from indirect evidence.

THE PRODUCTION OF GINGIVAL INFLAMMATION

The bacteria of the dental plaque do not appear to invade the tissues, but chemicals produced by the metabolism of bacteria in the plaque act as irritants to provoke an inflammatory response.

First, bacterial enzymes may attack the intercellular material of the crevicular epithelium. As stated hyaluronidase is produced by several of the oral flora, streptococci and diphtheroids in particular, and this can break up the hyaluronic acid of the intercellular ground-substance. This action could facilitate the penetration of mucopolysaccharidases, collagenases and proteases into the gingival corium. Such an invasion has not actually been demonstrated; also we do know that such an enzyme as collagenase can be formed by the tissues themselves (Fullmer and Gibson, 1966) as well as by bacteria such as *Bacteroides melaninogenicus*.

Immune Response

Many plaque metabolites are theoretically capable of tissue irritation and therefore of the provocation of an inflammatory response, but many of them also have potent antigenic properties. The immune response to antigen stimulation may be favourable initially and lead to inactivation of bacterial irritation both within the gingival crevice and in the tissues. However repeated exposure to the bacterial antigen may produce an immediate hypersensitivity response which results in tissue damage. Immunoglobulins are produced by the host in relation to specific antigen stimulation, and immunoglobulins are then found in the circulating blood, tissue spaces and on cell surfaces. The belief that immunological mechanisms are involved in the production of gingival inflammation is based on:

1. the presence in the gingival corium of lymphocytes and plasma cells which produce immunoglobulins.
2. the presence of immunoglobulins in inflammatory exudate from the crevice and in the gingival tissues.
3. a raised serum antibody titre to plaque bacteria where there is periodontal disease.
4. circulating antibodies are produced in response to endotoxin from *Bacteroides melaninogenicus*.

Endotoxins are important bacterial antigens. They are lipopolysaccharides derived from the cell wall of Gram-negative bacteria and it has been shown that when endotoxin is injected intramucosally regional lymph nodes show specific antibodies after which an infiltration of lymphocytes and plasma cells appear at the injection site (Berglund, Rizzo and Mergenhagen, 1969).

A possible pattern of activity worked out by Mergenhagen, Tempel and Snyderman (1970) is as follows:

Plaque antigens in the gingival corium stimulate lymphoid tissue (in regional lymph nodes and elsewhere) to produce immunocytes which accumulate at the site of irritation in the gingiva. These produce specific antibodies which form antigen-antibody complexes. The altered antibody then activates the complement system which goes on to release a variety of products which stimulate phagocytosis, increase vascular permeability and smooth muscle contraction, alter cell membranes, generate leukocyte chemotactic factors and lyse antibody-sensitized cells, *i.e.* changes typical of an inflammatory response. These changes also cause increased permeability of the tissue to further penetration by plaque antigens and the action of

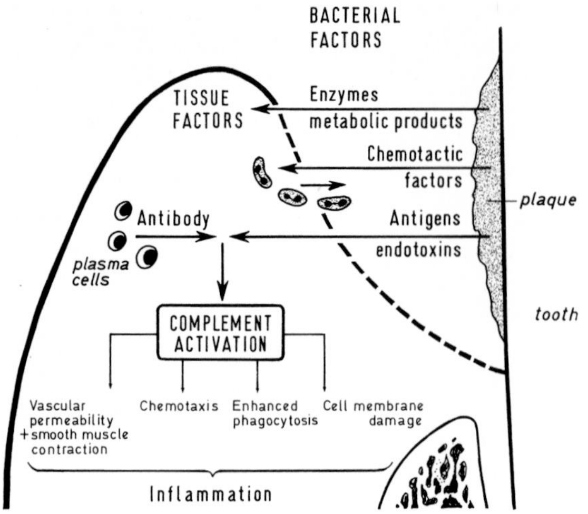

FIG. 41.—Diagram illustrating the role of complement in the production of gingival inflammation by bacterial plaque. (After Dr S. E. Mergenhagen.)

the polymorphonuclear leucocytes could release further tissue-damaging enzymes (Fig. 41). Thus while the bacterial plaque persists a self-perpetuating cycle of events produces a chronic inflammation.

Cell-mediated Immunity

In contrast to the activation of antibody which appears to rely on the transportation of antigen to lymphoid tissue, a more immediate mechanism is now believed to play an important role in the production of chronic gingival inflammation. This is the cell-mediated form of immunity. Small lymphocytes can initiate immune reactions that are mediated not by circulating antibody but by direct cellular activity. This was first demonstrated by Landsteiner and Chase (1942) who showed that contact hypersensitivity induced in guinea pigs by picryl chloride could be transmitted to normal guinea pigs by injecting living peritoneal exudate cells from the hypersensitive animal, but not by anti-serum. Histological analysis shows that in these lesions the essential change is a chronic inflammatory infiltrate consisting of large and small mononuclear cells. 'T' lymphocytes that have been sensitized by previous contact with the antigen *in vivo* can be stimulated to transform *in vitro* into lymphoblasts upon re-encountering the specific antigen. During this transformation process factors are produced which

1. inhibit macrophage mobility.
2. direct mononuclear migration.
3. inhibit proliferation of susceptible adjacent tissue cells, and
4. lyse the host's own tissue cells through a cytotoxic effect.

Lymphocytes are activated by plaque deposits *in vitro* and are evident *in vivo* in periodontal disease. Their products may well participate in the destructive mechanism of this disease (Horton, Leikin and Oppenheim, 1972).

It should be evident from this account that a very important change has taken place in thinking about disease; this is that the tissue changes found in disease, including chronic periodontal disease, represent a function of the *host response to irritation* rather than simply a function of the infecting agent.

RELATED ENVIRONMENTAL FACTORS

A number of environmental but non-bacterial factors may contribute to the initiation and progression of periodontal disease. These are listed as follows:

1. Food impaction
2. Carious cavities
3. Faulty restorations
4. Badly designed partial dentures
5. Orthodontic appliances
6. Lack of adequate function
7. Malalignment of teeth
8. Direct trauma
9. Failure to replace missing teeth
10. Mouth-breathing or lack of lip-seal

Most of these are regarded as predisposing or aggravating factors, *i.e.* factors which encourage bacterial stagnation or tend in some way to debilitate the gingiva so that bacterial effects are more likely.

Food Impaction

Food impaction is the forceful wedging of food against the gingiva between teeth. If the dento-gingival anatomy is normal food impaction is unlikely to occur. Where tooth shapes or relationships deviate from normal, food shedding becomes less efficient and food impaction is more likely to occur. Damage to the gingiva is then caused by both physical trauma and the products of plaque

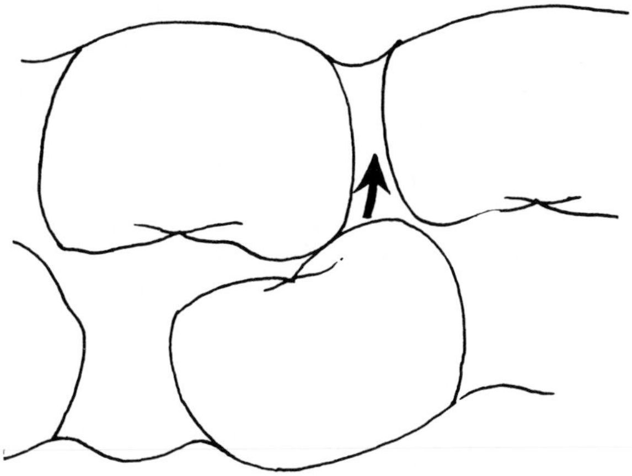
A

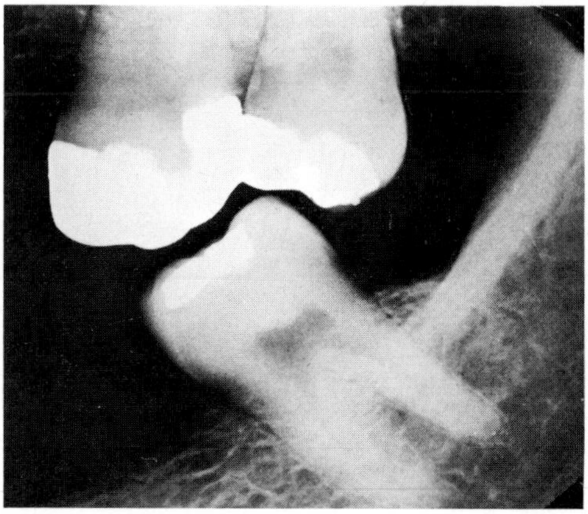
B

FIG. 42.—(*A*) Plunger cusp. (*B*) Bitewing radiograph showing the production of a plunger cusp by failure to replace missing teeth and subsequent tipping of molars.

and food stagnation. The most severe form of food impaction is caused by the 'plunger cusp' (Fig. 42).

Carious Cavities

Cervical cavities aid food stagnation, interproximal cavities also encourage food stagnation and by destroying contact areas and marginal ridges promote food impaction (Fig. 43). In these situations both caries and periodontal disease have bacterial plaque as the common aetiology and successful treatment of either disease requires the treatment of both. Adequate restorations cannot be inserted in the presence of gingival inflammation and unless good restorative work is carried out periodontal treatment must be ineffective.

Faulty Restorations

(a) *Overhanging Edges* (Fig. 44). There is no evidence that the restorative materials normally used in the mouth can of themselves cause gingival

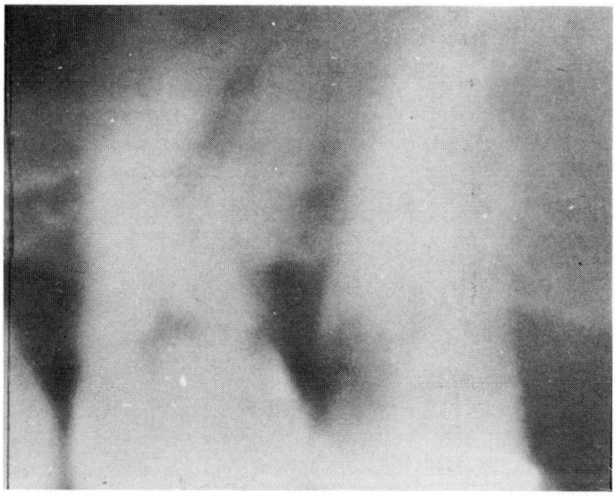

FIG. 43.—Periodontal destruction in relation to interproximal cavity.

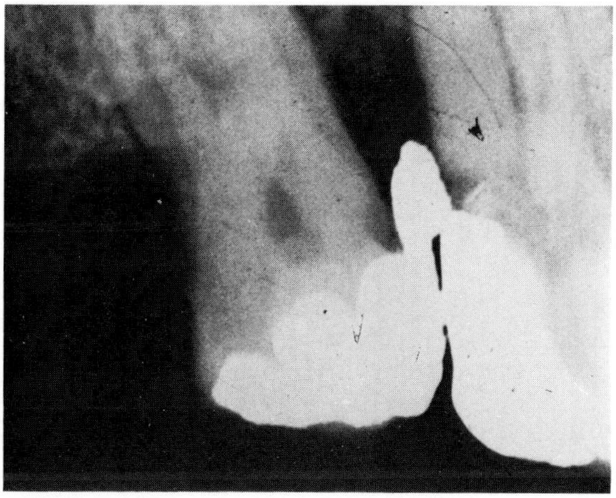

FIG. 44.—Overhanging edges of amalgam fillings (somebody else's dentistry!).

irritation, and there is no evidence to support the theory that the rough overhanging edge of a filling acts as a mechanical irritant as the gingival margin moves against it. A rough edge of any filling material will collect plaque; this is the irritant. Carefully carved highly polished restorations do not collect plaque, and therefore do not cause gingival irritation. Acrylic crowns have often been indicted as causing gingivitis (Fig. 45). Acrylic itself is not irritant to the gingiva but, because of shrinkage, acrylic crowns often have rough edges and a lute between the crown and the tooth preparation in which debris collects and stagnates.

(b) *Badly Contoured Restorations.* The contact point and marginal ridges act in food shedding to protect the interdental area from food impaction and stagnation. If the tooth contour is not properly restored, food shedding may be inefficient and food stagnation is likely to take place (Fig. 46). The badly contoured restoration may also have overhanging edges, and these two factors are probably responsible for a great deal of the gingival disease in young people.

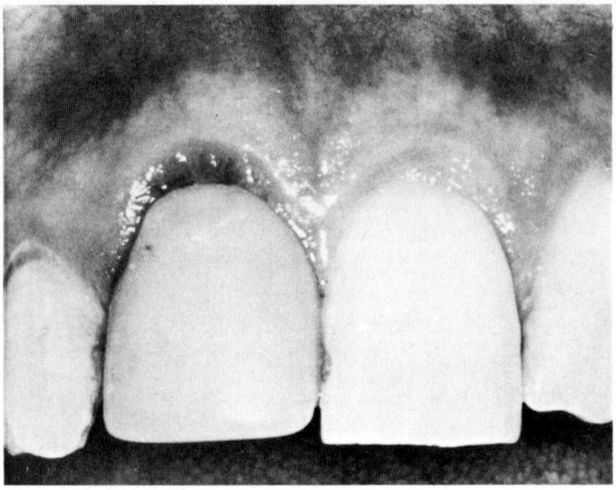

FIG. 45.—Gingival inflammation in relation to the edge of badly fitting porcelain crown.

Badly Designed Partial Dentures

These may cause gingival damage in several ways. They are foreign objects in the mouth and as such they tend to collect food debris so that special attention must be paid to keeping the appliances and abutment teeth clean.

Whenever the soft tissues are required to bear the load of an appliance the tissues tend to give and the appliance to sink into the mucosa. If abutment teeth are not adequately clasped the denture will tip. The gingival margin is subject to considerable pressure and may even be nipped between the denture and the teeth as masticatory forces are intermittently exerted. After a time almost all entirely tissue-borne partial dentures,

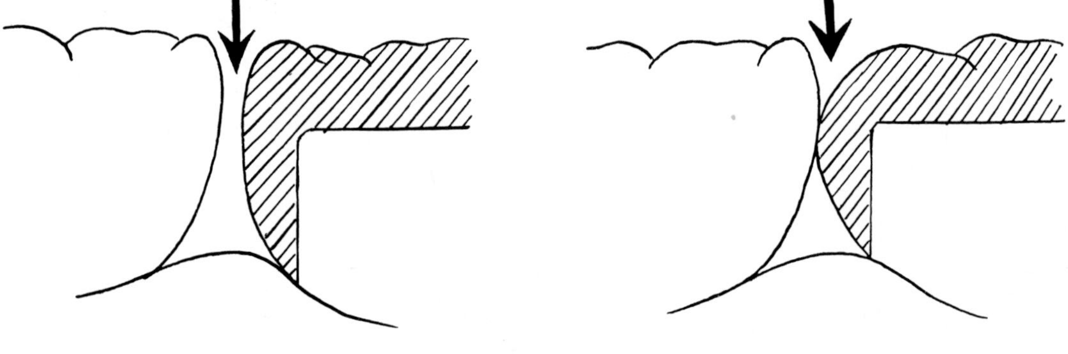

A *B*

FIG. 46.—Inefficient food shedding caused by badly contoured restorations. (*A*) Contact point not restored. (*B*) Marginal ridge not reproduced.

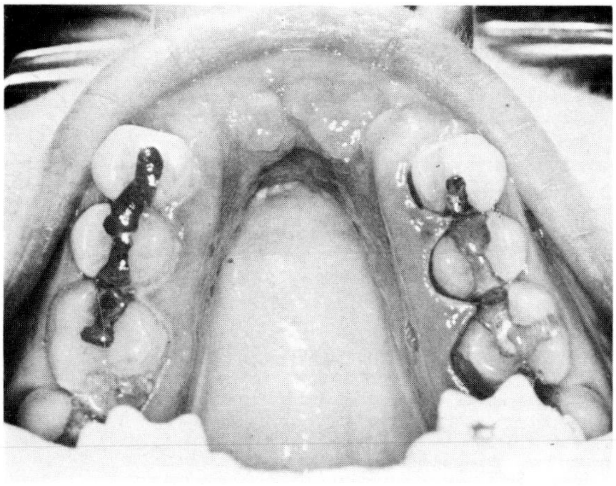

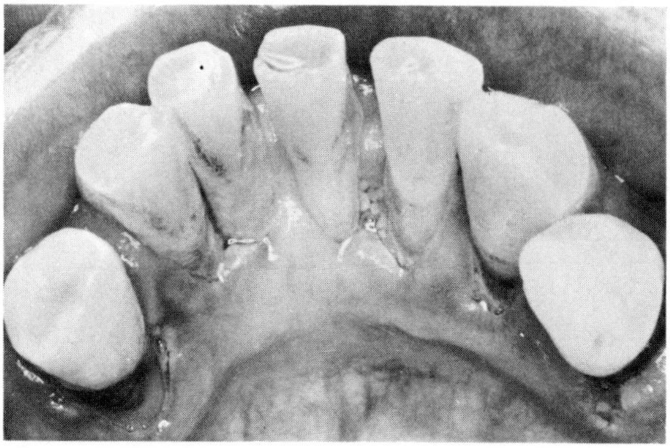

FIG. 47.—Gingival damage brought about by 'gum-stripping' dentures.

even those initially well-fitting, move away from the teeth so that there is a gap between the teeth and the appliance. The traumatized gingival margin may become inflamed and swell into this gap, food debris collects and subgingival calculus forms, so that further tissue abuse occurs. Both periodontal disease and cervical caries may be initiated in this way (Fig. 47).

Finally, if partial denture design is not carefully thought out the stresses on abutment teeth may be excessive (Fig. 48). The optimal direction for force on a tooth is axial; deviations from this line may cause damage to the periodontal fibres. Poor clasp design may result in quite strong horizontal forces acting on the tooth. If the gingivae are healthy these excessive forces are usually absorbed by the tissues but where gingival irritation and inflammation is already present these forces act to accelerate the progress of tissue damage (see Chapter 13).

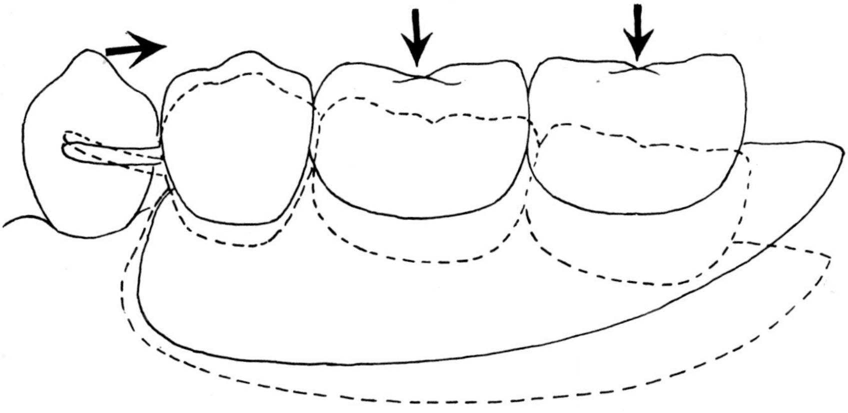

FIG. 48.—Forces exerted by a badly designed partial lower free-end saddle denture on abutment tooth.

Orthodontic Appliances

Removable appliances present some of the problems of the partial denture. The bands of a fixed orthodontic appliance are extremely difficult to keep clean. Without assiduous attention to the maintenance of good oral hygiene, food debris and plaque must collect about the bands with resultant gingival irritation, and production of gingival inflammation (Fig. 49). If such a condition goes untreated in a young patient progression of inflammation into deeper tissues is likely.

Mechanical Irritation and Lack of Adequate Function

Teeth and gingivae in function are subjected to the friction of food bolus passing over them. Although there is some controversy over this issue it seems likely that if hard and fibrous foods are eaten regularly their scouring effect may help to keep the teeth clean (Egelberg, 1965), but this effect cannot be relied upon to remove plaque from the gingival crevice. Hard foods also provide functional stimulus to the epithelium, the periodontal ligament and the alveolar bone.

Separating the effects of mechanical irritation from those of bacterial stagnation is impossible in the human being, and even in animal experiments in which the consistency of the diet has been changed we cannot really identify the effects of stagnation, mechanical irritation and mechanical stimulus.

Soft and pappy foods have little cleansing action; instead they tend to accumulate and stagnate about the gingival margin. Several studies have shown that soft foods appear to produce more periodontal disease in the laboratory animal than hard foods (Ivy, Morgan and Farrell, 1931; King and Gimson, 1947). On the other hand comparison of a hard coarse diet with the same diet in a finely powdered state yields conflicting results. Thilander (1961) found that the coarse diet in the rat produced more rapid and severe periodontal breakdown than the powdered diet and he concluded that this was due to the impaction of hard particulate matter into the gingival pocket. The only reliable way of separating the bacterial from the mechanical component would seem to be by using the germ-free animal.

Non-functional teeth rapidly become the site of plaque, debris and calculus accumulation (Fig. 50). This may happen in cases of anterior open bite, where some teeth are missing, or where teeth in both jaws are present but for some reason, often because a tooth is sensitive, the patient refrains from eating on that side.

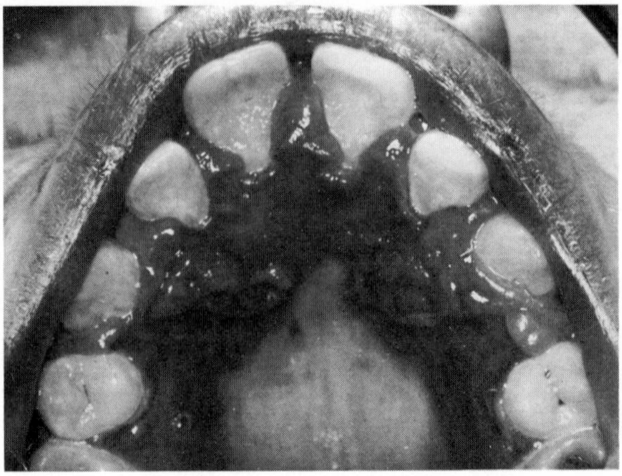

FIG. 49.—Gross inflammation under removable orthodontic appliance.

The tongue plays an important role in the removal of debris from about the teeth and from the vestibule. Some individuals are insensitive to the presence of debris and make no effort to use the tongue, or anything else, to remove it. The term 'self-cleansing' has been applied to places in the mouth where anatomical and functional factors prevent plaque accumulations.

Tooth Malalignment

Clinical observation leads to the impression that tooth malalignment encourages inflammation (Fig. 51) either by (i) predisposing towards the accumulation of bacterial plaque and making cleaning more difficult, or (ii) by producing poor 'food-shedding' which may result in mechanical irritation of the tissue. There is also the opposite idea that the gingivae suffers from not receiving adequate stimulus (Wheeler, 1938). Gianelly (1970) states explicitly 'a major contributing factor in periodontal disease is tooth position', and although a certain amount of orthodontic treatment is encouraged by this idea, the evidence for this assumption is conflicting. Some investigators find a correlation between prevalence of gingival disease and malalignment (Rosenzweig, 1960; Sutcliffe, 1968): others find no correlation (Beagrie and James, 1962; Gould and Picton, 1966).

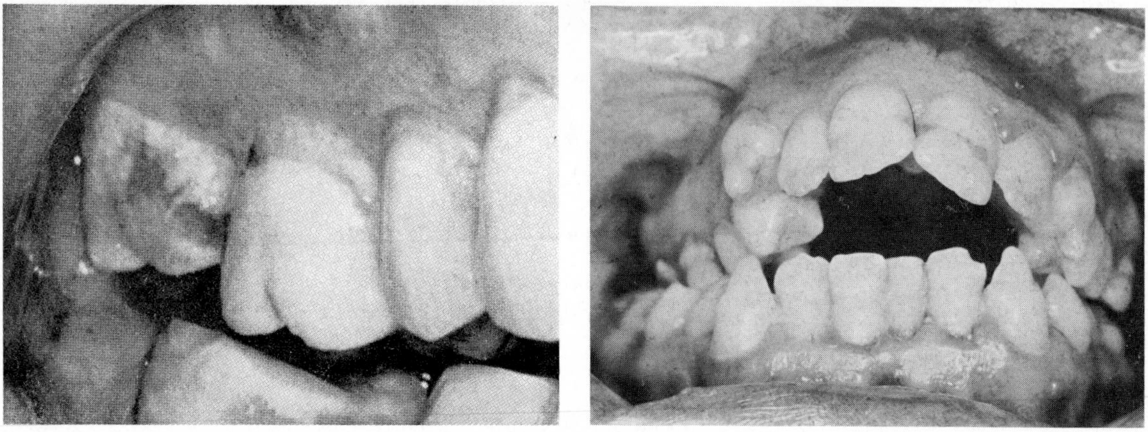

A *B*

FIG. 50.—(*A*) Non-functional molar as site of calculus deposition. (*B*) Generalized subgingival calculus around incisor teeth in a case of anterior open bite where the rest of the mouth is comparatively clean.

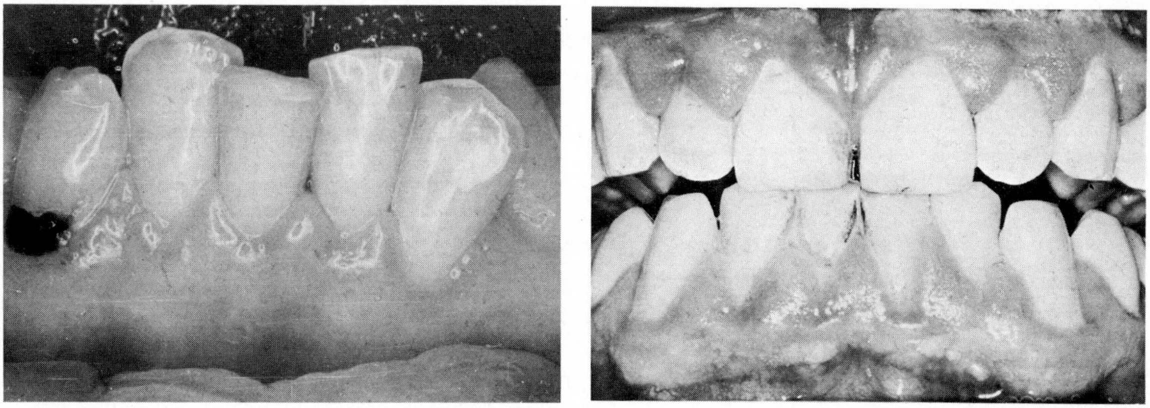

A *B*

FIG. 51.—(*A*) Gingival inflammation associated with malalignment of teeth. (*B*) Split papillae associated with poor oral hygiene and crowding of incisor teeth.

Probably the most exhaustive study in this field is that described by Alexander and Tipnis (1970) who in examining groups of dental students and patients did find some relationship between gingival inflammation and tooth irregularity. It is interesting to note that while there was no statistically significant correlation in the presumably highly motivated dental student group, there was a significantly higher degree of inflammation associated with tooth irregularity in the 200 patients who were, presumably, not so well motivated about oral hygiene.

These findings could be interpreted to mean that where oral hygiene is good tooth position makes little or no difference, but where oral hygiene is poor tooth malalignment becomes a significant factor. By the same token where oral hygiene is very poor and plaque has accumulated around both straight and malaligned teeth gingival inflammation is general.

Direct Trauma

Direct trauma to the gingivae, apart from food impaction, is not a common cause of gingival disease. Occasional hard or sharp particles in food, fish bones, for example, may injure the gum margin and even cause a gingival abscess, but they do not cause chronic gingivitis.

Incorrect tooth-cleaning techniques, such as the careless use of woodsticks, may damage the gingiva. Incorrect and too vigorous use of the toothbrush, particularly when it is used like a scrubbing brush, may damage the gingiva and produce gingival recession but rarely chronic gingival inflammation. By far the most important feature of an incorrect brushing technique is the failure to remove plaque.

Gingival damage and chronic inflammation may result when teeth make contact with gingiva in the opposing jaw (Fig. 52). This is quite common in cases of Angle Class II malocclusion with a very deep overbite so that the lower incisors strike the gingivae palatal to the upper incisors, or upper incisors strike the lower gingivae. Both recession and inflammation result, and the recession sometimes produces a little plateau of tissue behind the upper incisors which interferes with food shedding and causes food stagnation against the already traumatized tissue (Fig. 53). Similarly a gum flap over a lower third molar may be traumatized by an upper molar.

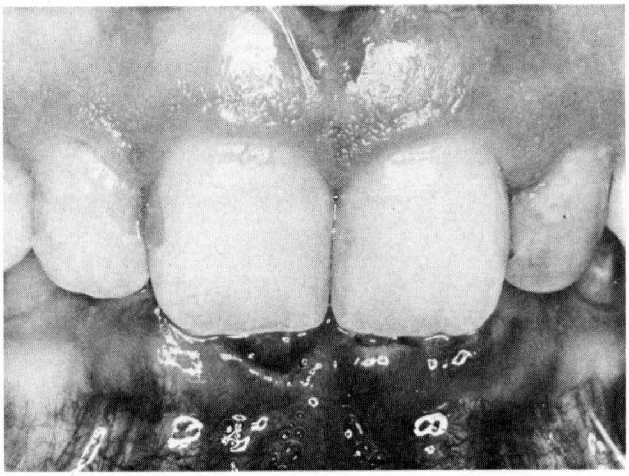

A

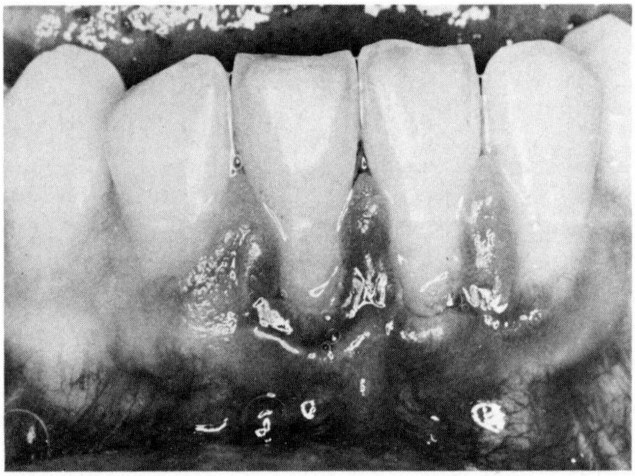

B

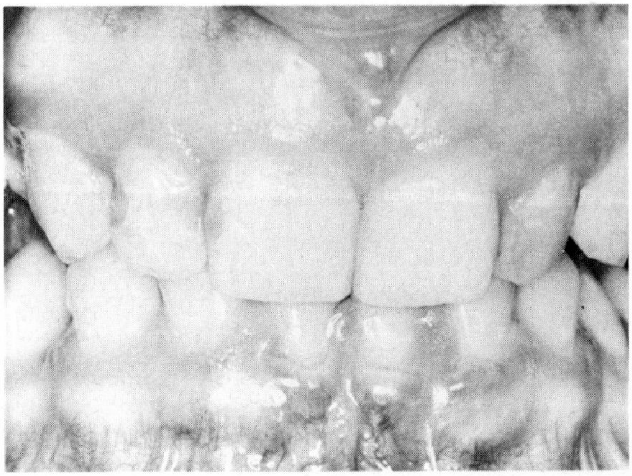

C

FIG. 52.—Gingival inflammation and destruction produced by impingement of upper incisors on lower labial gingivae in a case of deep overbite. (*A*) Overbite. (*B*) Gingival damage. (*C*) Resolution of inflammation when bite is opened by appliance.

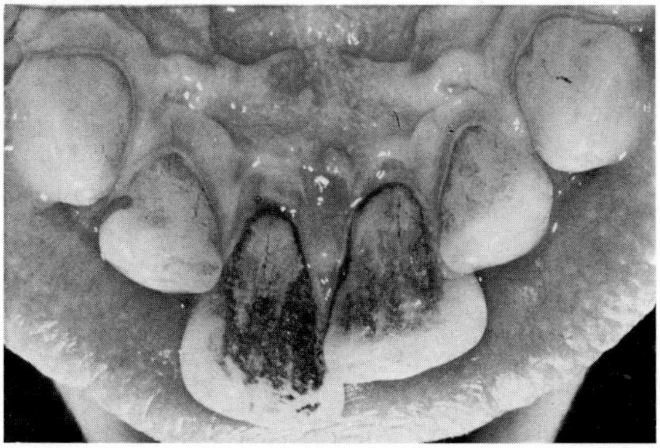

FIG. 53.—Inflammation of gingivae palatal to upper incisors caused by lower incisors in a case of deep overbite.

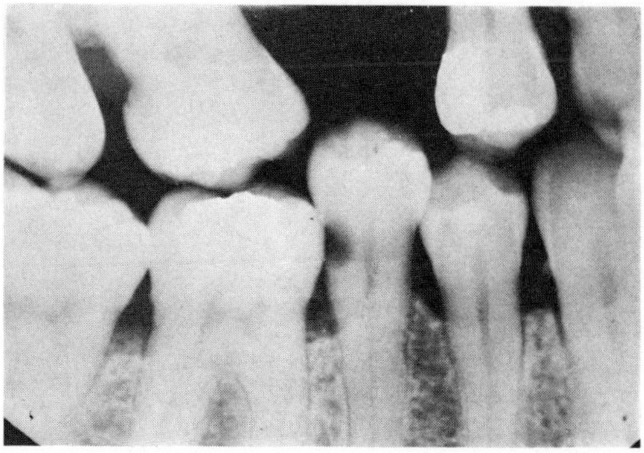

FIG. 54.—Bitewing radiograph demonstrating the movement of teeth and abnormal contact relationships resulting from failure to replace a tooth.

Failure to Replace Missing Teeth

The removal of a tooth disturbs the balance of forces which exists when teeth are in normal function. The result is tooth movement, and this initiates a complex of events:

(a) Opposing teeth overerupt.
(b) Teeth on either side of the gap tilt.
(c) Tooth contacts in both jaws become abnormal, food-shedding becomes inefficient and food-impaction and stagnation results.
(d) In the absence of the cleansing action of normal, food-shedding becomes inefficient debris.
(e) With tooth movement occlusal disharmonies are produced which may result in abnormal occlusal stresses (Chapter 13).

The net result is often gingival irritation and inflammation and, in time, periodontal breakdown and frequently cervical caries (Fig. 54).

Lack of Lip-seal

The term 'mouth-breathing' is commonly used when a patient's lips are held apart in repose even though he may be breathing through his nose. Whether or not the patient does, in fact, breathe through his mouth, it appears to be the lack of lip-seal which is important in relation to gingival health. The mechanism is uncertain but it seems possible that with the lips apart the gingivae in the front of the mouth are not bathed in saliva. The effects are two-fold:

(a) The normal cleansing action of the saliva

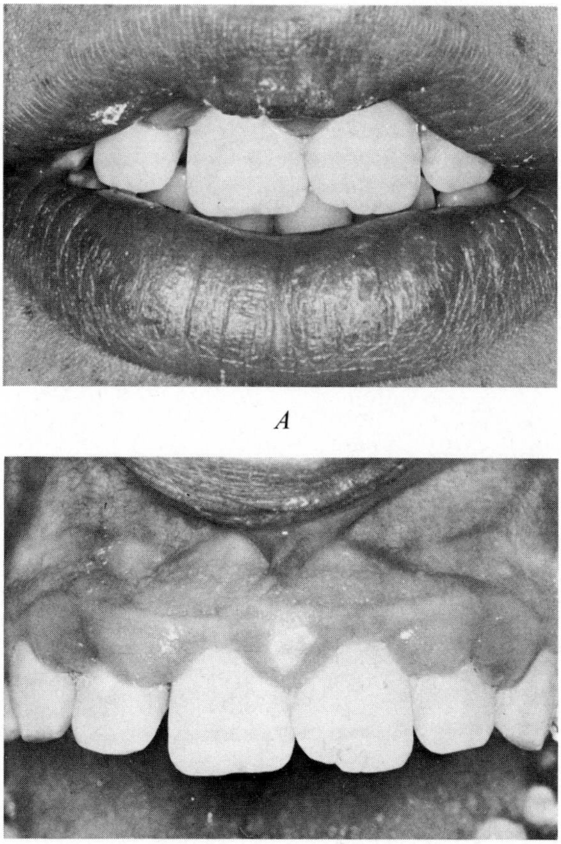

A

B

FIG. 55.—(*A*) Lip-apart posture in girl of sixteen. (*B*) Associated gingival swelling clearly restricted to the exposed area.

flow is absent and plaque accumulates on the labial aspect of the anterior teeth.

(b) The drying out of the epithelium lowers the resistance of the tissue.

Therefore a gingivitis results from the irritation of debilitated tissue by plaque. Characteristically this gingivitis is restricted to the upper anterior region, and mouth-breathing can often be diagnosed because of this localization (Fig. 55).

HOST FACTORS

Two individuals may be exposed to the identical environmental change such as a change in the temperature, humidity, altitude or diet and respond in completely different ways. We assume that age, nutrition, hormonal status and general health must influence tissue behaviour but the nature of that influence is obscure. We have to acknowledge that to date host factors are largely undefined. They may be divided into local and general factors.

LOCAL FACTORS

These represent characteristics of the oral tissues and specifically the gingivae at the time the environmental change is operating.

These factors have been discussed fully by Brandtzaeg (1966), and are summarized as follows:

1. A reduction in the flow of saliva over the gingiva must reduce both the mechanical action of the fluid flow and the effects of the anti-bacterial constituents.
2. The degree of keratinization or parakeratinization of the gingiva affects the facility with which toxic materials are able to diffuse through the gingival epithelium into the underlying corium.
3. The constant renewal of crevicular epithelium, the migration of cells to the surface and their subsequent desquamation acts as a self-cleansing mechanism which helps remove foreign bodies from the gingival crevice. Therefore factors which influence this cell turnover must have a significant effect on tissue response.
4. Plasma proteins produced by crevicular epithelium help maintain adhesion to the tooth. Proteolytic enzymes produced by bacteria and polymorphonuclear leucocytes destroy plasma proteins and thereby reduce adhesion.
5. Gingival fluid or exudate flushes out particulate matter and dilutes toxins. It contains lysozyme which destroys bacterial cell walls.
6. Indigenous oral flora may protect the tissues from attack by exogenous bacteria.

GENERAL FACTORS

Age

A number of changes take place in the periodontal tissues of the older individuals. Possibly the most important of these is the change in the periodontal blood vessels. Arteriosclerosis may occur in arteries and arterioles with decreased vessel diameter and reduced arterial blood flow (Grant and Bernick, 1970).

The gingiva becomes more fibrous but less well keratinized (Wentz, Maier and Orban, 1952).

The periodontal fibre bundles become thicker and less cellular. Ground substance reduces in amount and basement membranes may be thicker. These changes could be caused by the reduced blood supply. Areas of hyaline degeneration and calcification have been described in the aged periodontium (Grant and Bernick, 1970).

Cementum deposition continues throughout life and therefore it is thicker in the older individual (Zander and Hurzeler, 1958), but its rate of deposition slows down.

Alveolar bone shows changes typical of age changes in all other bone. Bone activity continues but the proportion of resorption to deposition increases with resultant osteoporosis (Manson and Lucas, 1962). This seems likely to occur earlier in women than men (Ward and Manson, 1973). Nevertheless in the absence of disease those bone changes which compensate for attrition and thus maintain the vertical facial dimension continue into senility.

It was believed that apical migration of the attachment epithelium with age was a physiological phenomenon. This was called 'passive eruption'. It is now generally believed that this epithelial migration with its exposure of root is pathological, due to inflammation and mechanical irritation. In an examination of Eskimos, Williams (1943) found that the gingival margin stayed at the amelo-cemental junction no matter how much attrition was present.

The relationship between periodontal disease

and age is obscure. Epidemiological studies show a direct correlation between the severity of periodontal destruction and age but this probably only reflects the persistence of a progressive disease which starts at a much earlier age. Indeed it is possible that age makes the *initiation* of periodontal disease less likely. Tissue reactivity is reduced, the inflammatory reaction is more subdued and it seems likely that the immune responses are well developed (see Prognosis, p. 207).

Nutrition

At one time nutritional deficiencies were considered to play a primary role in the aetiology of periodontal disease. The current belief is that nutritional deficiencies must change host factors so that the reaction to bacterial plaque is altered.

Severe periodontal destruction occurs in individuals on an ample diet but epidemiological studies do show greater severity of disease at each age level in Asian and African populations than in European. This could be due to nutritional deficiency or to poor oral hygiene, both of which reflect socio-economic status.

Theoretically a deficiency of any essential nutrient must affect periodontal status but there is little clear evidence of the importance of any specific nutritional element including Vitamin C. Usually multiple rather than specific deficiencies occur and such is the interdependance of the metabolism of the various dietary elements that even apparently controlled animal experiments are not necessarily valid. In Nigeria well-fed children have better periodontal health than badly nourished children irrespective of oral hygiene status and this appears to be associated with a protein-calorie deficiency (Enwonwu and Edozien, 1970). Acute ulcerative gingivitis occurs in West African children but rarely in European children (Emslie, 1963).

Vitamin C is essential for collagen production and therefore for normal cell turnover and repair. There is considerable debate about its optimal intake. Patients with zero plasma ascorbic acid may show no sign of scurvy. The clinical manifestations of scurvy include gingival inflammation and bleeding but it is believed that some gingival irritation, *i.e.* plaque, is essential to this response.

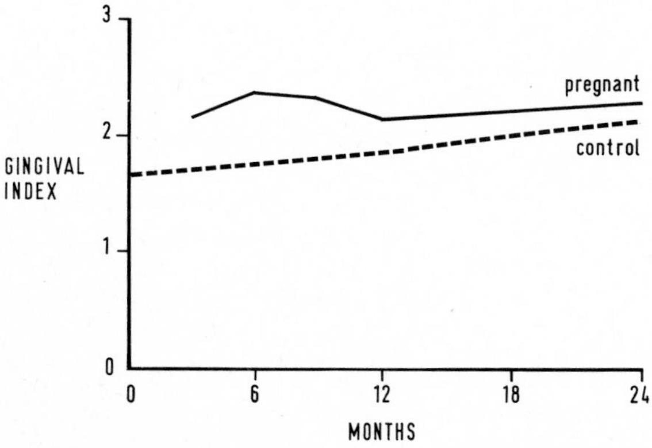

FIG. 56.—Gingival inflammation in a group of pregnant women compared with a control group. (By courtesy of Dr D. W. Cohen.)

HORMONAL STATES

Sex Hormones

Changes in the level of sex hormone activity do appear to alter tissue structure and tissue response to irritation. Increased levels of progesterone produce dilatation of gingival capillaries, increased capillary permeability and gingival exudate. Oestrogen also produces changes in the keratinization of gingival epithelium and alters the degree of polymerization of ground-substance. Injection of oestrogen seems to stimulate bone formation in animals. Testosterone also stimulates bone deposition. Changes in sex hormone are manifested in puberty, menstruation and pregnancy as altered responses to gingival irritation and plaque. In pregnancy there is a reduction in gingival keratinization and an increase in epithelial glycogen and therefore probably a reduction in the effectiveness of the epithelial barrier. Because of the vascular change there is a more ready and florid response to such irritation. Cohen *et al.* (1971) show significantly more gingival inflammation and horizontal tooth mobility in pregnant women than in non-pregnant women of the same ages (Fig. 56).

Diabetes

There do not appear to be any oral changes which are specific to diabetes but the presence of an ineffectively controlled diabetes does seem to alter tissue response in many individuals. There appears to be more rapid bone destruction and increased tendency to abscess formation. Healing is usually retarded. In artificially-induced diabetes in animals generalized osteoporosis occurs. Glavind, Lund and Löe (1968) investigated the periodontal condition of controlled diabetics as compared with a group of non-diabetics and found that up to the age of 30 years the rate of periodontal destruction is the same for diabetics and non-diabetics. Between 30 and 40 years of age the diabetics show a slightly increased amount of breakdown, and diabetics with more than ten years' history show greater periodontal destruction than patients with less than ten years' history of diabetes (Fig. 57). Also those diabetics with retinopathy show greater periodontal breakdown than those without retinal changes.

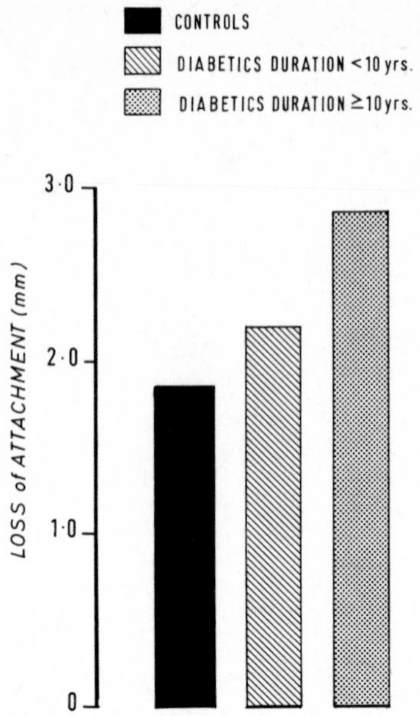

Fig. 57.—Periodontal destruction in diabetic patients aged 20–40 years compared with controls. Destruction is greatest in patients suffering diabetes for longer than ten years. (By courtesy of Dr H. Löe.)

Altered Immune Response

The role of the immune responses in periodontal disease is gradually being elucidated (Lehner, 1972). It seems likely that both humoral and cell-mediated immunity mechanisms are involved. There is evidence that in juvenile periodontitis (periodontosis) the rapid tissue breakdown manifests a failure in lymphocyte transformation which may be genetic or developmental (Chapter 18).

GINGIVITIS→PERIODONTITIS

We have come to accept the transition from chronic gingivitis to chronic periodontitis as involving no more than the spread of inflammation from superficial to deeper tissues. This idea is summarized in the statement that the cause of chronic periodontitis is inadequate control of chronic gingivitis (Manson, 1970). Does the persistence of inflammation in the gingiva, given time, inevitably result in destruction of the deeper tissues or do other factors play an essential role? As Waerhaug (1966) points out, innumerable epidemiological studies demonstrate a strong correlation between oral hygiene and gingivitis, periodontitis and bone destruction, and where large population samples have been examined there is found a linear correlation paralleled only by the linear correlation between periodontal destruction and age. This appears to indicate that no new factor enters into the situation. However, Russell's Periodontal Index (1957), which has been the most extensively used epidemiological instrument, does not allow one to identify the earliest stage in the transition from gingivitis to periodontitis and the more precise Periodontal Disease Index (Ramfjord, 1959) relies on the identification of the amelo-cemental junction which is not always easy and may be impossible in the presence of calculus. Thus, any interruption which may be present in this straight line correlation is not discerned, and even if we accept this correlation for the large group, there is individual variation within the group.

Goldman (1957) and others have described the event which delineates the reversible gingivitis from the irreversible periodontitis as a break in integrity of the transseptal fibres which allows apical migration of the crevicular epithelium. Ramfjord and Kohler (1959) state that the alveolar crest fibres and the most coronal Sharpey's fibres inserted into cementum are the most stable under various forms of occlusal stress. In the past decade considerable attention has been focused on actual and potential agents of collagen fibre destruction. The aetiological factors we should now be attempting to identify are not only those capable of breaking down collagen or connective tissue ground substance but also those factors capable of inhibiting collagen or ground substance formation. Tissue changes are cell-mediated and if collagen fibres are broken and not immediately reformed this points to some interference with fibroblasts and their progenitors. Melcher (1962) has described degeneration of the fibroblast which accompanies disintegration of periodontal fibre bundles in chronic gingivitis. However, the lesion in chronic periodontitis is not so much a lesion of the periodontal ligament as of the ligamentous attachment to the tooth. One of the characteristics of this lesion is that it is usually well circumscribed and fibre bundles quite close to the base of the pocket are intact even when their orientation is altered. Thilander (1961) examined the early stages of chronic periodontitis by light microscope and electron-microscope and found that dissolution of the collagen fibres began just apical to the epithelial attachment with early disappearance of the cementoblasts between the most coronal marginal bundles. In a few cases he found thickening of the collagen bundles with corresponding cementum hyperplasia. This destruction of the connective tissue attachment just below the epithelial attachment was explained by Fleischmann and Gottlieb (1920) and Gottlieb (1923) as a loss of vitality of cementum caused by some metabolic change but they do not seem to have related this to the oral flora. Later Fish (1950) and others suggested that the destruction of the collagen bundles was caused by enzymes produced by the microorganisms of the pocket. The fact that the periodontal lesion is irreversible indicates that the break in attachment of collagen fibres to cementum is not repaired. This can only be because the cell responsible for maintaining the integrity of the attachment is inactive and not being replaced. Cementum mediates the attachment of periodontal ligament to dentine and as Thilander (1961) has shown in the early lesion there is both a break between the ligament and cementum and breakdown of the dentino-cementum junction. It seems reasonable to propose that the essential factor in the progression of gingivitis to periodontitis is death of the most coronal cementoblasts, that is those cells which lay on the surface of the 'acellular' cementum near the enamel-cementum junction, and interference with their differentiation from any progenitor cells in the adjacent connective tissue. However there is as yet little evidence for this hypothesis, and the transition of chronic gingivitis to chronic periodontitis has yet to be explained.

REFERENCES

ALEXANDER, A. G. and TIPNIS, A. K. (1970). The effect of irregularity of teeth and the degree of overbite and overjet on the gingival health. *Brit. dent. J.*, **128**, 539.

ARNO, A., WAERHAUG, J., LOVDAL, A. and SCHEI, O. (1958). Incidence of gingivitis as related to sex, occupation, tobacco consumption, toothbrushing and age. *Oral Surg.*, **11**, 587.

ASH, M. M. JNR., GITLIN, B. N. and SMITH, W. A. (1964). Correlation between plaque and gingivitis. *J. Periodont.*, **35**, 424.

BAER, P. N. and Lieberman, J. E. (1959). Observation on some genetic characteristics of the periodontium in three strains of inbred mice. *Oral Surg.*, **12**, 820.

BEAGRIE, G. S. and James, G. A. (1962). The association of posterior tooth irregularity and periodontal disease. *Brit. dent. J.*, **113**, 239.

BERGLUND, S. E., RIZZO, A. A. and MERGENHAGEN, S. E. (1969). The immune response in rabbits to bacterial somatic antigen administered via the oral mucosa. *Arch. oral Biol.*, **14**, 7.

BRANDTZAEG, P. (1966). Local factors of resistance in the gingival area. *J. periodont. Res.*, **1**, 19.

COHEN, D. W., SHAPIRO, J., FRIEDMAN, L., KYLE, G. C. and FRANKLIN, S. (1971). A longitudinal investigation of the periodontal changes during pregnancy and fifteen months post-partum, Part II. *J. Periodont.*, **42**, 653.

EGELBERG, J. (1965). Local effect of diet on plaque formation and development of gingivitis in dogs. III. Effect of frequency of meals and tube feeding. *Odont. Revy*, **16**, 50.

EMSLIE, R. D. (1963). Cancrum oris. *Dent. Practit.*, **13**, 481

ENWONWU, C. O. and EDOZIEN, J. C. (1970). Epidemiology of periodontal disease in Western Nigerians in relation to socio-economic status. *Arch. oral Biol.*, **15**, 1231.

FISH, E. W. (1950). Problems of paradontal disease. *Brit. dent. J.*, **88**, 139.

FLEISCHMANN, L. and GOTTLIEB, B. (1920). Beiträge für Histologie und Pathogenese der Alveolar-Pyorrhoe. *Öst. Z. Stomat.*, **18**, 43.
FULLMER, H. M. and GIBSON, W. (1966). Collagenolytic activity in gingivae of man. *Nature*, **209**, 728.
GIANELLY, A. A. (1970). Orthodontic considerations in periodontal therapy. *J. Periodont.*, **41**, 119.
GLAVIND, L., LUND, B. and LÖE, H. (1968). The relationship between periodontal state and diabetes duration, insulin dosage and retinal changes. *J. Periodont.*, **39**, 341.
GOLDMAN, H. M. (1957). Behaviour of transseptal fibres in periodontal disease. *J. dent. Res.*, **36**, 249.
GOTTLIEB, B. (1923). Die diffuse Atrophie des Alveolar Knochens: zweitere Beiträge für Erkenntiss des Alveolarschwundes und dessen Wiedergutmachung durch Zementwachstum. *Z. Stomat.*, **21**, 195.
GOULD, M. S. E. and PICTON, D. C. A. (1966). The relation between irregularities of the teeth and the degree of overbite and overjet on the gingival health. *Brit. dent. J.*, **121**, 20.
GRANT, D. and BERNICK, S. (1970). Arteriosclerosis in periodontal vessels of ageing humans. *J. Periodont.*, **41**, 170.
HORTON, J. E., LEIKIN, S. and OPPENHEIM, J. J. (1972). Human lymphoproliferative reaction to saliva and dental plaque deposits: an *in vitro* correlation with periodontal disease. *J. Periodont.*, **43**, 522.
IVY, A. C., MORGAN, J. E. and FARRELL, J. I. (1931). Effects of total gastrectomy. *Surg. gynec. Obstet.*, **53**, 611.
KING, J. D. and GIMSON, A. P. (1947). Experimental investigations of paradontal disease in the ferret and related lesions in man. *Brit. dent. J.*, **83**, 126, 148.
LANDSTEINER, K. and CHASE, M. W. (1942). Experiments on the transfer of cutaneous sensitivity to simple compounds. *Proc. Soc. exp. Biol. Med.*, **49**, 688.
LEHNER, T. (1972). Cell-mediated immune responses in oral disease: a review. *J. oral Path.*, **1**, 39.
LÖE, H., THEILADE, E. and JENSEN, S. B. (1965). Experimental gingivitis in man. *J. Periodont.*, **36**, 177.
MANSON, J. D. and LUCAS, R. B. (1962). Microradiographic study of age changes in the human mandible. *Arch. oral Biol.*, **7**, 761.
MANSON J. D. (1970). Periodontics for the Dental Practitioner, 2nd ed. Henry Kimpton, London.
MELCHER, A. H. (1962). Pathogenesis of chronic gingivitis. I. The spread of the inflammatory process. *Dent. Practit. dent. Rec.*, **13**, 2.
MERGENHAGEN, S. E., TEMPEL, T. R. and SNYDERMAN, R. (1970). Immunologic reactions and periodontal inflammation. *J. dent. Res.*, **49**, Suppl. to No. 2, 256.
RAMFJORD, S. P. (1959). Indices for prevalence and incidence of periodontal disease. *J. Periodont.*, **30**, 51.
RAMFJORD, S. P. and KOHLER, C. A. (1959). Periodontal reaction to functional occlusal stress. *J. Periodont.*, **30**, 95.
ROSEBURY, T. (1947). Nature and significance of infection in periodontal disease. *Amer. J. Orthodont. oral Surg.*, **33**, 658.
ROSENZWEIG, K. A. (1960). Gingivitis in children of Israel. *J. Periodont.*, **31**, 404.
ROVIN, S., COSTICH, E. R. and GORDON, H. A. (1966). The influence of bacteria and irritation in the initiation of periodontal disease in germfree and conventional rats. *J. periodont. Res.*, **1**, 193.
RUSSELL, A. L. (1957). Social factors associated with the severity of periodontal disease. *J. dent. Res.*, **36**, 922.
SAXE, S. R., GREEVE, J. C., BOHANNAN, H. M. and VERMILLION, J. R. (1967). Oral debris, calculus and periodontal disease in the beagle dog. *Periodontics*, **5**, 217.
SCHEI, O., WAERHAUG, J., LÖVDAL, A. and ARNO, A. (1959). Alveolar bone loss as related to oral hygiene and age. *J. Periodont.*, **30**, 7.
SCHUESSLER, C. F., FAIRCHILD, J. M. and STRANSKY, I. M. (1945). Penicillin in the treatment of Vincent's infection. *J. Amer. dent. Ass.*, **32**, 551.
SOCRANSKY, S. S. and GIBBONS, R. J. (1965). Required role of Bacteroides melaninogenicus in mixed anaerobic infections. *J. infect. Dis.*, **115**, 247.
SOCRANSKY, S. S. (1970). Relationship of bacteria to the etiology of periodontal disease. *J. dent. Res.*, **49**, Suppl. to No. 2, 203.
SUTCLIFFE, P. (1968). Chronic anterior gingivitis: An epidemiological study in school children. *Brit. dent. J.*, **125**, 47.
THILANDER, H. (1961). Periodontal disease in the white rat. (Experimental studies with special reference to some aetiologic and pathogenetic features.) Thesis, *Trans. Roy. Sch. Dent. Stockholm & Umea*, No. 6.
WAERHAUG, J. (1956a). Effect of rough surfaces upon gingival tissue. *J. dent. Res.*, **35**, 323.
WAERHAUG, J. (1956b). Effect of zinc phosphate cement fillings on gingival tissues. *J. Periodont.*, **27**, 284.
WAERHAUG, J. (1966). Epidemiology of periodontal disease. *In* World Workshop in Periodontics. (Ramfjord, S. P. *et al.*, eds). University of Michigan, p. 181.
WARD, V. W. and MANSON, J. D. (1973). Alveolar bone loss in periodontal disease and the metacarpal index. *J. Periodont.*, **44**, 763.

WENTZ, F. M., MAIER, A. W. and ORBAN, B. (1952). Age changes and sex differences in the clinically 'normal' gingiva. *J. Periodont.*, **23**, 13.
WHEELER, R. C. (1938). Etiology, treatment and prevention of chronic gingival irritation around porcelain jacket crowns. *J. Amer. dent. Ass.*, **25**, 1742.
WILLIAMS, C. H. M. (1943). Investigation concerning the dentitions of the Eskimos of Canada's Eastern Arctic. *J. Periodont.*, **14**, 34.
ZANDER, H. A. and HURZELER, B. (1958). Continuous cementum apposition. *J. dent. Res.*, **37**, 1035.

5. Epidemiology of Periodontal Disease

Casual observation and clinical experience tells us something about the prevalence and distribution of disease and can also suggest causal factors and predisposing conditions. However, such data is not reliable and in fact can be misleading. Two major problems need to be overcome to obtain a valid picture of a disease. First, there is considerable variation between individuals both in health and in disease so that a large number of individuals may need to be examined before any general description of a disease can be given. Second, the subjective element in the assessment of a clinical state must be reduced to a minimum so that reliable standards are established from which valid comparison can be made. In order to achieve this end, one attempts to reduce examination to simple and objective and therefore easily reproducible observations to which numbers can be assigned. Clear definition of single clinical features is attempted by asking simple questions such as: Is the interdental papilla red? Yes or No; Does it bleed on touch? Yes or No; If a probe is scraped across the tooth surface does it come away with a deposit? Yes or No. Prevalence refers to the number of such specific items collected from an individual or population at a specific time; incidence refers to the number of items found to occur during a given period of time. Epidemiology is the scientific study of the occurrence and distribution of disease within population groups.

In studies of periodontal disease one needs to know:

1. How many individuals suffer from disease.
2. The severity of the disease.
3. Associated factors to be studied.

To this end a number of indices have been devised which allow us to assess gingivitis, periodontal destruction, bone loss and the state of oral hygiene. Among the most commonly used indices are the following.

GINGIVAL INFLAMMATION INDICES

1. P-M-A (Schour and Massler, 1948)
The P-M-A index was probably the first successful attempt to design a numerical system for recording periodontal conditions. The three letters stand for papillary (P), marginal (M), and attached gingiva (A). From clinical experience it was postulated that periodontal disease starts in the interdental papillae (P), spreads to the marginal area (M), and then in severe cases to the attached gingiva (A). Thus, the location of the inflammatory process to some extent indicates the severity of the condition. Within each of these three areas the severity of the inflammation can also be indicated on a scale running from 0 to 4.

- 0 – No gingivitis.
- 1 – Mild inflammation with slight change in colour and little loss of contour.
- 2 – Moderate inflammation with swelling, glazing and redness. Tendency to bleed on slight pressure. Papillae or margins become blunted or rounded. Slight extension of inflammation to adjacent tissue.
- 3 – Severe inflammation with more swelling and redness, pocket formation, spontaneous bleeding. Involvement of the adjacent tissues. Slight degeneration.
- 4 – Very severe inflammation any degree more severe than the above including ulceration and sloughing as in acute ulcerative gingivitis.

In its original form only the labial gingivae of the six lower front teeth were examined. The scores for P, M and A can be added and this sum divided by the number of teeth included can be taken as representing the gingival status of that individual. The data may also be presented as the percentage of individuals having one or more inflamed gingival units, or as the average number of P-M-A units per person. For prevalence studies each P-M-A unit is scored 0 or 1 for absence or presence of inflammation respectively and the intensity scores are not considered.

2. Gingival Index (Löe and Silness, 1963)
The gingival index system (GI) is based on the same principles as the P-M-A index. The severity of the condition is indicated on a scale running from 0 to 3 as follows:

- 0 – Normal gingiva.
- 1 – Mild inflammation, slight change in colour, slight oedema. No bleeding on probing.
- 2 – Moderate inflammation, redness, oedema and glazing. Bleeding on probing.
- 3 – Severe inflammation, marked redness and oedema, ulceration. Tendency to spontaneous haemorrhage.

The mesial, distal, buccal and lingual gingival units are scored independently. For clinical trials this index is very sensitive, particularly in the early stages of gingival inflammation.

The P-M-A and GI are reversible indices, *i.e.*, their values return to zero with the disappearance of disease. Thus they represent assessments of *active* disease. Irreversible indices assess the permanent damage caused by active disease.

PERIODONTAL DESTRUCTION INDICES

1. Periodontal Index (P.I.) (Russell, 1956)
All teeth present are examined; the criteria used in this index are as follows:

- 0 – Negative: there is neither overt inflammation in the investing tissues nor loss of function due to destruction of supporting tissues.
- 1 – Mild gingivitis: there is an overt area of inflammation in the free gingivae, but this area does not circumscribe the tooth.
- 2 – Gingivitis: inflammation completely circumscribes the tooth, but there is no apparent break in the epithelial attachment.
- 6 – Gingivitis with pocket formation: the epithelial attachment has been broken and there is a pocket (not merely a deepened gingival crevice due to swelling in the free gingivae). There is no interference with normal masticatory function; the tooth is firm in its socket, and has not drifted.
- 8 – Advanced destruction with loss of masticatory function: the tooth may be loose; may have drifted; may sound dull on percussion with metallic instrument; may be depressible in its socket.

  RULE: When in doubt, assign the lesser score.

This index has been applied with success to large population groups. Its limitation is that its scoring for periodontal destruction is so heavily weighted that it is not possible to distinguish the early stages of a chronic periodontitis.

2. Periodontal Disease Index (PDI) (Ramfjord, 1959)
The periodontal disease index introduced by Ramfjord is a development of the Russell index. As mentioned above, one weak point in the latter index is that there is no provision for distinguishing between slight and extreme pocket deepening. The Ramfjord index is particularly designed for assessing the extent of pocket deepening below the cemento-enamel junction. Scoring is as follows:

- 0 – Health.
- 1 – Mild to moderate inflammatory change not extending all around tooth.
- 2 – Mild to moderate inflammatory change extending all around tooth.
- 3 – Severe gingivitis, characterized by marked redness, tendency to bleed, ulceration.
- 4 – 3 mm apical extension of crevice from enamel-cement junction.
- 5 – 3–6 mm extension.
- 6 – Over 6 mm extension.

Another feature of the PD1 is that only six teeth, 6|14, 41|6, are selected for examination and measurement. The data from these teeth have been found to be representative of the dentition as a whole, and their average score is the score of the patient. Separate measurements are made from the amelo-cemental junction to the gingival margin and for the distance from the gingival margin to the bottom of the pocket. These are added or subtracted to arrive at the tooth score. Thus if the gingival margin is on cementum the score is negative. When first used the measurements were made on all the surfaces of the specified teeth, and the most unfavourable score was assigned to the tooth. Modification of the method has shown that the score of the mesial surface can be taken as representative of all the surfaces of the tooth. A limitation of the method centres on the difficulty of identifying the amelo-cemental junction particularly where deposits of calculus are present.

ORAL HYGIENE INDICES

1. The Simplified Oral Hygiene Index (Greene and Vermillion, 1960)
The oral hygiene index is a composite index based on an oral debris score and a calculus score. The following surfaces are selected for examination: the facial surfaces of the upper first molars and the upper right and lower left incisors, the *lingual* surfaces of the lower first molars. Each surface, buccal or lingual, is considered to encompass half the circumference of the tooth. All surfaces are first examined for debris and then for calculus.

Oral debris is the soft foreign matter loosely attached to the teeth. The following scoring system is used:

0 – No debris or stain present.
1 – Soft debris covering not more than one-third of the tooth surface.
2 – Soft debris covering more than one, but not more than two-thirds of the exposed tooth surface.
3 – Soft debris covering more than two-thirds of the exposed tooth surface.

Calculus scores are assigned according to the same criteria as for debris scores, with the addition that individual flecks of subgingival calculus are given score 2, and a continuous heavy band of subgingival calculus is given score 3.

The debris score and calculus score are totalled and divided by the number of surfaces examined to give the oral hygiene score.

2. Plaque Index (Silness and Löe, 1964)
Criteria for scoring are:

0 – No plaque.
1 – Film or plaque, visible only by removal on probe or by disclosing.
2 – Moderate accumulation of deposits within the pockets or on the margins which can be seen with the naked eye.
3 – Heavy accumulation of soft material filling the niche between gingival margin and tooth surface. Interdental region is filled with debris.

This index has been used together with the Gingival Index to provide precise evidence of the relationship between plaque and gingival inflammation.

A bone destruction score has also been devised by Schei *et. al.* (1959). This utilizes intra-oral radiographs and indicates the *proportion* of tooth-supporting bone which has been lost. A mean value for the mouth = sum of individual tooth scores/number of teeth.

PREVALENCE OF GINGIVITIS

A large number of studies of gingivitis have been carried out in many parts of the world. These studies usually concentrate on young people as in the adult the condition is complicated by the presence of periodontal destruction and by tooth loss from accidents, caries and periodontal disease.

Gingival inflammation is found to appear at the age of four or five. Prevalence and severity seem to go hand in hand and when the permanent teeth erupt, there is a rapid increase in both factors so that by the age of 14 over three-quarters of individuals have some inflammation. A number of studies demonstrate this high prevalence: 90% in 12–14-year-old Dundee school-children (King, 1945); 98% in New York children aged 1–14 (McCall, 1933); 92% of American boys and 97% of Indian boys aged 11–17 (Greene, 1960); 99% of Nigerian children (Sheiham, 1968); 99.7% in Surrey children (Sheiham, 1969); 95.5% in 15-year-old boys and 85.5% in 15-year-old girls in York, England (Murray, 1969). Before 14 years the prevalence seems to be slightly greater in girls, but after that it is greater in boys. This may be related to earlier puberty in girls or to differences in oral hygiene habits. Following puberty there is a decline in prevalence (Fig. 58) and a striking decline in severity, but in young adults the prevalence increases again until it has been recorded at 100% in young men of 17–22 (Barnard and Bradley, 1966; Lightner *et al.*, 1967).

PREVALENCE OF PERIODONTAL DESTRUCTION

The prevalence and severity of periodontal destruction increases with age. Pocketing has been found in 9% of children aged 11–15 (Miller and Seidler, 1942), but usually chronic perio-

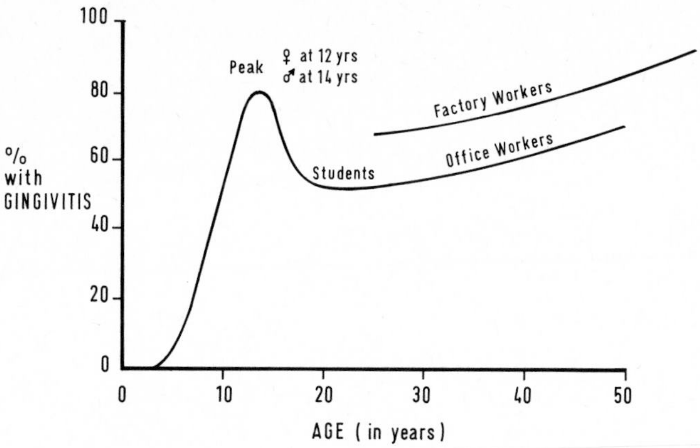

FIG. 58.—The prevalence of gingival inflammation in 10,000 individuals. (By courtesy of Dr M. Massler.)

dontitis is associated with adults. In the 19–26 year group it has been found to affect 24–69% and by the age of 45 it affects virtually 100% of the population (Marshall-Day, Stephens and Quigley, 1955) (Fig. 59).

Pocketing seems to be less severe in women at all ages (Johnson, Kelly and Van Kirk, 1965), and it is probable that this reflects better personal hygiene in women.

There do appear to be racial differences in the prevalence of periodontal destruction. Prevalence and severity are greater in Negroes than in Caucasions at all ages (Russell, 1957a). In the U.S.A. P.I. scores for white men and women are 1.21 and 0.81 respectively comparing with P.I. scores of 1.77 and 1.41 for Negro men and women (Johnson *et al.*, *ibid.*). The same amount of destruction is found at an earlier age and the transition from chronic gingivitis to chronic periodontitis appears to take place at an earlier age in Asiatic people than in Europeans (Lilienthal and Amerena, 1966). However this may be a reflection of socio-economic factors which in turn determine both nutritional status and oral hygiene habits. The apparent differences between racial groups may be explained by differences in oral hygiene habits, and there is some evidence that people with a high income and educational level have better oral hygiene and less periodontal disease than poorer and less well educated people (Russell, 1957b). Studies do not show any well defined relationship between periodontal destruction and nutritional status except in areas of severe Vitamin A and protein deprivation (Russell, 1963). The most important factor determining the prevalence and severity of periodontitis and gingivitis is oral hygiene (Schei *et al.*, 1959; Greene, 1963; Russell, 1967).

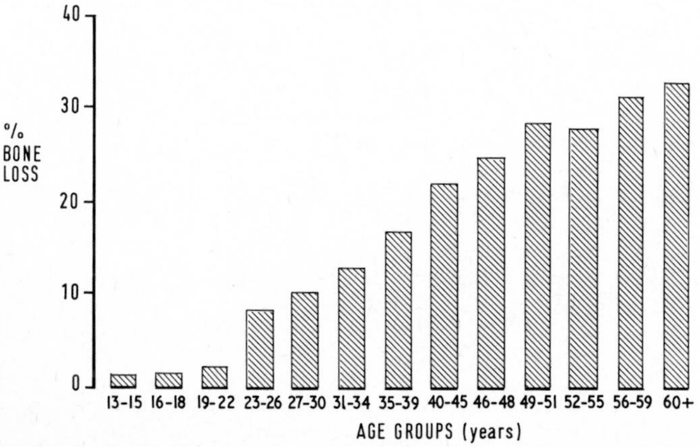

FIG. 59.—The increase of alveolar bone resorption with age. (After Dr C. D. Marshall-Day.)

Factors which predispose to plaque accumulation and retention such as amalgam filling overhangs are associated with greater periodontal destruction (Gilmore and Sheiham, 1971). The evidence relating malocclusion to either gingivitis or periodontitis is equivocal: some studies show a correlation, others do not (see page 38). It seems possible that malalignment can be a contributory factor where oral hygiene is only fairly good but, as stated, its effect is not significant where oral hygiene is either very good or very bad.

The large number of epidemiological studies carried out confirm that although other factors may play a part in the aetiology of periodontal disease poor oral hygiene, *i.e.* the presence of bacterial plaque, is the most important factor.

REFERENCES

BARNARD, P. D. and BRADLEY, D. I. (1966). Dental conditions of senior dental students. *Aust. dent. J.*, **11**, 338.

GILMORE, N. and SHEIHAM, A. (1971). Overhanging dental restorations and periodontal disease. *J. Periodont.*, **42**, 8.

GREENE, J. C. and VERMILLION, J. R. (1960). The simplified oral hygiene index. *J. Amer. dent. Ass.*, **68**, 7.

GREENE, J. C. (1960). Periodontal disease in India: report of an epidemiologic study. *J. dent. Res.*, **39**, 302.

GREENE, J. C. (1963). Oral hygiene and periodontal disease. *Amer. J. publ. Hlth*, **53**, 913.

JOHNSON, E. S., KELLY, J. E. and VAN KIRK, L. E. (1965). Selected dental findings in adults by age, race and sex. United States 1960–62. U.S. Dept. Health, Education & Welfare, National Center for Health Statistics. Series 11, No. 7, 1.

KING, J. D. (1945). Gingival disease in Dundee. *Dent. Rec.*, **65**, 9, 32, 55.

LIGHTNER, L. M., O'LEARY, T. J., DRAKE, R. B., CRUMP, P. P., JIVIDEN, G. J. and JUNGHAUS, J. A. (1967). The periodontal status of incoming Air Force Academy cadets. *J. Amer. dent. Ass.*, **75**, 111.

LILIENTHAL, B. and AMERENA, V. (1966). Adaptation of Knutson's 'working estimate' in surveys of gingivitis and periodontitis. *Arch. oral. Biol.*, **11**, 293.

LÖE, H. and SILNESS, J. (1963). Periodontal disease in pregnancy. I. Prevalence and severity. *Acta odont. scand.*, **21**, 533.

MCCALL, J. O. (1933). The periodontist looks at children's dentistry. *J. Amer. dent. Ass.*, **20**, 1518.

MARSHALL-DAY, C. D., STEPHENS, R. G. and QUIGLEY, L. F. (1955). Periodontal disease: prevalence and incidence. *J. Periodont.*, **26**, 185.

MILLER, S. C. and SEIDLER, B. B. (1942). Relative alveoclastic experience of the various teeth. *J. dent. Res.*, **21**, 365.

MURRAY, J. J. (1969). Gingivitis in 15-year-old schoolchildren from high fluoride and low fluoride areas. *Arch. oral. Biol.*, **14**, 951.

RAMFJORD, S. P. (1959). Indices for prevalence and incidence of periodontal disease. *J. Periodont.*, **30**, 51.

RUSSELL, A. L. (1956). A system of classification and scoring for prevalence surveys of periodontal disease. *J. dent. Res.*, **35**, 350.

RUSSELL, A. L. (1957a). Some epidemiological characteristics of periodontal disease in a series of urban populations. *J. Periodont.*, **28**, 286.

RUSSELL, A. L. (1957b). A social factor associated with the severity of periodontal disease. *J. dent. Res.*, **36**, 922.

RUSSELL, A. L. (1963). International nutrition surveys: A summary of preliminary dental findings. *J. dent. Res.*, **42**, 233.

RUSSELL, A. L. (1967). Epidemiology of periodontal disease. *Int. dent. J.*, **17**, 282.

SCHEI, O., WAERHAUG, J., LOVDAL, A. and ARNO, A. (1959). Alveolar bone loss as related to oral hygiene and age. *J. Periodont.*, **30**, 7.

SCHOUR, I. and MASSLER, M. (1948). Prevalence of gingivitis in young adults. *J. dent. Res.*, **27**, 733.

SHEIHAM, A. (1968). The epidemiology of chronic periodontal disease in Western Nigerian children. *J. periodont. Res.*, **3**, 257.

SHEIHAM, A. (1969). The prevalence and severity of periodontal disease in Surrey schoolchildren. *Dent. Practit.*, 19, 232.

SILNESS, J. and LÖE, H. (1964). Periodontal disease in pregnancy. II. Correlation between oral hygiene and periodontal condition. *Acta odont. scand.*, **22**, 121.

6. Prevention of Periodontal Disease

Rationale

Having accepted the progression:

Dental plaque → chronic gingivitis → chronic periodontitis, it follows that the prevention of periodontal disease centres on the prevention of plaque deposition or removal of plaque before it can produce gingival inflammation.

The mechanism of the adhesion of the acquired pellicle and of bacteria to the tooth surface is under investigation and it seems possible that the surface reactions involved may be altered by a number of agents including the fluoride ion. However, these studies are in their infancy and our efforts must concentrate on plaque removal once it has been deposited, plus the correction of those factors which encourage plaque retention.

At one time it was believed that tooth surfaces could be cleaned naturally by hard and fibrous foods, apples, carrots, celery, sugar cane, etc., but many studies have shown that such natural cleaning agents have no effect on the plaque deposits in the sheltered regions of the gingival margin (Emslie, 1967; Löe, 1970). Therefore it is necessary to resort to artificial methods of plaque removal.

It must also be emphasized that a great deal of chronic periodontal disease is iatrogenic, that is, produced by incorrect dental treatment which encourages plaque deposition and makes its removal difficult or impossible.

The practitioner's obligations are therefore two-fold:

1. to practice sound dentistry, and
2. to educate his patients in oral hygiene techniques.

SOUND DENTAL TECHNIQUES

All dental procedures, apart from the construction of full dentures, can affect the periodontal tissues for good or ill. Fortunately, the periodontal tissues are capable of considerable adjustment to varying conditions, and in some individuals even real abuse is tolerated. But all tissues have a threshold of tolerance beyond which irritation causes breakdown. This breakdown is usually the result of a summation of factors acting on the tissues. Seen in isolation some of these factors may seem trivial and incapable of causing more than minor irritation, but within the context of the mouth in function even the most minor irritation may assume significance.

Throughout this text emphasis is placed on careful examination of the mouth in order to define factors which initiate and encourage the progress of periodontal disease, but it seems worthwhile at this point to stress certain simple yet important practical points. Restorations should restore physiological tooth form and tooth relationships, and hence normal function. Overhanging margins can be avoided by the careful use of matrix bands and wedges. Accurately placed contact points and marginal ridges should achieve efficient food shedding. Occlusal relationships should be checked in all mandibular excursions to avoid occlusal stress.

Appearance usually dictates that a lost anterior tooth should be replaced, but if appearance is not a factor to be considered the decision as to whether replacement is necessary may be very difficult to make. Many factors must be taken into account. It would be unrealistic to suggest that every missing tooth be replaced, if only because the replacement such as a partial denture may be a greater evil than the absence of a tooth. In every situation the advantages and disadvantages of replacement need to be weighed against each other. Certainly if proximal teeth begin to drift or incline, or if opposing teeth overerupt, the missing tooth should be replaced immediately. It is bad practice to wait until gross changes have taken place. Regular critical appraisal of the situation should indicate whether changes are beginning to take place; in this respect food impaction, slight tooth mobility, or tooth sensitivity on percussion represent warning signals.

Care should be taken in the design of partial dentures so that they do not become the agent of complete tooth loss. The appliance should make minimum contact with the gingival margin and should be tooth-borne. As many teeth as possible should be used as abutments with the load distributed as closely as possible along the long axis of the abutment tooth. Appliances, like restorations, should occlude properly in all mandibular excursions.

ORAL HYGIENE

The fundamental requirement of any aid to oral hygiene is that it is capable of removing plaque without causing damage to the soft and hard tissues, or to restorations.

Methods of plaque removal are mechanical and chemical.

MECHANICAL CLEANING

There are a variety of mechanical devices for cleaning teeth, the most important of which is the toothbrush.

There is considerable debate about the qualities a toothbrush should possess; whether it should be nylon or bristle, soft or hard, large or small has been the subject of much research and conflicting results.

Requirements for a satisfactory toothbrush are as follows:

1. It should be small enough to be manipulated properly everywhere in the mouth, yet not so small that it has to be used for a long time and with extreme care in order to obtain complete coverage of the dentition. A head length of about 2.5 cm is satisfactory for the adult (Fig. 60), and a smaller brush with a head length of 1.5 cm is suitable for a child. Scully and Wade (1970) report better results using a short-headed brush.
2. The bristles should be of even length (about 1 cm long) so that they function simultaneously. A convex- or concave-shaped brush with bristles of different length will not clean a flat surface without excessive pressure on some of the bristles, which might cause gingival injury (Fig. 61). Bristles which are too short will fail to reach the interdental areas; they may also be rather rigid and traumatize the gingivae.
3. The texture should permit effective use without causing tissue damage. A very soft bristle will not clean effectively and, except for a short time after gingival surgery, a brush of medium stiffness should be used. A hard bristle brush may be useful in the case of a heavy smoker, but it is essential that the individual using a hard brush has tough gingivae and knows how to use the brush so that the tissues are not injured.

There has been some controversy about the relative merits of nylon and bristle in this respect, and the nylon brush has been viewed as potentially harmful. The defect of some of the nylon brushes used in the past lay not so much in the material of the bristles, but in their diameter and resilience. These two factors plus the number of bristles per tuft determine the hardness of a brush. As the bristle diameter is increased the potential for damaging the gingivae also increases.

Bay, Kordel and Skougaard (1967) report significantly better removal of plaque by nylon brushes than bristle brushes. However, any brush is capable of damaging the tissues if used incorrectly.

4. The brush must be easy to keep clean. Densely packed tufts will tend to collect debris and toothpaste at the base of the bristle. The multitufted brush in which the tufts are fairly close together but made up of fewer bristles provides a firm and effective head which is at the same time easy to keep clean.

Toothbrushes which have been found satisfactory include the Wisdom medium nylon multituft short head and the Gibbs hard nylon short head. The Wisdom brush head is 30 mm long and 9.5 mm wide with bristle length 12.00–12.7 mm. It has 45 tufts each of 34 bristles.

Method of Toothbrushing

A large number of brushing techniques have been devised. Greene (1966) has divided them into seven groups based on the movement of the brush. These are: 1. Vertical, 2. Horizontal, 3. Roll, 4. Vibratory (Charters, Stillman, Bass), 5. Circular (Jones), 6. Physiological (Smith), 7. Scrub Techniques.

With such a confusing proliferation of techniques it is essential to present the patient with a simple and straightforward account of a plaque control technique so that he can evolve one which suits him best.

Requirements of a Satisfactory Toothbrushing Technique

1. The toothbrushing technique should clean

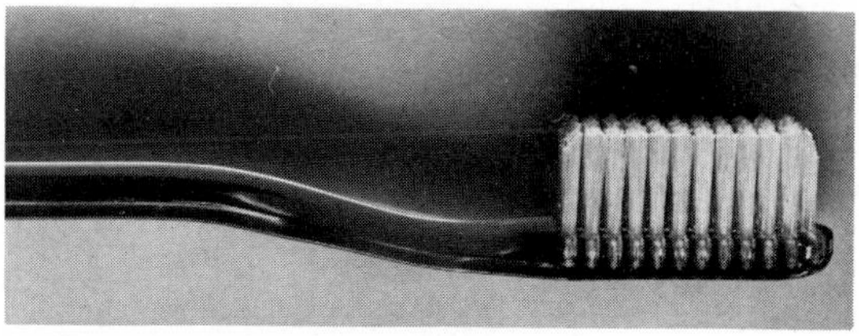

FIG. 60.—A satisfactory toothbrush design.

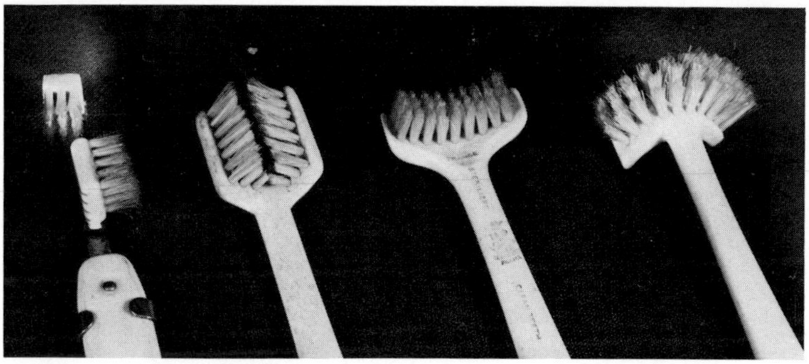

A

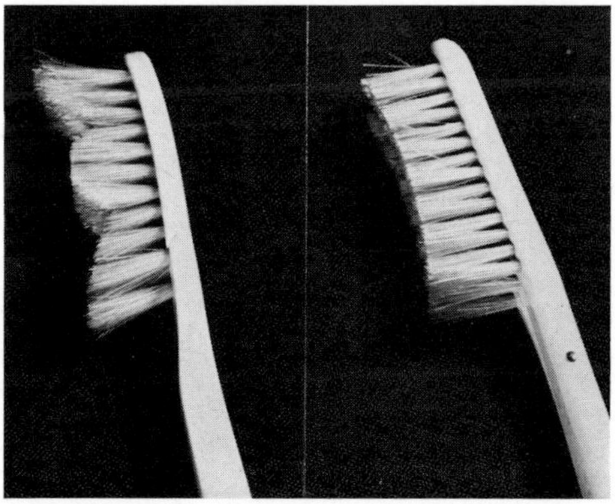

B

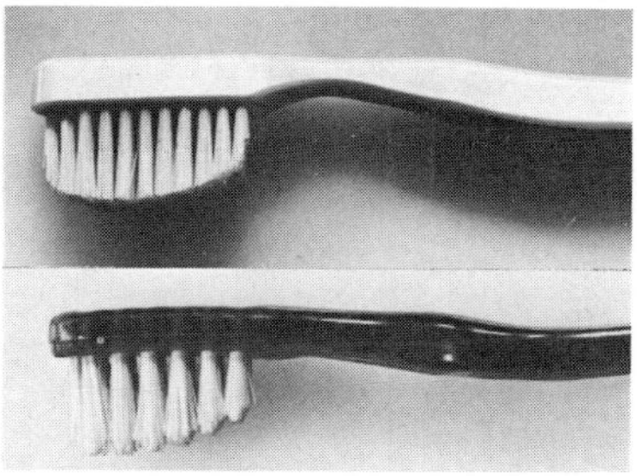

C

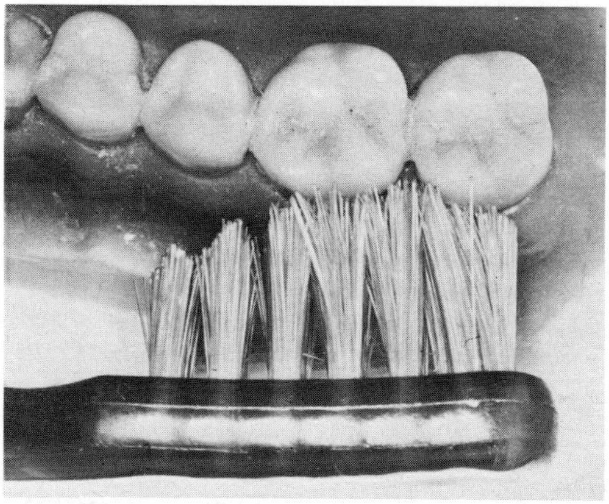

D

FIG. 61.—Unsatisfactory toothbrush designs.
(*A*) Four antique brushes.
(*B*) Brushes that are too large, and with bristles of uneven length.
(*C*) Convex heads.
(*D*) A convex head fails to reach more than one interdental area at a time unless excessive pressure is exerted on the brush.

efficiently all tooth surfaces, most particularly the area of the gingival crevice and especially the interdental region. Any vigorous technique will clean the convex tooth surfaces but may leave debris at the gingival margin, and the patient is deceived into believing that his technique is efficient. This is one reason why in so many apparently clean mouths there is a marginal gingivitis, and in most mouths the truth is revealed only by careful examination and the use of a disclosing agent.
2. The movement of the bristles should not injure the tissues. The vertical and horizontal scrubbing techniques may cause gingival damage and recession.
3. The technique must be relatively simple and fairly rapid.
4. It must be well organized so that each part of the mouth is brushed in turn and no area is overlooked. In the average mouth using a small-headed brush each quadrant can be divided into 3 sections; posterior, middle and anterior (Fig. 62).

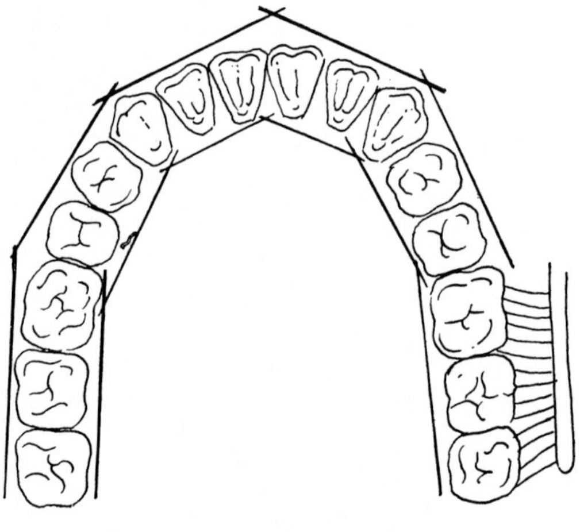

FIG. 62.—Each jaw can be divided into six segments.

5. It must fit in with the patient's capabilities. Each patient needs individual advice as to the best method for him to use.

It is advisable to teach the patient a definite technique initially as this forms a base from which he can go on to develop his own personal technique. The disclosing agent regularly used (twice a week) provides the only reliable test of that technique and the admonishment to 'get the red off' provides the simplest and clearest incentive.

For the sake of simplicity only two techniques will be described.

Other than the horizontal scrubbing method two of the most commonly recommended methods are the roll technique and the Bass technique.

The Roll Technique

This is a relatively gentle technique very suitable in the post-surgical phase.

The sides of the brush must be placed firmly against the buccal aspect of the teeth and gingivae, with the back of the brush at the level of the biting surface of the teeth and with the bristles parallel to the long axis of the teeth. Then the brush must be rotated (down in the upper jaw, and up in the lower jaw) so that the side of the bristles firmly sweeps the surface of the tooth and gums (Fig. 63). Eight strokes are given to the buccal

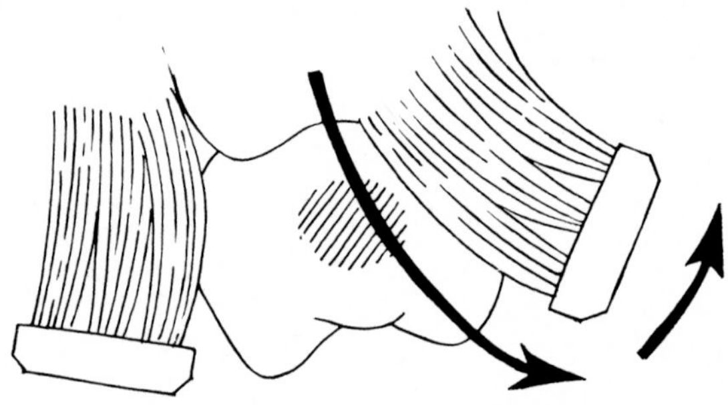

FIG. 63.—The modified Stillman technique. The rotatory movement is firm and deliberate, so that pressure is maintained on the gingiva and tooth surface and the bristles are forced into the interdental area.

aspect and eight to the lingual. The brush is moved methodically from one section to the next. Anterior palatal and lingual surfaces in narrow arches may be cleaned with the brush held vertically (Fig. 64). When all buccal and lingual surfaces are brushed, the biting surfaces can be cleaned with a rotary movement.

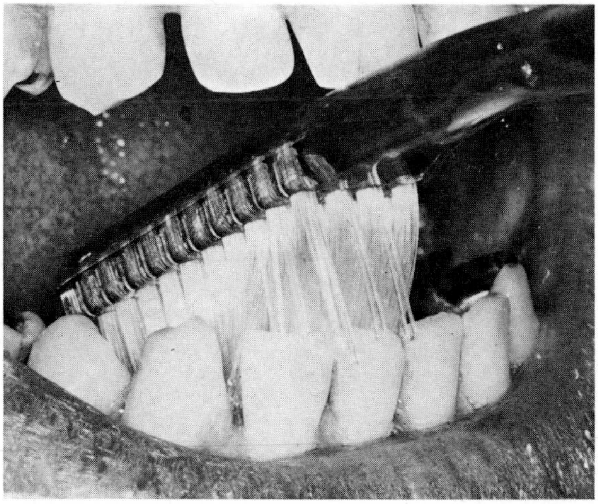

FIG. 64.—If the anterior segment of the arch is too narrow to apply the brush horizontally, a vertical position can be used.

The Bass Technique

This is one of the so-called 'sulcular' (or crevicular) techniques in which an attempt is made to clean the gingival crevice.

In this method the brush is held so that the bristles are at 45° to the long axis of the teeth with the bristle ends pointing into the gingival crevice and across the gingival margin (Fig. 65). The brush is pressed towards the gingivae and moved slightly backwards and forwards with a vibratory or very small circular movement. Each area is taken in turn. Providing the toothbrush head is small the gingival crevice in every region of the mouth can be reached.

Although the roll technique is the method most frequently recommended the horizontal scrub technique has been found more effective in plaque removal. The latter is however likely to be more traumatic. If used correctly a Bass-type technique for crevicular cleaning can be very effective. It is not particularly difficult or time consuming.

Frequency of Brushing

Theoretically one needs to clean teeth once every other day to keep gingivae healthy (Löe, 1970). However, few individuals clean so well that all the plaque is removed every time they brush. Therefore it seems advisable to try to remove all the plaque by cleaning at least twice a day; after breakfast and before bed are the usually recommended times. Where there is food impaction it may be necessary to clean after each meal for the sake of comfort.

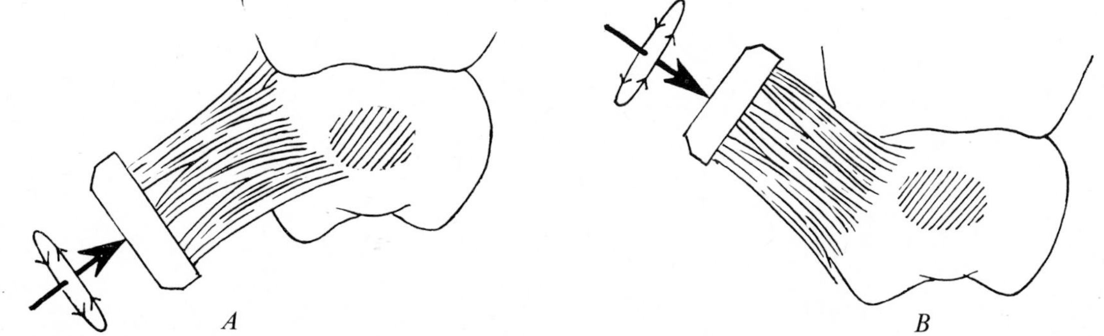

FIG. 65.—Alternative techniques.
(*A*) Bass method (sulcular or crevicular technique). The bristles point apically at about 45° to the tooth axis. Pressure is applied and a slight jiggling movement is made with the brush so that the gingivae are stimulated. This technique is not recommended where the tissue is at all fragile. (*B*) Charters method. The movement is the same as that used in the Stillman method but the bristles point in an occlusal direction. This technique is useful for dislodging debris from between the teeth.

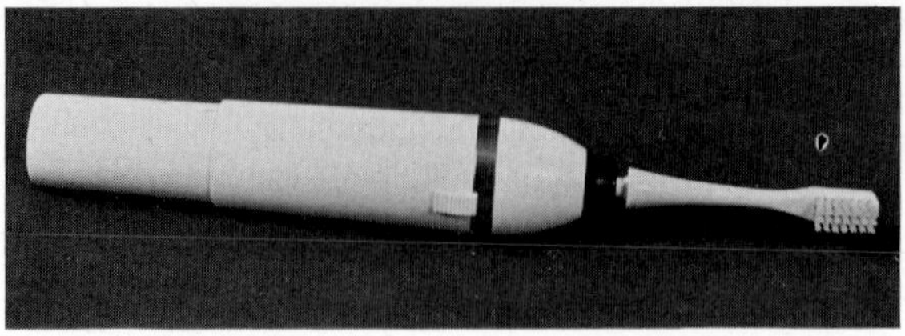

FIG. 66.—Automatic toothbrush. (By courtesy of Teledyne Aqua Tec.)

The Automatic Toothbrush

There are a number of designs of automatic toothbrush (Fig. 66). Four types of movement are available, 1. Reciprocating, 2. Vibrating, 3. Arcuating and 4. Rotating. The reciprocating and arcuating types are the most commonly used; there is little evidence comparing the effectiveness of these two types.

There have been many studies comparing the effectiveness of the hand and automatic brushes and the results appear to depend on the subjects studied rather than on the technique used.

Well-informed individuals such as dental students, etc., use the manual toothbrush as effectively as the automatic brush (McKendrick, Barbenel and McHugh, 1968). Physically and mentally handicapped people certainly derive greater benefit from the automatic brush (Huff and Taylor, 1965). For the *uninstructed* patient the automatic brush is as effective or more effective in plaque removal than the manual brush (Lobene, 1967).

When first introduced there was some apprehension about whether the automatic brush would damage the tissues, but little or no such damage has been found.

There was also a great deal of scepticism about the possible value of the automatic brush but experience has confirmed their place in the armamentarium of oral hygiene aids.

The well-designed automatic toothbrush cleans as effectively as a conventional brush used correctly. As most people do not use the conventional brush correctly the automatic brush in the hands of most people may be more effective than the conventional brush, especially as access to difficult areas may be easier with the small head of the automatic brush. What is more, many people, and particularly children, find the well-designed automatic brush pleasant to use and enjoy the resultant cleanliness which is obtained with such little effort. For these reasons the use of the brush is likely to be regular and even frequent. Once the patient is accustomed to the pleasure of a clean mouth it is likely that even if he returns to the conventional brush he will use it more efficiently than before. In this way the automatic brush can play an effective part in patient training.

It is also very usefully employed by handicapped individuals, especially children, whose mouths often suffer severely from poor oral hygiene.

INTERDENTAL CLEANING

The interdental area is the most important site of plaque collection and the most inaccessible to the toothbrush. Neither the manual nor the automatic brushes are effective in removing interdental plaque, therefore a variety of devices have been developed as aids to supplement the toothbrush. These include the dental woodstick, the interspace brush, and dental floss and tape.

The Dental Woodstick

The original advocates of dental woodsticks suggested that regular interdental massage improved keratinization and therefore resistance to irritation. This supposition has never been established, but the woodstick is certainly more effective than the toothbrush in removing bacterial plaque from the interdental area (Morch and Waerhaug, 1956). They are usually made from soft wood, triangular in cross-section and taper to a point. Certain conditions are essential for their use:

1. There must be interdental spaces. If the stick is pushed between teeth where a healthy interdental papilla fills the interproximal

space, tissue damage is inevitable.

2. The mouth must be clean and the tissue healthy. Rubbing inflamed gingivae over subgingival calculus is only likely to exacerbate the gingivitis.
3. The stick must be used at the correct angle following the normal contour of the interdental papilla (Fig. 67). In too many cases the stick is held horizontally and used like a saw so that the papilla atrophies, and the interdental space increases in size and becomes a food trap, so that even more assiduous use of woodsticks is necessary.

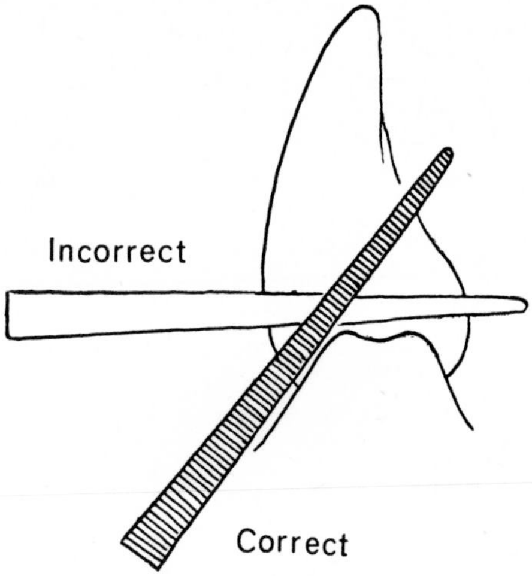

FIG. 67.—The dental woodstick should be used at an angle following that of the gingival contour.

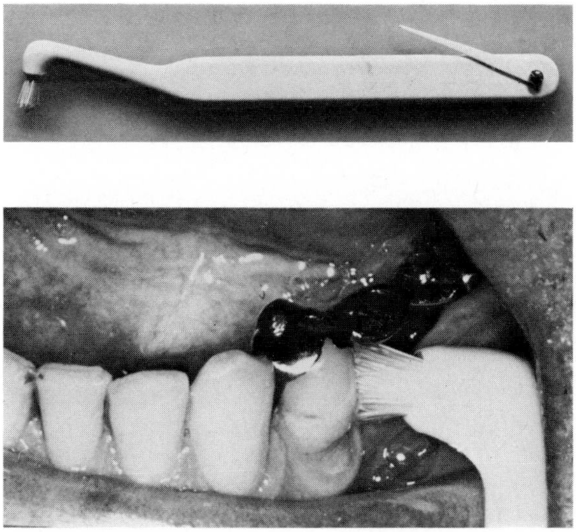

FIG. 68.—The Interspace brush for use in areas difficult to reach with a larger brush, for example behind a bridge pontic.

The Interspace Brush

This is a single tufted brush which is an extremely valuable adjunct to the ordinary toothbrush and can be used for cleaning all areas of the mouth (Fig. 68). It is very useful for cleaning areas difficult of access such as around irregular teeth, in spaces created by missing teeth and around bridge pontics.

Dental Floss

Both waxed and unwaxed dental floss are used for removing interproximal plaque and debris. Unwaxed floss is thin and therefore slips more easily through interdental contacts. The use of floss can be very effective in plaque removal when used by the careful and conscientious patient. It is a time-consuming procedure and one which needs to be carefully taught, otherwise gingival damage can result (Fig. 69). It is also essential to remove all calculus and rough margins of restorations before a patient is allowed to use floss, otherwise the floss will break and the gingivae will be irritated.

Some patients find a flat dental tape easier to use and this is especially effective in removing plaque from bridge abutments and pontics (Fig. 70).

Irrigating Devices

A large number of unsubstantiated claims have been made for water irrigators. They remove food debris from the mouth but they will not remove bacterial plaque. They can be useful supplements to the toothbrush and are particularly useful in the immediate post-operative phase where the tissue is sensitive and the toothbrush painful in use. If used carelessly damage to the soft tissue may result (O'Leary *et al.*, 1970).

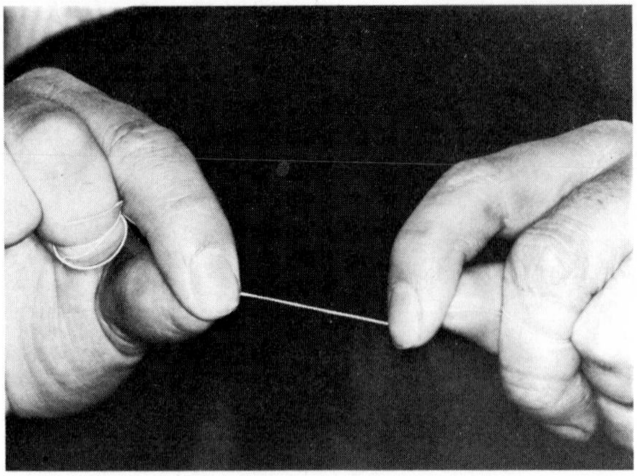

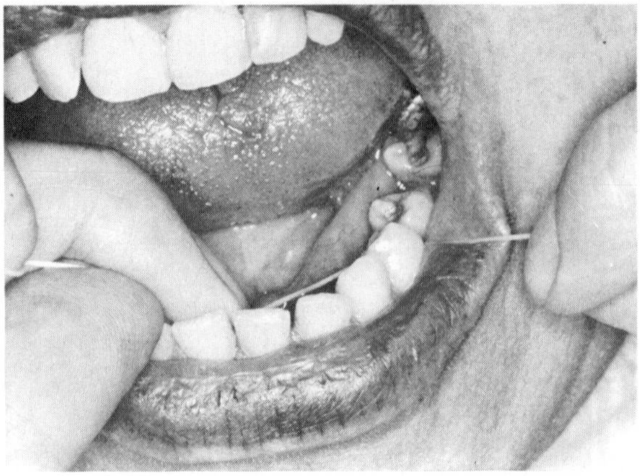

FIG. 69.—Handling of dental floss for interproximal cleaning.

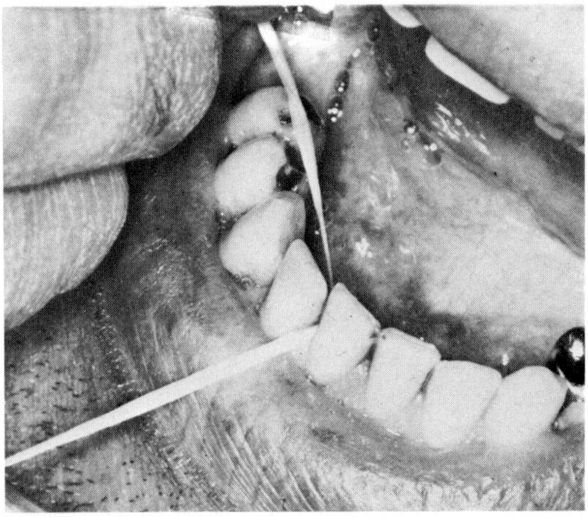

FIG. 70.—Flat dental tape being used to polish interproximal surfaces.

Toothpaste

Two important functions are served by toothpaste and dentifrices:

1. Their detergent and abrasive action aid the toothbrush in the removal of plaque.
2. Their refreshing taste and smell encourage the more frequent use of the toothbrush.

Although many toothpastes contain some agent with a specific therapeutic role there seems to be little evidence to recommend any one product as being more effective than another in the prevention of periodontal disease. Toothpowders can be more effective than pastes in the removal of stain, but because they are abrasive their constant or vigorous use should be avoided.

Toothpastes containing sugar or sodium perborate should be avoided.

CHEMICAL CLEANING

Achieving a high standard of oral hygiene by mechanical means is not easy. It depends on constant perseverance and a measure of dexterity, characteristics which not all individuals possess. Therefore attempts are being made to develop methods of chemical control to supplement or even replace mechanical cleaning.

Action against the formation and retention of plaque may be made in several ways:

1. **Suppression of the oral flora.** Stralfors (1962) has calculated that 99.9% of oral bacteria must be killed to inhibit plaque formation. Suppression of the oral flora can be obtained by using broad-spectrum antibiotics, but this is a transient effect and accompanied by possible hazards. Resistant strains may

develop, Monilia may proliferate and sensitivity reactions may be produced. More specific attacks may be made using for example Vancomysin which is active against Gram-positive bacteria. This has been shown to be an effective plaque inhibitor in hamsters (Keyes *et al.*, 1966) but other studies show only a temporary reduction in human plaque (Jensen *et al.*, 1967).

Daily rinses with 0.2% aqueous solutions of chlorhexidine reduce the salivary bacterial count and inhibit plaque formation over prolonged periods (Rindom Schiøtt *et al.*, 1970). When used in these concentrations chlorhexidine does not appear to be a tissue irritant nor does it delay wound healing, but it has a very bitter taste which is difficult to mask and tends to discolour teeth and fillings. However, the long-term effects of this treatment are not known.

2. **Inhibition of plaque forming factors.** Plaque-forming streptococci produce insoluble extracellular polysaccharides, mainly dextrans. A number of agents, sodium lauryl sulphate, amine fluorides and dextranase (Bowen, 1968) appear to interfere with plaque production *in vitro* and in animal studies, but so far results in humans have been variable.
3. **Inhibition of bacterial colonization of tooth surface.** The chemical composition of plaque appears to vary with the surface on which the plaque grows. Plaque on silicate fillings is not identical with plaque on tooth surface (Norman *et al.*, 1971). Inhibition of artificial plaque by chemical agents also appears to depend on the surface upon which the plaque is grown. Therefore alteration in the nature of the surface might influence plaque formation. Many disinfectants effective against oral bacteria do not affect plaque growth, but complete plaque inhibition appears to follow when a 0.2% aqueous solution of chlorhexidine digluconate is used as a mouthwash (Löe and Rindom Schiøtt, 1970). Topically applied chlorhexidine does not affect the number of salivary micro-organisms, but it does seem to prevent their colonizing the tooth surface (Davies *et al.*, 1970). Where subgingival plaque and calculus are present chlorhexidine produces little improvement in gingival condition, but it has been shown to prevent the development of gingival inflammation where the usual cleaning procedures have been withdrawn.
4. **Dissolution of established plaque.** 0.2% chlorhexidine mouthwash dissolves newly formed plaque and considerably reduces the amount of old plaque accumulation.
5. **Inhibition of plaque calcification.** A number of agents have been used to attempt to interfere with calculus formation; pancreatin mucinase and other proteolytic enzymes incorporated in toothpastes, powder and chewing gum have demonstrated some calculus inhibiting effect. Vitamin C is said to have crystal inhibiting properties.

In summary, the use of chlorhexidine, and possibly other cationic disinfectants, appears to offer the greatest promise in plaque control (Fig. 71), but further study of its toxicity and long-term effects must be carried out. At the moment it appears to provide a valuable adjunct to mechanical cleaning, to be used for limited periods of time where gingival inflammation is to be treated.

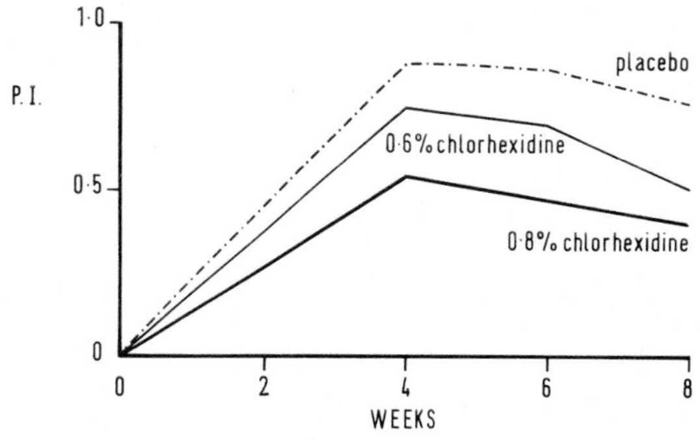

FIG. 71.—Mean plaque index scores after brushing with chlorhexidine-containing dentifrices. (By courtesy of Dr P. Gjermo.)

PATIENT EDUCATION

The mechanics of prevention are straightforward. It is easy enough to tell a patient that he must clean his teeth in a certain way at least twice a day, have a scaling twice a year, finish his meals with fresh fruit, take his toothbrush to the office, and rinse his mouth after eating. To have the patient act on these suggestions is a different matter. In order to obtain his co-operation the patient has to be made to feel that it is all worthwhile. He must be educated to the point of view that teeth are worth preserving for life, and that they can be preserved for life if he is prepared to co-operate fully in maintaining good oral hygiene.

Instruction in oral hygiene techniques should be given to all patients, not only to those who have already developed periodontal disease. It is in the long term the most valuable service the dentist can render his patient. Instruction is most effective if tailored to the needs of the patient.

Motivation of Children

A number of methods of teaching children have been tried. An informed individual is much more likely to be co-operative, and attempts have been made to improve the oral hygiene of children by giving them illustrated talks on the subject.

Parfitt, James and Davis (1958) instructed one group of 11–15 year-old children by lectures and films, but found little difference in gingival condition compared with an uninstructed group. Another study compared the effects of instruction given by school teachers and dentists, and concluded that effective motivation can be produced only when instruction is given by a well informed and authoritative teacher, *i.e.* a dentist or one of a dental team, but not by a layman. In other studies children have been given practical toothbrushing instruction in groups to produce a definite improvement in oral hygiene and a reduction in gingival inflammation, but when instruction terminated there was relapse to the initial condition (Lindhe and Koch, 1966). The use of disclosing tablets for mouth care appears to provide a further stimulus to effective care. The greatest co-operation and benefit is derived where toothbrushing is supervised daily, but again once supervision is withdrawn the children revert to old habits. Remotivation at intervals is essential. Instruction of parents may be the most effective way of teaching their children. Creating positive attitudes within the family group is likely to produce the most permanent effects.

Motivation of Adults

A number of studies have been carried out on adult groups and on individual adults. Individual instruction in which there is two-way communication between teacher and pupil has been proved to be the most effective method, but this is very time-consuming. The solution, particularly if effective public health measures are to be instituted, would seem to be the enlargement of the dental team to include ancillary workers trained to carry out oral hygiene instruction. The dental hygienist and dental nurse should be thoroughly equipped for this responsibility.

Several arguments can be employed to obtain patient co-operation:

1. **Impaired function.** No appliance can function as efficiently as the healthy dentition.
2. **Effect on general health.** Toxins from a periodontal lesion are absorbed along two paths; from the pocket directly into the tissues, and indirectly via the digestive system. Although no connection has been established between periodontal disease and any systemic disease, it is possible that where other pathology exists, for example gastric ulcer, the existence of oral sepsis may aggravate the condition.
3. **Social handicap.** Periodontal disease produces halitosis, the social effects of which are sufficiently well advertised to make further comment unnecessary. Dirty teeth and periodontal disease also make the mouth visually unpleasant.
4. **Personal hygiene.** Concern about oral hygiene is linked with concern for personal cleanliness and hygiene in general. It is unlikely that an individual who is unconcerned about personal cleanliness will be very conscious of, or concerned about, calculus or food debris in his mouth.

   Most patients do not realize that their mouths are dirty. Many even feel offended when this is suggested. When the true situation is pointed out and instruction in oral hygiene is given, the patient who is concerned about personal hygiene is most likely to co-operate.
5. **Personal disfigurement.** The idea of physical disfigurement is repellant to most people. Many primitive people associate teeth with virility, and most of us, at least unconsciously, associate loss of teeth with loss of youth. Yet so many people accept tooth loss, a form of disfigurement, with complete resignation. The reasons would seem to be at least partly socio-economic. It seems possible that with an increasing standard of living a higher value will be placed on the dentition and on oral hygiene.

A Method of Instruction

It is a good habit to introduce the subject of oral hygiene even before a scaling is carried out. The patient is given a hand-mirror to follow the inspection of his mouth and is shown any inflammation, pocketing, stain, materia alba, bacterial plaque, calculus or food debris present. To press home the point a piece of calculus or debris is removed and shown to the patient with some remark about the smell and bacterial content of such debris. The dentist must tailor his remarks to suit the individual. A girl of eighteen may respond to the idea that her mouth smells or is ugly; a man of forty to the idea that every mouthful of food is contaminated by the dirt in his mouth.

It must be stressed that the most important factor, the plaque, is light coloured and almost invisible. Its presence is however effectively demonstrated with a disclosing solution or lozenge (Fig. 72). These agents are essentially non-toxic dyes such as basic fuchsin or erythrosin together with some form of soluble vehicle and flavouring agent. They are absorbed by plaque and also stain the oral mucosa but this discolouration disappears after a few hours.

At a previous appointment the patient is advised to bring his toothbrush for the dentist's inspection and comment, on the next visit. In general a short-head medium nylon multituft brush is recommended, as consistently good results have been obtained with this type of brush (Fig. 60).

The patient is asked to brush his teeth in the surgery so that obvious shortcomings can be pointed out. Common errors include scrubbing very vigorously, which may produce gingival recession and tooth abrasion; missing out lingual and palatal surfaces, particularly of posterior teeth; trying to brush the buccal aspect of posterior teeth with the mouth wide open; or using a technique such as the conventional horizontal stroke which cleans labial and lingual surfaces but fails to reach the interproximal surfaces.

Once the patient has recognized the faults in his usual technique he is ready to be shown a better method. It is not essential for the patient to follow rigidly any prescribed technique of toothbrushing; if he is aware of the need for the removal of all plaque and debris he may devise his own technique providing it does not injure the tissues. As stated when a disclosing tablet has been used the patient is merely instructed to 'get the red off'. Nevertheless, a definite technique is demonstrated initially to provide a foundation for patient education.

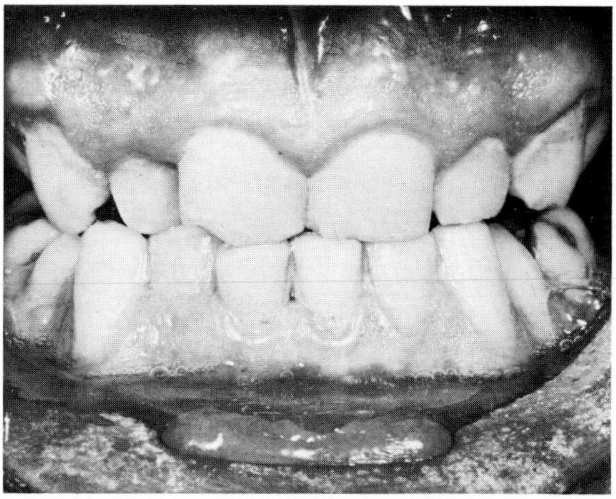

A

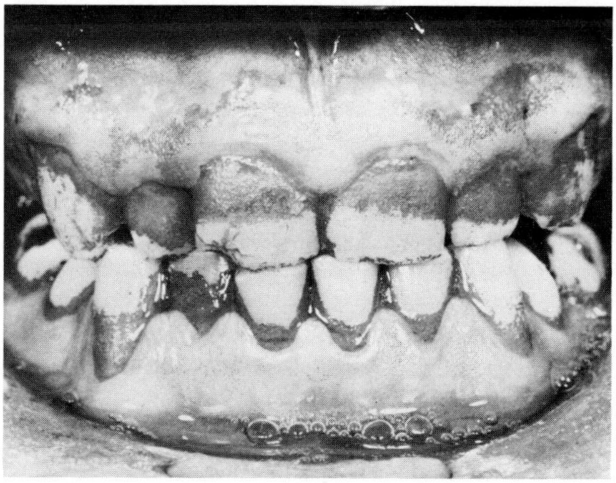

B

FIG. 72.—(*A*) Appearance before rinsing with disclosing solution. (*B*) After staining plaque with a 6 per cent basic fuschin solution.

Demonstration

Models and a toothbrush are useful to the initial demonstration of the actual technique advised. The demonstration may be carried out before or after scaling. The need for a properly organized method of cleaning is stressed.

In the average mouth, using a small-headed brush, each quadrant may be divided into three sections; posterior, middle, and anterior (Fig. 62). Start at the most posterior tooth in one jaw and proceed methodically around the mouth. The roll or Bass technique can be demonstrated on the model and then by the operator using the patient's brush in *the patient's mouth*. The patient is then given the brush and a hand-mirror and requested to demonstrate his technique in his mouth to the teacher. Only by actually witnessing the patient cleaning his own teeth can the teacher be sure that his or her technique is adequate. It may be time-consuming but there is no satisfactory alternative to this procedure.

At this stage the patient may find that certain areas present a special problem which requires the dentist's attention and advice; awkward areas may require the use of a special brush, such as the Interspace brush (Fig. 68). Other techniques than the one described may be used, but it is better to describe one technique only in the first place to avoid confusing the patient. One technique used well is better than a mixture of techniques used inefficiently; if the described technique appears to be inadequate then another method must be tried. The use of an interdental cleaner, usually the woodstick, is then demonstrated. Finally the patient is then instructed to complete the act of cleaning by sucking water vigorously between the teeth and expelling it. It is surprising how many patients cannot wash out their mouths efficiently. Often it helps to ask the patient to wash out making a lot of noise.

Visually, and by tactile inspection with his tongue, the patient can find out if he has completed the brushing efficiently. If he feels it is not satisfactory in any area he must repeat the brushing in that area. Some disclosing solution may be given to the patient for home use.

Follow-up

The patient should return with a toothbrush two weeks later and be given a hand-mirror to watch the inspection of his mouth. Both he and the dentist will be able to see any change in the condition of the tissues and whether he is properly maintaining cleanliness; after that a disclosing agent can be used. If the teeth are not as clean as they should be, the patient must demonstrate the way he is using the brush and any mistakes should be corrected.

It may be necessary to repeat the whole procedure two weeks later, but usually if the patient is concerned about his mouth there will be obvious improvements (Figs. 73 and 74).

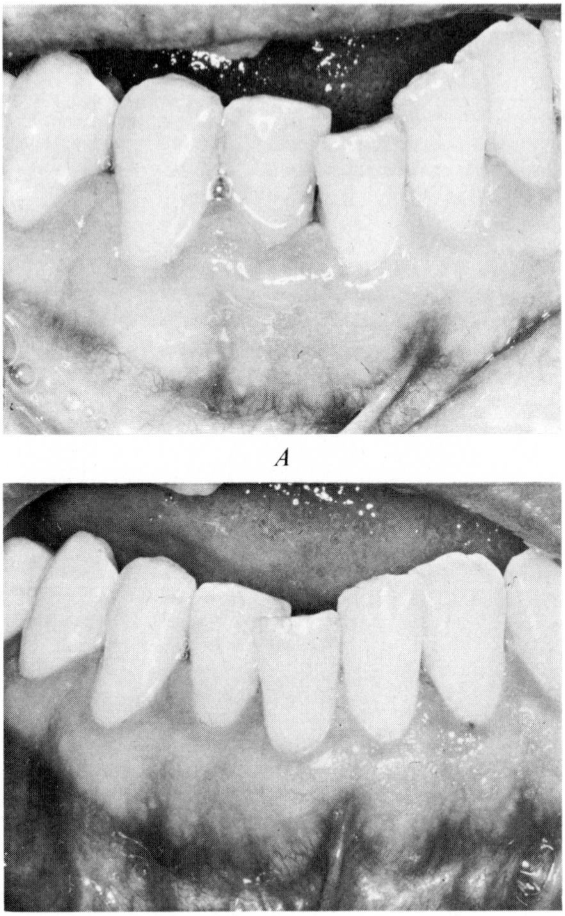

A

B

FIG. 73.—(*A*) Chronic gingivitis due to poor oral hygiene. (*B*) Two months after scaling and instruction in oral hygiene techniques. Note reduction in papillary swelling.

When the patient is not co-operating it will also be obvious, and it is perfectly justifiable to dismiss him as being insufficiently concerned.

The following points must be stressed:

1. Very few patients will acquire a correct brushing technique from one lesson.
2. A stock brush and model may be adequate for the first demonstration, but subsequently the patient must demonstrate his technique

in his mouth. It should never be taken for granted that the patient can brush satisfactorily until he demonstrates in the surgery that he can do so.

3. All techniques should be simple. Difficult or prolonged technique may work with the occasional enthusiast but will be discarded by others who have more than their teeth to occupy their thoughts. Anyone advocating more than five minutes mouth-cleaning night and morning shows himself to be out of contact with reality. Five minutes is a long time; two minutes seems to be the maximum that the average patient will tolerate as an acquired habit.
4. Teaching should be individual as far as possible. Class instruction is necessary in schools and clinics, but merely serves to give a broad outline of technique and is never matched to the patient's individual requirements. There is no substitute for chairside demonstration given either by the dentist, his nurse, or his hygienist.
5. Even when the technique has been learned satisfactorily by the patient, a check should be made at regular intervals.

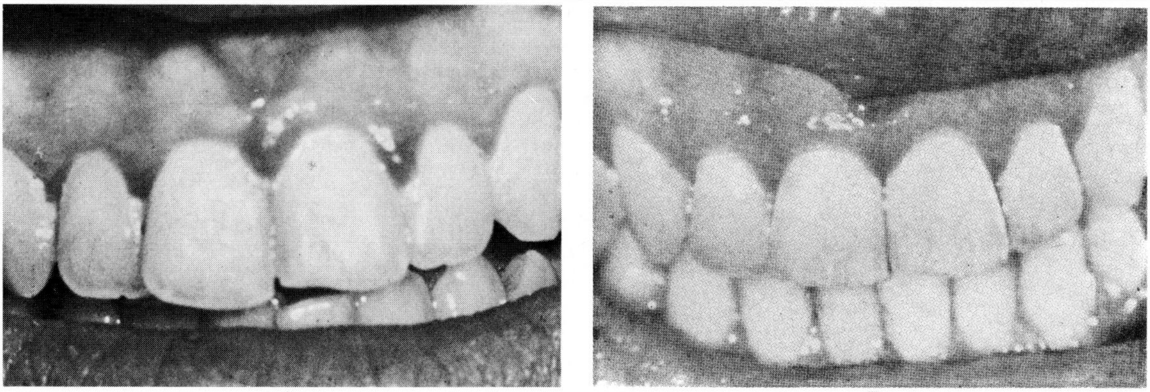

A *B*

FIG. 74.—(*A*) Chronic gingivitis due to poor oral hygiene. (*B*) After using an electric toothbrush for three weeks as the only treatment.

REFERENCES

BAY, I., KARDEL, K. M. and SKOUGAARD, M. R. (1967). Quantitative evaluation of the plaque-removing ability of different types of toothbrushes. *J. Periodont.*, **38**, 526.

BOWEN, W. H. (1968). Effects of dextranase on cariogenic and non-cariogenic dextrans. *Brit. dent. J.*, **124**, 347.

DAVIES, R. M., JENSEN, S. B., RINDOM SCHIØTT, C. and LÖE, H. (1970). The effect of topical application of chlorhexidine on the bacterial colonization of the teeth and gingiva. *J. periodont. Res.*, **5**, 96.

EMSLIE, R. D. (1967). Prevention in periodontal disease. *Int. dent. J.*, **17**, 320.

GREENE, J. C. (1966). Oral health care for prevention and control of periodontal disease. *In* World Workshop in Periodontics. Univ. Michigan Press, Ann Arbor, Mich.

HUFF, G. C. and TAYLOR, P. P. (1965). Clinical evaluation of toothbrushes used in pedodontics. *Texas dent. J.*, **83**, 6.

JENSEN, S. B., LÖE, H., RINDOM SCHIØTT, C., THEILADE, E. and MIKKELSEN, L. (1967). The effect of vancomycin and polymyxin B on experimental gingivitis in man. *J. periodont. Res.*, **2**, 242 (Abstr.).

KEYES, P. H., ROWBERRY, S. A., ENGLANDER, H. R. and FITZGERALD, R. J. (1966). Bio-essays for medicaments for the control of dentobacterial plaque, dental caries, and periodontal lesions in Syrian hamsters. *J. oral. Ther.*, **3**, 157.

LINDHE, J. and KOCH, G. (1966). The effect of supervised oral hygiene on the gingiva of children. Progressional inhibition of gingivitis. *J. periodont. Res.*, **1**, 260.
LOBENE, R. R. (1967). The effect of an automatic toothbrush on periodontitis. *J. oral. Ther.*, **3**, 284.
LÖE, H. (1970). A review of the prevention and control of plaque. *In* Dental Plaque (McHugh, W. D., ed.). Livingstone, Edinburgh, p. 259.
LÖE, H. and RINDOM SCHIØTT, C. (1970). The effect of mouthrinses and topical application of chlorhexidine on the development of dental plaque and gingivitis in man. *J. periodont. Res.*, **5**, 79.
MCKENDRICK, A. J. W., BARBENEL, L. M. H. and MCHUGH, W. D. (1968). A two-year comparison of hand and electric toothbrushes. *J. periodont. Res.*, **3**, 224.
MORCH, T. and WAERHAUG, J. (1956). Quantitative evaluation of the effect of toothbrushing and toothpicking. *J. Periodont.*, **27**, 183.
NORMAN, R. D., VIRMANI, R., SWARTZ, M. L. and PHILLIPS, R. W. (1971). The effects of restorative materials on plaque composition. IADR Prog. Abstracts, No. 162, p. 93.
O'LEARY, T. J., SHAFER, W. G., SWENSON, H. M., NESLER, D. C. and VAN DORN, P. R. (1970). Possible penetration of crevicular tissue from oral hygiene procedures: 1. Use of oral irrigating devices. *J. Periodont.*, **41**, 158.
PARFITT, G. J., JAMES, P. M. C. and DAVIES, H. C. (1958). A controlled study of the effect of dental health education on the gingival structures of school children. *Brit. dent. J.*, **104**, 21.
RINDOM SCHIØTT, C., LÖE, H., JENSEN, S. B., KILIAN, M., DAVIES, R. M. and GLAVIND, K. (1970). The effect of chlorhexidine mouthrinses on the human oral flora. *J. periodont. Res.*, **5**, 84.
SCULLY, C. M. and WADE, A. B. (1970). The relative plaque-removing effects of brushes of different lengths and texture. *Dent. Practit.*, **20**, 244.
STRALFORS, A. (1962). Disinfection of dental plaques in man. *Odont. T.*, **70**, 183.

7. Chronic Gingivitis

The aetiology of chronic gingivitis (described in Chapter 4) can be stated as the metabolic products of bacterial plaque in persistent contact with the gingival margin and the vulnerable gingival crevice. The tissue response to this irritation takes the form of a subacute or chronic inflammation which manifests itself at a clinical level as a gingivitis.

Histopathology

The tissue response is a mixed response in which there are two elements, inflammation and repair. The inflammatory component consists of the usual vascular changes with exudation of serum and leucocytes plus the recruitment of various inflammatory cells. As stated earlier, the disruption of the tissue is caused not only by the irritant but by the tissue response to the irritant. The site of the initial lesion may be the gingival crevice or the interdental col. In the interdental region the inflammation spreads through the corium of the col area. Inflammatory cells, plasma cells, lymphocytes and macrophages, and inflammatory exudate infiltrate the area. Vessels are dilated and packed with red cells; some vessels become thrombosed and small areas of necrosis are found in the corium. The presence of bacteria has also been demonstrated in the superficial tissue. The inflammatory exudate spreads between fibre bundles and along the superficial layers of the periodontal ligament which loses its characteristic structure and becomes amorphous and infiltrated with inflammatory cells. The inflammatory process spreads to the corium of neighbouring areas of gingiva along the transseptal fibres and extends through these fibres to the vicinity of the alveolar periosteum. In a severe gingivitis the collagen bundles are broken up so that the gingival fibre apparatus may be almost completely replaced by inflammatory elements. The ground substance also undergoes disaggregation. When the gingival fibres are broken up the gingiva loses its normal tone and can be separated easily from the tooth surface. This loss of tone plus inflammatory swelling gives rise to the 'gingival' or 'false' pocket (Fig. 75). The crevicular epithelium proliferates

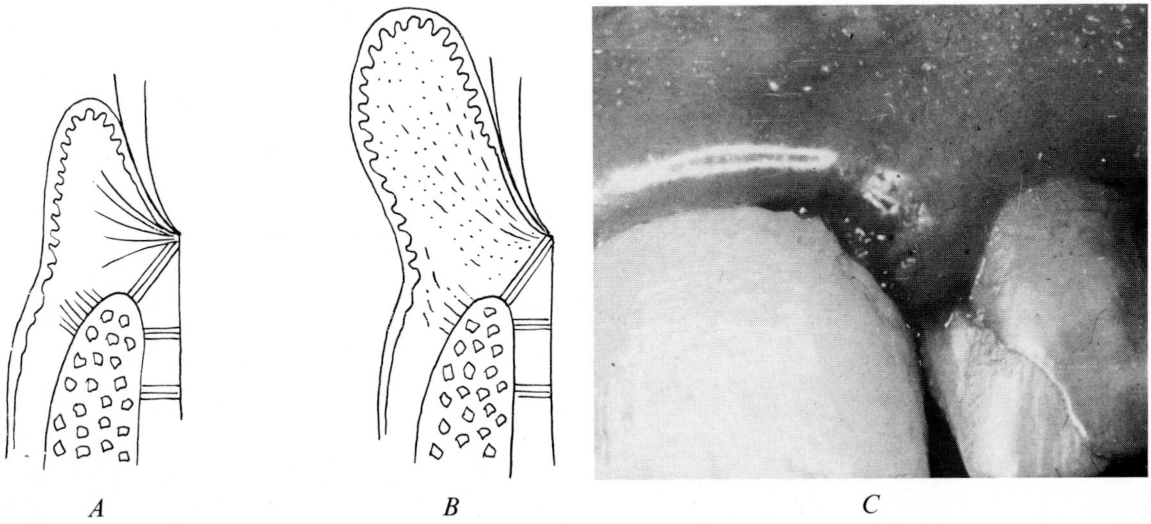

FIG. 75.—(*A*) A healthy gingival margin with the tissue forming a tight collar around the neck of the tooth and the crevicular epithelium attached at the amelocemental junction. (*B*) A 'gingival' or 'false' pocket formed by swelling of the gingival margin. The crevicular epithelium is attached at the amelocemental junction. (*C*) An inflamed interdental papilla which is red, swollen and smooth.

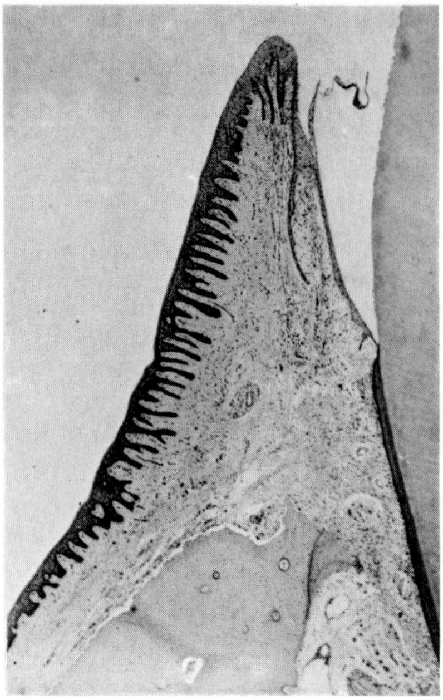

A

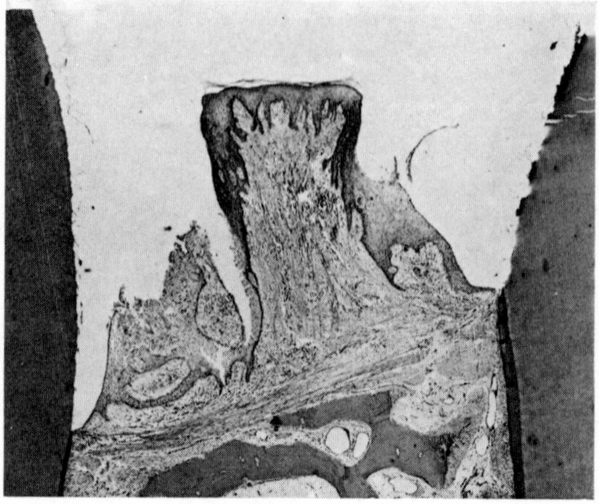

B

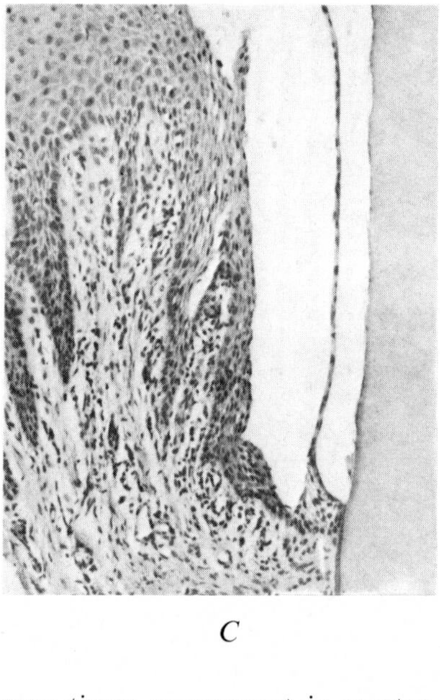

C

FIG. 76.—(*A*) Very early stage of gingival inflammation and epithelial proliferation in human specimen. (*B*) Section through the interdental papilla of same specimen showing much more marked inflammatory infiltration and epithelial proliferation. (*C*) Higher power showing epithelial proliferation, inflammatory infiltrate and base of crevice at amelo-cementum junction.

Note that transseptal ligament is intact.

irregularly in the form of cords and loops (Fig. 76). There is intracellular oedema and cell degeneration so that the epithelial barrier breaks down in small areas with consequent bleeding on pressure.

At the same time there is some formation of fibrous connective tissue, *i.e.* repair. The proportion of the two components, inflammatory infiltration and fibrous tissue formation, varies and it is likely that many systemic factors dictate this variation. In the young the response is almost entirely inflammatory, the gingivae becoming soft, red and swollen. In other cases, particularly in the adult and where the condition is of long-standing, the fibrous tissue component is greater and the tissue may be swollen but firm and pink. This variation is very important from a clinical point of view. Where the inflammatory component is dominant removal of the irritant may be followed by resolution of the inflammation and reorganization of the fibre apparatus so that the morphology of health is reinstated: thus the condition is reversible. Where there is a considerable fibrous tissue component the condition is not completely reversed merely by removing the irritant; the fibrous tissue is not completely resorbed and the gingiva remains thick so that food-shedding may be impaired and irritation maintained.

CLINICAL FEATURES

As stated earlier there is considerable variation in the reaction of any tissue to a change in its environment and therefore of the gingivae to irritation. In some individuals symptoms may be absent and tissue changes not obvious, therefore the diagnosis of chronic gingivitis depends upon careful examination in which even the smallest departure from health is detected.

1. **Gingival bleeding** is the most common complaint and *always* indicates pathology. It may be very slight and occur only on toothbrushing. It may occur on eating hard food like apples, and sometimes, especially in adolescents and young adults, the gingivae may bleed readily on the slightest irritation or pressure so that the patient complains of finding blood on the pillow on awaking.

2. **Unpleasant taste.** When gingivae bleed, the patient may notice the taste of blood. A very unpleasant taste may be experienced when the patient sucks at an interdental space which is the site of stagnation. In some individuals the senses dull easily and even with very dirty mouths many patients do not complain of any unpleasant taste.

3. **Halitosis.** Some unpleasant smell usually accompanies gingival disease and this is often the reason for the visit to a dentist. The smells of decomposing blood, tobacco, or gross debris and gingival disease may have to be distinguished from those originating elsewhere than the mouth. These derive from diseases of the respiratory tract and the exhalation of metabolic products associated with

(a) systemic disease; diabetes, uraemia, etc.
(b) pathology of the digestive tract
(c) items of diet such as garlic, onion and peppermint.

4. **Discomfort and pain.** These are not common features of chronic gingivitis. The absence of pain and discomfort is perhaps the main reason for overlooking periodontal disease until it is at an advanced stage. A patient may suffer soreness on toothbrushing, and because of this he brushes more lightly and less frequently; plaque and food debris accumulate and make the condition worse. Only when acute inflammation supervenes, as when a gingival or periodontal abscess develops, is real pain experienced.

5. **Altered gingival appearance.** Changes in gingival appearance are defined according to colour, size, shape, consistency and surface characteristics. It is important to keep in mind the appearance of the gingivae in health; healthy gingivae are firm and pale pink (except where there is physiological pigmentation), the surface is streamlined and contiguous with the tooth surface, the margins are knife-edged, scalloped and hug the tooth surface, stippling and sluiceways are well marked (Fig. 77). Deviations from this usually denote disease. There are two components of the gingival reaction to irritation: (a) inflammation; and (b) fibrous tissue production. The gingival appearance is determined by the amount and ratio of these two reactions. Generally the more long-standing the irritation the greater the fibrous tissue component. In the mildest case of gingivitis (chronic marginal gingivitis) inflammation may be restricted to the interdental papillae or extend along the gingival margin which becomes red or blue-red and slightly swollen with a smooth glossy surface (Fig. 78). If the inflammation becomes

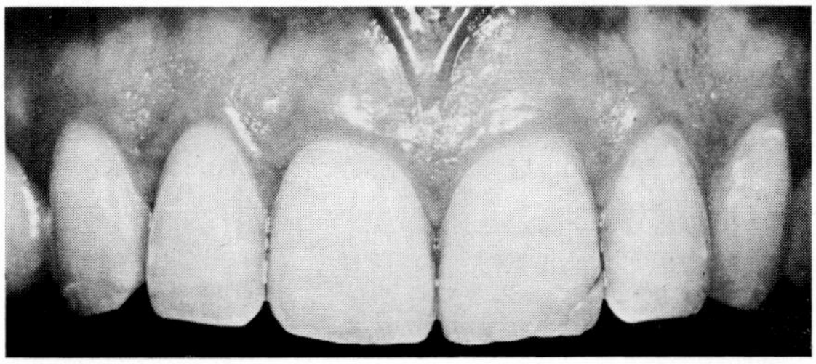

FIG. 77.—Healthy gingivae in a 20-year-old woman.

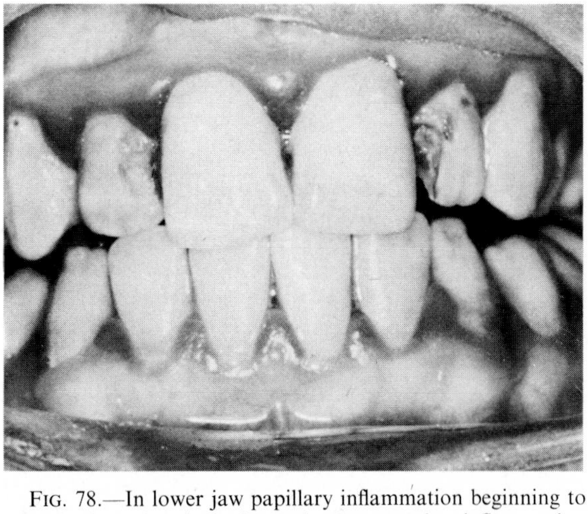

FIG. 78.—In lower jaw papillary inflammation beginning to spread along the gingival margin. In upper jaw inflammation more diffuse and spreading across attached gingiva.

more diffuse and spreads into the attached gingiva the stippling disappears and almost the entire width of gingiva may be red, swollen, smooth and glossy (Fig. 79). In more severe cases the inflammation may spread across the zone of attached gingiva into the alveolar mucosa and obliterate the mucogingival line.

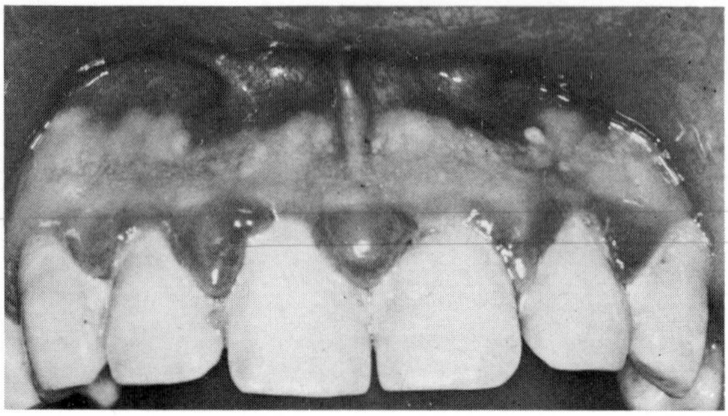

FIG. 79.—Marginal inflammation beginning to spread across zone of attached gingiva at |2.

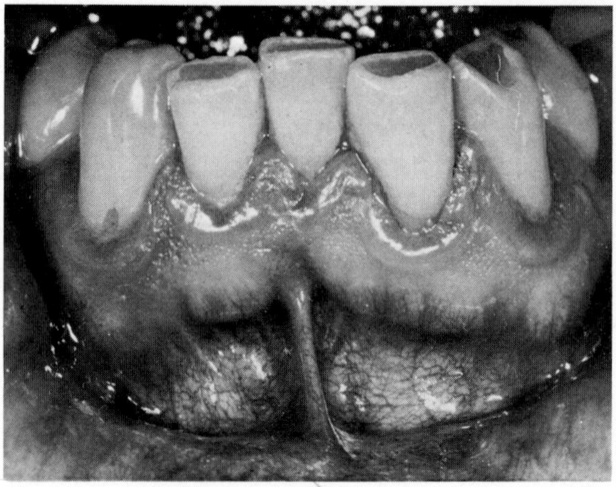

FIG. 80.—Abnormally shaped gingivae which are pink, firm and stippled, in a 39-year-old man.

Normally the most pronounced and obvious changes are seen in adolescents and young adults where inflammatory swelling may be considerable with the production of 'false' pocketing. In older adults the inflammatory process is usually minimal, and the gingivae although pink, firm and evenly stippled usually have an abnormal contour. The margins are thick and rounded, papillae enlarged and sluiceways absent (Fig. 80). In the older individual the changes described are often accompanied by gingival recession and root exposure.

The localization of gingival inflammation is usually associated with some obvious aetiological factor. This association often allows one to make an immediate diagnosis of the aetiological factors involved, invariably a plaque retentive factor.

For example:

(a) Inflammation restricted to lower incisor and upper molar regions – poor oral hygiene and supragingival calculus formation.
(b) Inflammation of palatal gingivae – upper partial denture.
(c) Inflammation in upper incisor region – lack of lip-seal (the area of inflammation is sometimes exactly delineated by the upper lip).
(d) Inflammation of isolated papillae – abnormal tooth contact or overhanging edges of fillings.
(e) Inflammation of gingivae on right side – an inefficient brushing technique used by a right-handed individual (Fig. 81).

Careful examination usually reveals a cause for the gingival inflammation. If no cause is apparent it is essential to use a disclosing solution

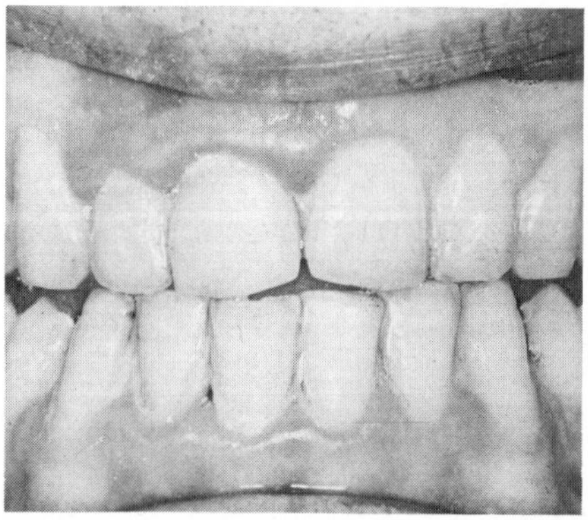

FIG. 81.—Gingival inflammation on right side in right-handed individual.

to reveal plaque that might otherwise be overlooked (Fig. 82).

All aetiological factors must be defined whenever possible. If they are not, treatment will be symptomatic and inevitably disease will recur.

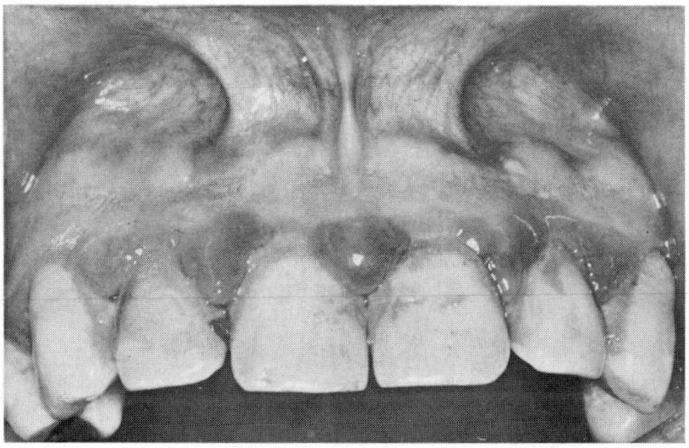

FIG. 82.—Patient in Fig. 79 after using disclosing lozenge.

TREATMENT OF CHRONIC GINGIVITIS

All periodontal treatment follows the same general plan:

(i) Remove the immediate cause of disease.
(ii) Correct predisposing factors.
(iii) Take preventive measures to avoid recurrence.

The outline for the treatment of chronic gingivitis is as follows:

1. Give instruction in oral hygiene techniques (see Chapter 6).
2. Scale and polish teeth.
3. Correct faulty restorations, prosthetic appliances and any other predisposing factor.
4. Perform gingivoplasty where the gingival contour is poor and not improved by scaling.
5. Re-appraise oral hygiene.
6. Recall regularly for inspection and scaling.

Scaling

This may be the most tedious yet one of the most important dental procedures. If it is to be effective as a form of treatment it must be thorough. Teeth are either perfectly clean or they are not clean. If calculus or plaque is left on the teeth gingival irritation and inflammation will persist. Therefore all plaque and calculus, both supragingival and subgingival, food debris and stain must be removed.

Each operator devises his own particular technique and uses the instruments he prefers, but certain conditions are essential:

(a) The technique must be methodical. The operator must work round the mouth and around each tooth in an orderly fashion so that no tooth surface is missed.
(b) The operator must have a secure finger rest so that the scaling instrument can be firmly applied, be moved with complete control and without risk of the instrument slipping and damaging the soft tissues.
(c) The correct instrument should be used, *i.e.* one which fits fairly well against the tooth surface to be cleaned, and for the removal of subgingival calculus one which is small enough to be inserted into the gingival crevice.
(d) Each stroke of the instrument should be deliberate and achieve something. It is easy to scratch around ineffectively.
(e) The root surface must not be damaged.

Supragingival calculus can be removed with several types of scaler. The Ivory C.I., Pickard and Cumine scalers all have their particular uses, but they are much too gross to be used in the removal of subgingival calculus (Fig. 83). Several instruments are available for this operation; curettes, periodontal hoes, Younger-Good scalers and Hygienist scalers (see Chapter 21 on Instruments).

Whichever instrument is used it is employed

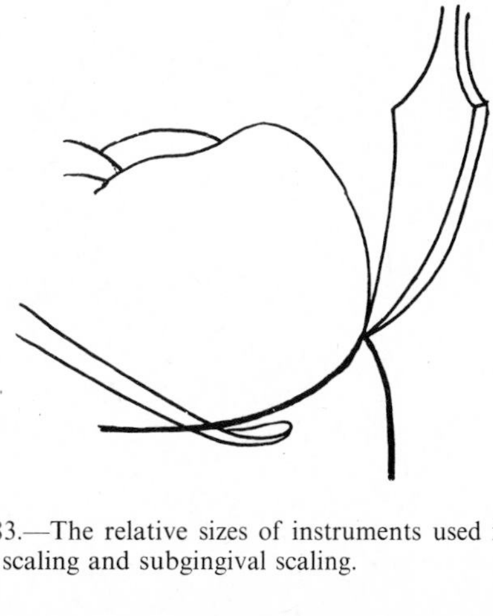

FIG. 83.—The relative sizes of instruments used for supragingival scaling and subgingival scaling.

first as a 'seeker' so that the calculus, particularly subgingival calculus, is detected by tactile sensation, and secondly to remove the calculus as effectively, expeditiously and atraumatically as possible.

In using the hoe for subgingival scaling the shank is held parallel to the tooth axis and inserted carefully into the gingival crevice alongside the tooth. The instrument should not be pressed against the tooth or it will impinge on subgingival calculus. When the instrument meets the resistance of the soft tissues it is pressed against the tooth surface so that a firm two-point contact is made, and then moved coronally. In this way the instrument passes the calculus on insertion and is brought with the calculus out of the crevice (Fig. 84). Curettes are also used in the same way for the removal of subgingival calculus. In cleaning a root surface it is important to apply the instrument, hoe or curette so that the cementum is not gouged (Fig. 85). These instruments may be used in this way all around the tooth except where the interdental space is very small (Fig. 86). Here Younger-Good or Hygienist scalers should be more effective.

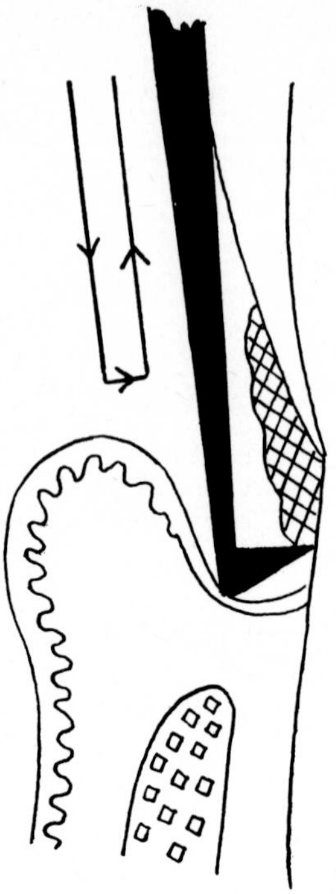

FIG. 84.—The periodontal hoe is inserted gently into the crevice, and on reaching the apical limit of the calculus is moved coronally while firm contact is maintained with the tooth surface.

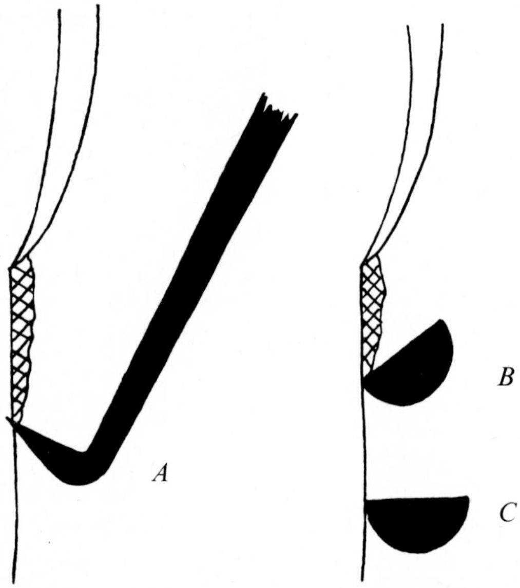

FIG. 85.—The instrument is applied to the tooth surface so that although firm contact is maintained and calculus is efficiently removed the root is not gouged.
(*A*) Incorrectly applied hoe. (*B*) Curette used inefficiently. (*C*) Curette correctly applied to tooth surface.

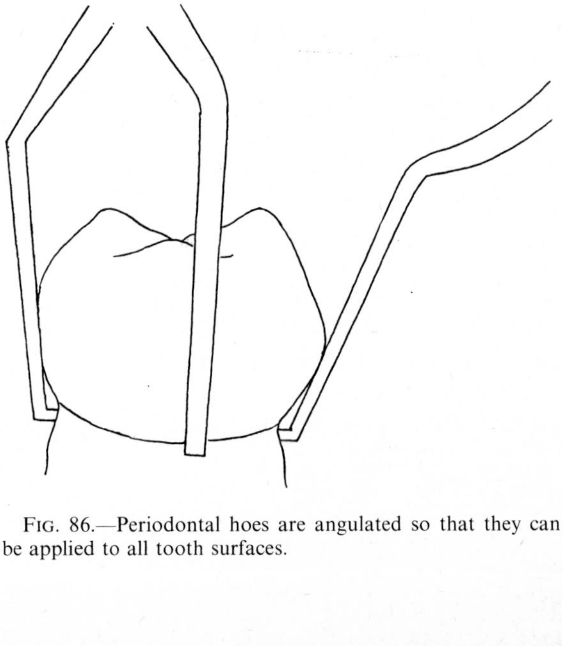

FIG. 86.—Periodontal hoes are angulated so that they can be applied to all tooth surfaces.

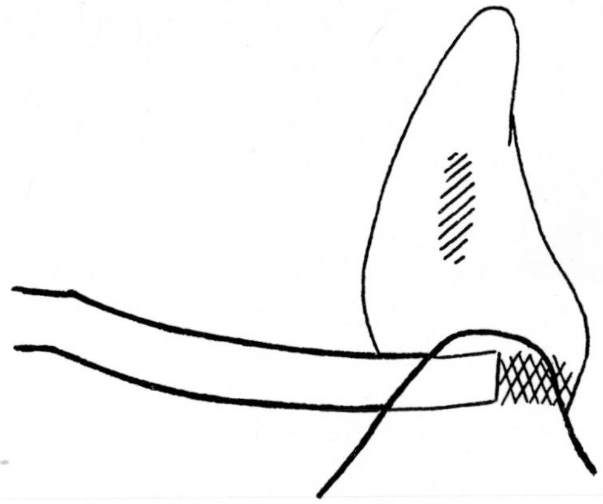

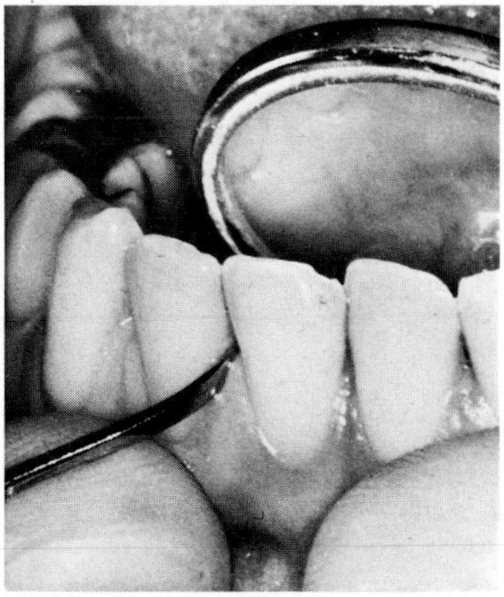

FIG. 87.—The periodontal chisel (also known as the 'push', 'watch-spring', or 'Zerfing' scaler) can be used to remove interproximal calculus providing there is an interdental space into which it can be inserted.

Interproximal surfaces may be inaccessible to all but the thinnest instruments. The 'watch-spring' scaler or periodontal chisel can be inserted into small spaces and, if used with care, remove calculus from these surfaces very effectively (Fig. 87). A secure finger rest is essential in pushing this instrument from the labial aspect between the teeth. It is a wise precaution to hold a mouth mirror lingual to these teeth so that the tongue is protected from the instrument's sharp edge.

When it is thought that all calculus has been removed, subgingival surfaces should be examined carefully with a Briault or Cross calculus probe. It is also helpful to blow warm air at the crevice; this removes saliva and separates the gingival margin from the tooth so that a view into the crevice is obtained.

The Ultrasonic Scaler (Fig. 88)

Ultrasonic instruments are now generally employed for the removal of both supragingival and subgingival calculus. They function according to the principles of magnetostriction whereby an alternating current alters the length of the instrument approximately one-thousandth of an inch 25,000 times a second. The motion of the instrument can fragment surfaces against which it is placed. Thus it can break up calculus as well as the lining of the gingival crevice. The tip of the instrument is kept under a continuous spray of water which has two functions (1) to keep the tip cool and (2) to produce a form of detergent phenomenon known as 'cavitation' which is effected by microscopic bubbles created by the contact of the vibrating tip with the water.

The effect produced by the instrument is related to the amplitude of movement of the tip, the pressure and angulation at which it is used, the sharpness of the tip and the length of time with which it is in contact with the surface.

In scaling a tip suitable for the shape of the surface is selected and used with a light stroking movement so that calculus is fragmented without damage to the tooth surface. Like all instruments it can produce damage if used clumsily, but when used carefully it is a very valuable addition to the

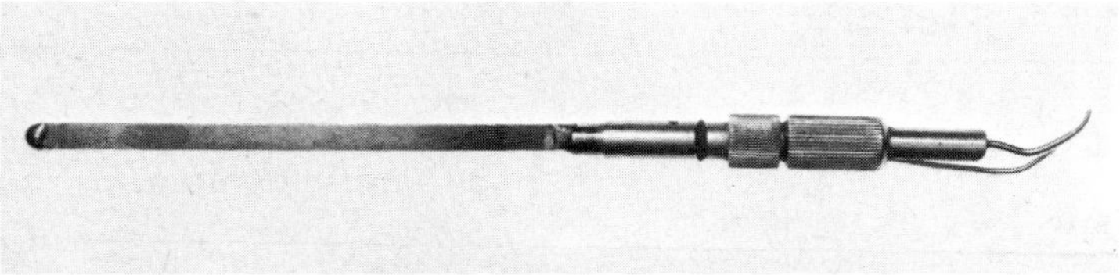

FIG. 88.—Ultrasonic curette used for scaling.

scaling armamentarium.

Its main limitation lies in the absence of any tactile sensation whereby the operator can detect the presence of calculus against the instrument. This means that all scaling must be completed with hand instruments.

Some patients find the use of the ultrasonic instrument very painful and of course it must be used with caution against ceramic restorations, especially gold bonded to porcelain.

Polishing

After scaling, teeth should be clean and smooth. Rough surfaces quickly become the site of plaque and calculus deposition, therefore polishing is essential. Stain and plaque are removed with small cup-shaped brushes or rubber cups, and a slightly abrasive polishing paste. Firm but intermittent contact is necessary so that the brush removes stain effectively without overheating the tooth. Sometimes stain adheres so strongly to the tooth surface that a scaler must be used to remove it. In this case it is important not to scratch the tooth surface; if this happens the scratched surface must be polished with an abrasive rubber wheel used with intermittent pressure to avoid overheating.

Finally, linen polishing strips can be used to polish interproximal surfaces. In cleaning interproximal areas one must avoid damaging the interdental papilla. If there is difficulty in inserting even a fine instrument or strip between the teeth it is more than likely that no space exists in which plaque may be present; in such cases this procedure should be avoided.

CORRECTION OF PREDISPOSING FACTORS

Correction of Faulty Restorations (See Chapter 20, page 241).

Small overhanging edges may be polished down with fine tapering burs, flame-shaped polishing burs, push-through scalers and polishing strips. In doing this one must try to avoid damaging the interdental papilla more than necessary. Large overhanging edges may be eradicated only by removal of the restoration and its replacement by a new correctly contoured restoration.

Marginal ridges may be cut into the occlusal surface of a restoration, but if the restoration is very badly shaped or the contact relationship is poor a new restoration is necessary. Matrix bands, wedges when necessary, and cellophane strips must be used correctly to obtain satisfactory restorations. Any gingival damage which might result from a deeply placed matrix band or wedge is likely to heal and is of less consequence than that which results from an overhanging margin.

Correction of Faulty Dentures

It would be out of place in this text to enlarge upon correct partial denture design. Nevertheless certain remarks are pertinent.

All partial dentures are potentially harmful. Even the most perfectly designed prosthesis is a foreign body resting against the gingival margin at some point and exerting pressures on some teeth. In designing a partial denture it is necessary to reduce contact with the gingival margin to a minimum, and to attempt to make those points of contact self-cleansing. It is also necessary to clasp and load teeth so that stresses are as nearly as possible in the long axis of the abutment teeth and to choose abutment teeth sound enough to bear the extra load. For this, accurate study models of the jaws and periapical radiographs of the teeth to be used as abutments are needed. Models should be surveyed and as many sound teeth as possible used as abutments, the wider the distribution of the load the less the individual tooth has to bear. Clasps must be designed so that horizontal pressures from the lingual aspect are counteracted by supporting labial arms. Multiple occlusal rests ensure axial support of the denture and protection for the gingivae. At the same time the denture must be highly polished and easy to keep clean. A well designed tooth-borne skeleton metal denture meets these requirements (Fig. 89).

Fixed Bridgework

Fixed bridgework should meet the requirements for both good restorations and good prostheses. Crowns and inlays must have well-fitting highly polished edges placed if possible coronal to the gingival margin (see Chapter 20). Pontics should be shaped to fit against the minimal area of alveolar ridge compatible with aesthetic requirements. They must not encroach upon the gingival margins of abutment teeth, and should be as self-cleansing as possible (Fig. 90). At the same time they should be comfortable to the tongue. A

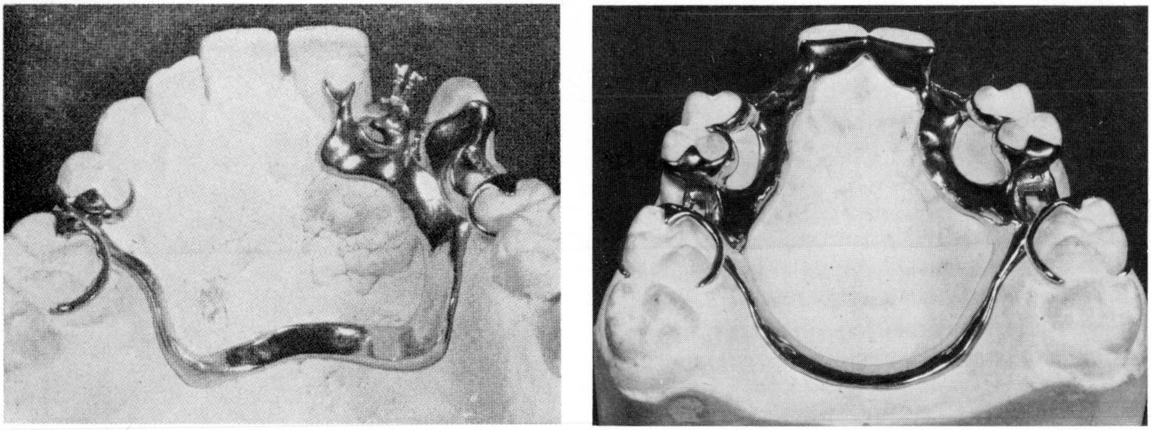

FIG. 89.—Skeleton chrome-cobalt dentures which make minimum contact with the gingival margin and are adequately tooth-borne.

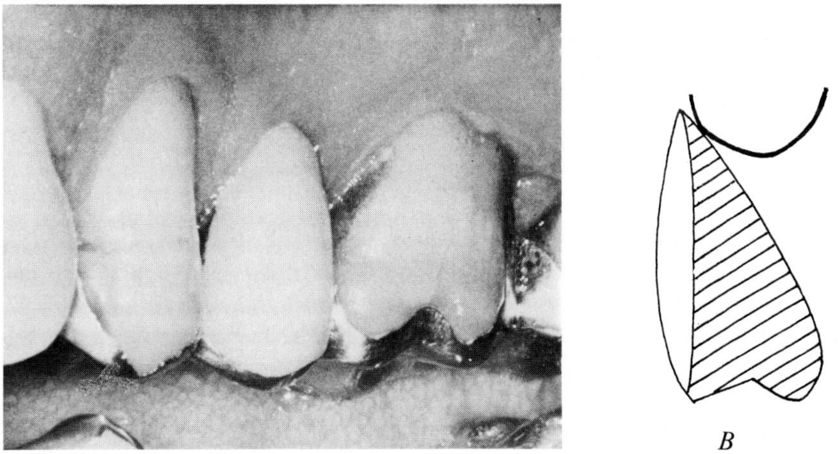

B

A

FIG. 90.—(*A*) A well-designed pontic which does not encroach on the gingival margin of the abutment teeth. (*B*) The relationship of pontic to ridge so that the area can be easily cleaned.

sanitary pontic may be self-cleansing but also cause tongue irritation. A pontic shape which is not too far removed from that of a normal tooth may be more comfortable for the patient.

Fixed Orthodontic Appliances

These may present a difficult problem. They can be difficult to keep clean and few children are sufficiently conscientious to keep them completely free of debris. Careful instruction in plaque control is essential. The regular use of a disclosing agent, say, once weekly, should be mandatory. This discipline and regular scaling may keep a gingivitis under reasonable control but its complete eradication may have to be delayed until the appliance has been removed. Often the gingiva in relation to an orthodontic appliance is extremely red and swollen (Fig. 91), and at first sight immediate removal of the orthodontic appliance would seem to be indicated. It should be remem-

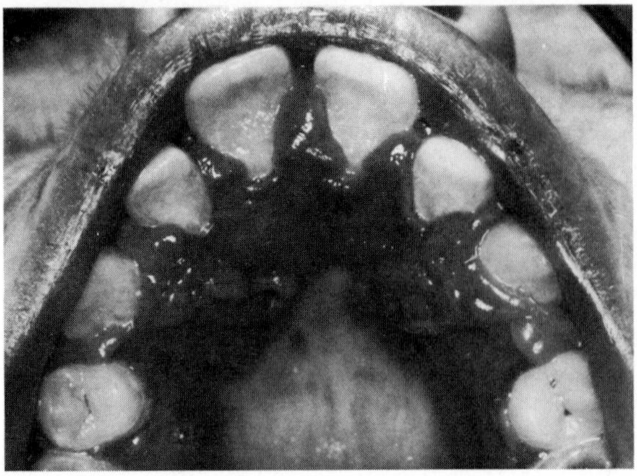

FIG. 91.—Inflammation under removable orthodontic appliance.

bered that fortunately the most exaggerated tissue reaction to irritation is the one which responds most rapidly, and often spectacularly, to an improvement in oral hygiene.

If the orthodontic appliance is badly constructed and ill-fitting then it must be removed and remade.

Treatment of Lack of Lip-seal

In many cases thorough scaling and instruction in oral hygiene techniques is sufficient treatment to restore the gingivae to health. To maintain the gingivae in health is more difficult. It is important that the patient understands his problem and realizes that he has to make an extra effort to keep his mouth clean. If this can be done the provision of a special appliance to be worn during sleep (the oral screen) (Fig. 92) will be unnecessary. A patient provided with an oral screen may regard it as the primary treatment tool and neglect oral hygiene as being of secondary importance. Even when an oral screen is provided, patients often do not persist with it for very long. The sometimes recommended expedient of sticking sellotape to the lips before bed is never tolerated. Smearing the gingivae with petroleum jelly does not appear to help.

Gingivoplasty

Gingivoplasty is the procedure of recontouring gingiva which has lost its physiological form. It is a gingivectomy with the limited aim of improving gingival contour without the necessity for the elimination of pockets.

When a gingivitis has been present for a relatively short time and distortion of gingival contour is due to inflammatory oedema, thorough scaling may produce resolution and a return to normal contour. In the presence of fibrotic changes which do not resolve on scaling, the gingivae may remain thick and rolled so that food shedding is inefficient and the resulting food stagnation may maintain gingival irritation. In these circumstances either the gingivitis does not resolve or it recurs quickly after scaling. In this case surgical reshaping of the gingiva, *i.e.* gingivoplasty, is indicated. It is important to keep the patient under observation for a few weeks after scaling; if the gingival contour remains abnormal gingivoplasty should not be delayed.

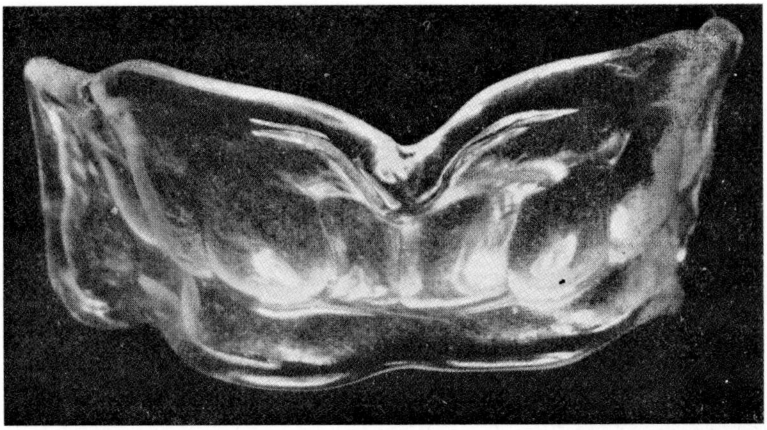

FIG. 92.—Oral screen.

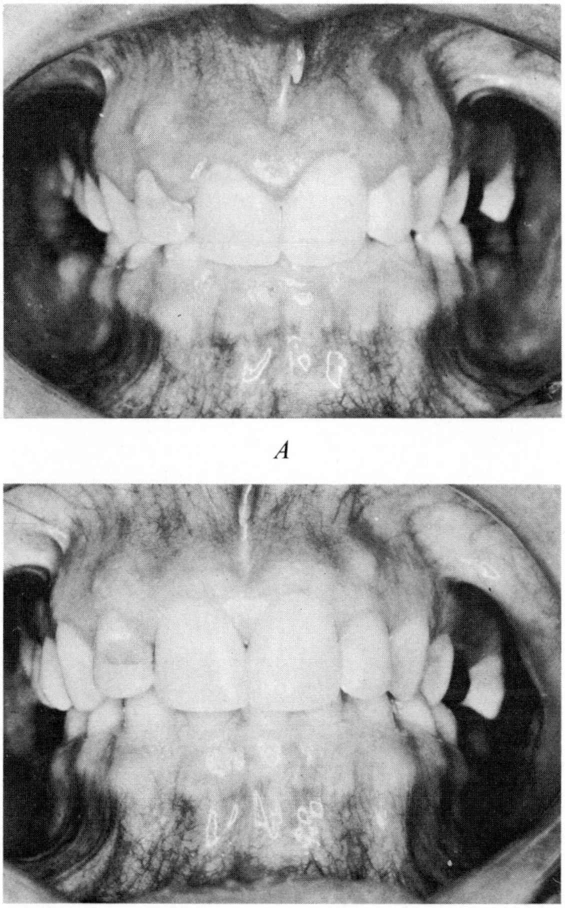

A

B

Fig. 93.—(*A*) Papillary swelling after several episodes of Vincent's disease. (*B*) After gingivoplasty.

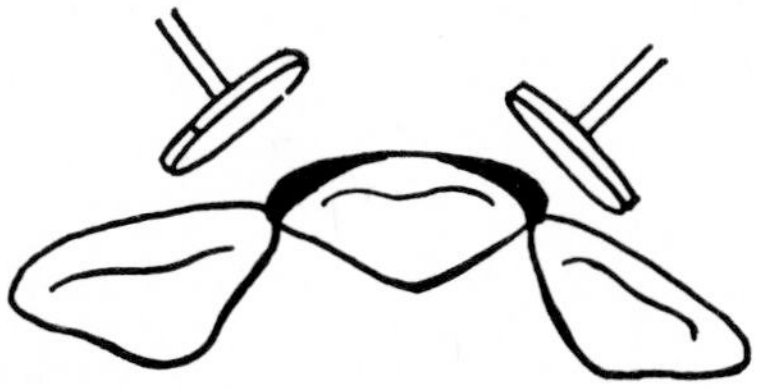

Fig. 94.—The reshaping of a labially placed incisor to improve food-shedding.

After one or more episodes of Vincent's disease (Chapter 19) the gingival contour may be completely distorted. Tissue destruction produces saucer-shaped defects which are areas of food impaction and plaque stagnation (Fig. 93*A*). Thus gingival irritation is perpetuated and chronic periodontal disease develops unless the gingival contour is improved. Gingivoplasty is required in a large percentage of cases of Vincent's disease (Fig. 93*B*).

The gingivae around irregular teeth often has an abnormal shape with thickened margins and absence of interdental sluiceways. Even after thorough scaling, difficulties in plaque control can maintain the condition; in this case gingivoplasty should be preceded where possible by modifying the tooth contour (Fig. 94).

A poor gingival contour may also reflect the abnormal shape of an alveolar bone margin affected by chronic inflammation.

The object of gingivoplasty is to produce a streamlined gingival contour with a knife-edged and scalloped gingival margin, and correctly shaped papillae with an interdental sluiceway.

The detailed management of gingivoplasty is described under 'Gingivectomy' (Chapter 9) but certain features may be described briefly at this point. Three techniques may be employed for removing gingival tissue: scalpel incision, diamond stone abrasion and electro-surgery.

Scalpel Incision

Several types of periodontal knife may be used; these include the Kirkland knife, Blake knife or a Swann-Morton scalpel with a No. 12 blade (this is the writer's preference for all labial and buccal surfaces) (Fig. 95). Whichever blade is preferred it must be very sharp and narrow enough to penetrate the tissues completely, particularly in interdental regions. The blade is held at about 45° and a continuous incision is made in such a position that the required gingival shape is produced (Fig. 96). The usual mistake is to make the incision in too coronal a position. It is often advisable to have an incision line in mind and then make the incision slightly apical to this. Once the excess gingival tissue has been removed the gingival contour can be further streamlined and interdental sluiceways accentuated by scraping the tissue with a rigid blade such as that of the Kirkland knife (Fig. 97). Thickened papillae may also be trimmed with fine nail clippers (Fig. 97*C*).

It is essential that the desired contour be produced at operation. Pressure from the periodontal dressing or energetic use of dental woodsticks cannot compensate for a poor recontouring technique.

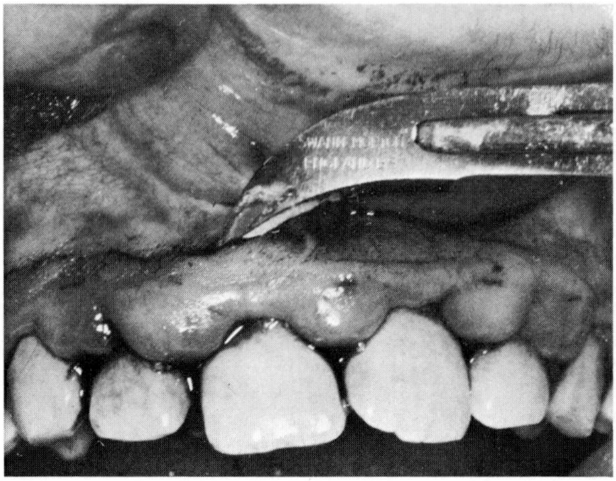

FIG. 95.—Gingivoplasty incision. Chronic hyperplastic gingivitis in a 17-year-old girl.

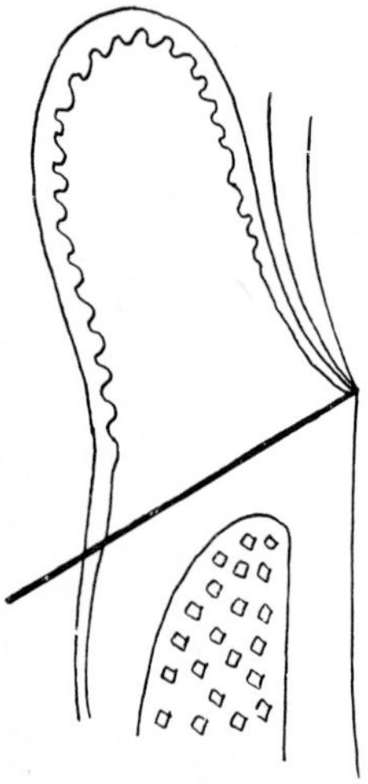

A

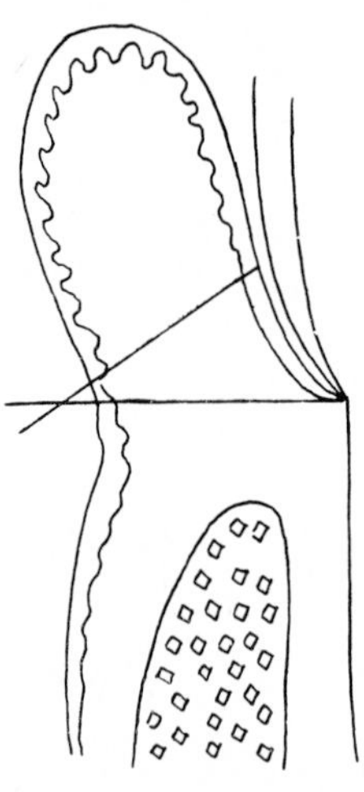

B

FIG. 96.—(*A*) The correct angle of a gingivoplasty incision. (*B*) Incorrect positions for incisions.

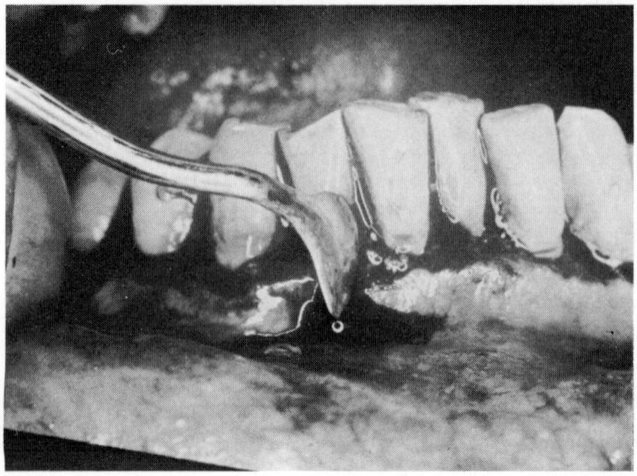

A

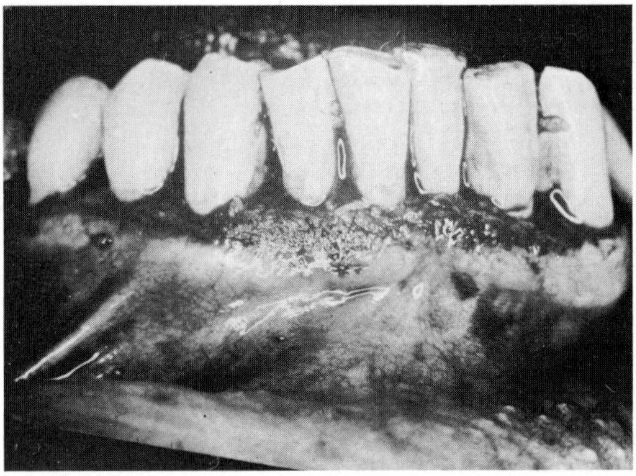

B

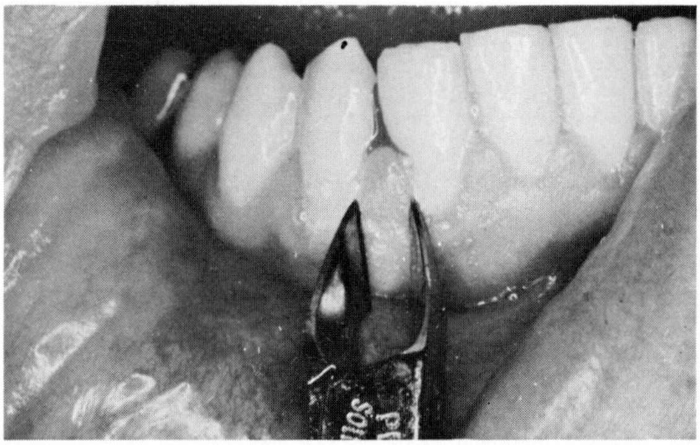

C

FIG. 97.—(*A*) Kirkland knife being used to improve gingival shape by scraping the tissue at the edge of the initial incision. (*B*) Streamlined shape produced. (*C*) Thickened papillae being trimmed with fine nail clippers.

Diamond Stone Abrasion

If the gingival tissues are fibrous and tough a rapidly rotating diamond stone can be used to reshape them easily and without tissue damage providing the instrument is used gently, under an efficient water spray. The technique is useful for reshaping thickened interdental papillae and in modifying a scalpel incision, but where the gingivae are very enlarged gingivoplasty by scalpel incision is to be preferred.

A rough diamond stone rotating at fairly high speed (30,000 r.p.m.), or a small cylindrical diamond stone in the air-turbine cuts the tissue effectively. A longer tapered fissure diamond stone (Fig. 98) may be used for shaping interdental papillae. The instrument is stroked lightly and intermittently across the tissue until the desired contour is produced (Fig. 99).

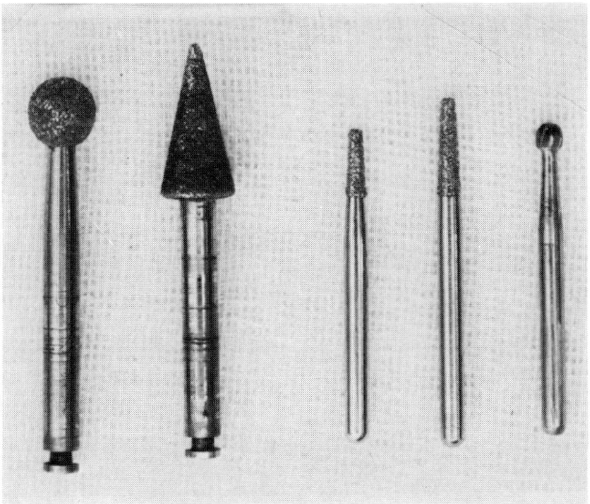

FIG. 98.—Rotary instruments used for reshaping gingivae (and bone). Dendia diamond instruments No. 5 round and No. 4 cone; Hi-Di friction grip diamond burs Nos. 551 and 554; tungsten carbide No. 5 round bur (for bone trimming).

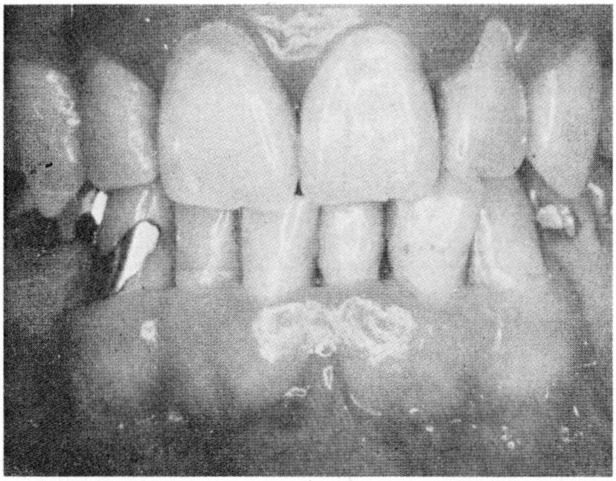

A

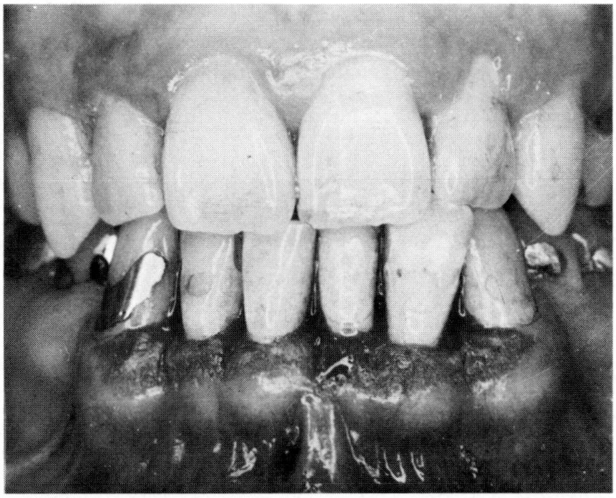

B

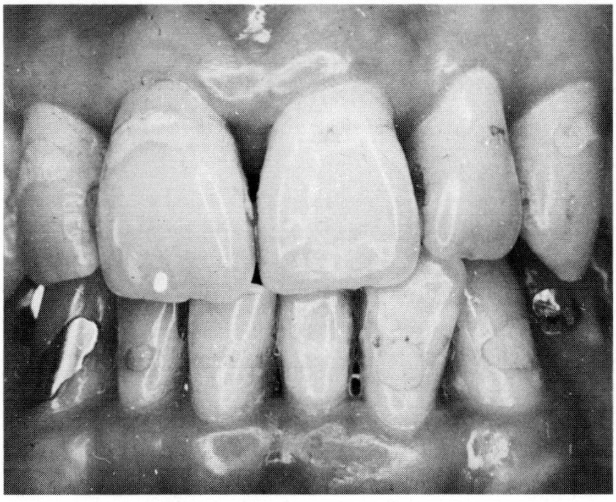

C

FIG. 99.—(*A*) Gingival distortion around lower incisors after Vincent's disease (22-year-old man). (*B*) After reshaping with rotary diamond burs. (*C*) Five weeks post-operation.

Electrosurgery

A bipolar or unipolar electrocautery may be used for removing gingival tissue. There are indications that post-operative discomfort is greater and that the healing time may be longer after electrosurgery than after a scalpel incision. Patients find the smell of burning tissue very disagreeable, and many are extremely apprehensive about the use of a hot instrument in the mouth. Therefore the scalpel is the instrument of choice and electrosurgery should be restricted to those cases where obvious advantages accrue from its use. It is best used for the removal of soft, haemorrhagic and movable tissue which is difficult to immobilize for incision with a scalpel, and for the removal of small localized flaps of movable tissue, as for example the flap distal to a partly erupted lower third molar, which may be difficult to remove completely with a scalpel. In using the instrument great care must be taken to ensure that it does not come into contact with a metal instrument or with any tissue other than that to be removed. To this end the area must be well packed off with swabs and the tongue protected with a wooden spatula. Direct vision is essential. In using the electrocautery very light intermittent stroking is made with the tissue. Prolonged application must be avoided as touching bone can produce necrosis.

After the correct gingival contour has been produced, whatever the technique used, all tissue

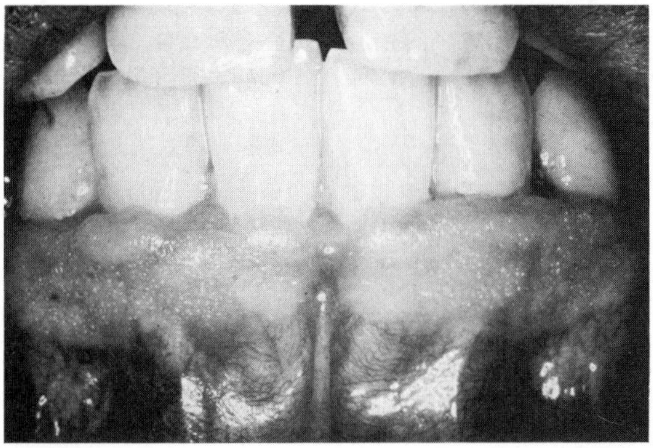

A

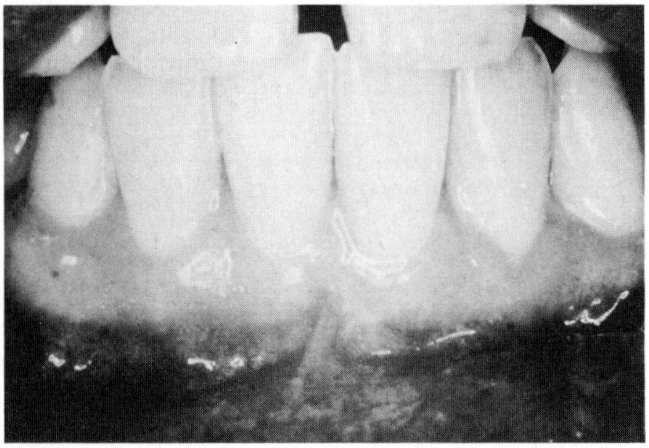

B

FIG. 100.—(*A*) After scaling thickened fibrous papillae remain which, if not further treated would soon become inflamed. (*B*) Several months after gingivoplasty the patient is maintaining an excellent standard of cleanliness and the gingival contour remains satisfactory.

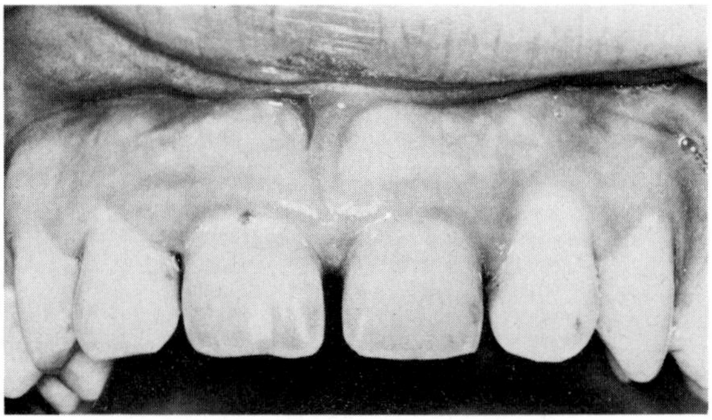

A

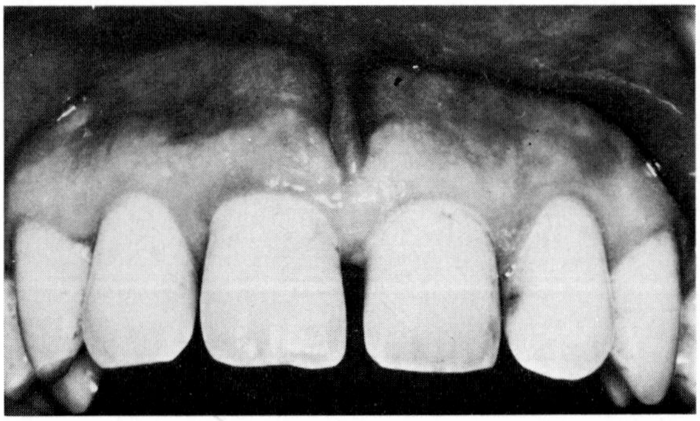

B

FIG. 101.—(*A*) Chronic hyperplastic gingivitis due to poor oral hygiene with deep gingival pocketing. (*B*) Three months post-gingivoplasty. Although a good surgical result was achieved the patient is not keeping his mouth clean and some gingival inflammation is appearing.

tags are removed with a sharp curette, and the exposed root surface is inspected for calculus. Often no calculus is present, particularly if the patient has previously received a scaling and is conscientiously carrying out a good oral hygiene regime.

When the teeth are clean, swabs are firmly placed on the wound to arrest bleeding and the periodontal dressing is applied (Chapter 9). Healing after gingivoplasty is usually uneventful. The dressing is kept in place for one week, and following its removal a strict regime of oral hygiene is instituted. For about one week copious and frequent mouth washes and a soft toothbrush are used, after which a normal routine of oral hygiene is instituted (Figs. 100 and 101).

RECOMMENDED READING

BODECKER, C. F. (1943). The difficulty of completely removing subgingival calculus. *J. Amer. dent. Ass.*, **30**, 703.

FRISCH, J., BHASKAR, S. and SHELL, D. D. (1967). Effect of ultrasonic instrumentation on human gingival connective tissue. *Periodontics*, **5**, 123.

GOLDMAN, H. M. (1950). Development of physiologic gingival contours by gingivoplasty. *Oral Surg.*, **3**, 879.

KERRY, G. J. (1967). Roughness of tooth surfaces after use of ultrasonic instrumentation and hand curettes. *J. Periodont.*, **38**, 340.

LÖVDAL, A., ARNO, A., SCHEI, O. and WAERHAUG, J. (1961). Combined effect of subgingival scaling and controlled oral hygiene on the incidence of gingivitis. *Acta odont. scand.*, **19**, 537.

SCHAFFER, E. M. (1964). Objective evaluation of ultrasonic versus hand instrumentation in periodontics. *Dent. Clin. N. Amer.*, March, p. 165.

8. Chronic Periodontitis

Chronic gingivitis and chronic periodontitis are sequential stages in chronic periodontal disease. The various manifestations of chronic periodontal disease represent milestones in the history of a disease which has its beginnings in gingival inflammation and ends in tooth loss. If the aetiology of chronic periodontitis is to be defined it must be inadequate control of chronic gingivitis.

The changes so far described are limited to the gingivae and with treatment are reversible. Gingival inflammation has been described as 'contained' (Goldman, 1942). It can also be described as 'extra-alveolar'. Even if gingival inflammation spreads by vascular pathways into alveolar trabecular spaces, thus inducing some internal bone resorption and rarefaction of alveolar crest, all the changes are reversible because all the tissues involved, epithelium, fibrous connective tissue and bone, have considerable powers of regeneration, and there is normally an ample reservoir of undifferentiated connective tissue cells from which new fibroblasts and osteoblasts can arise.

As long as the most coronal periodontal fibres remain intact and there is no apical migration of crevicular epithelium down the root the condition remains a gingivitis. If the chronic inflammation is not controlled it can progress into the deeper tissues. Once the most coronal periodontal fibres are disrupted and epithelial cells proliferate into the defect, the physiological seal between tooth and soft tissue breaks down and a 'periodontal' or 'true' pocket is formed (Fig. 102). Initially this is a histopathological lesion which cannot be detected clinically, but it represents an irreversible change. Once formed the periodontal pocket is a self-perpetuating lesion which cannot heal spontaneously. Its contents are inaccessible to the patient's routine cleaning procedures, and the accumulation of foreign material within the

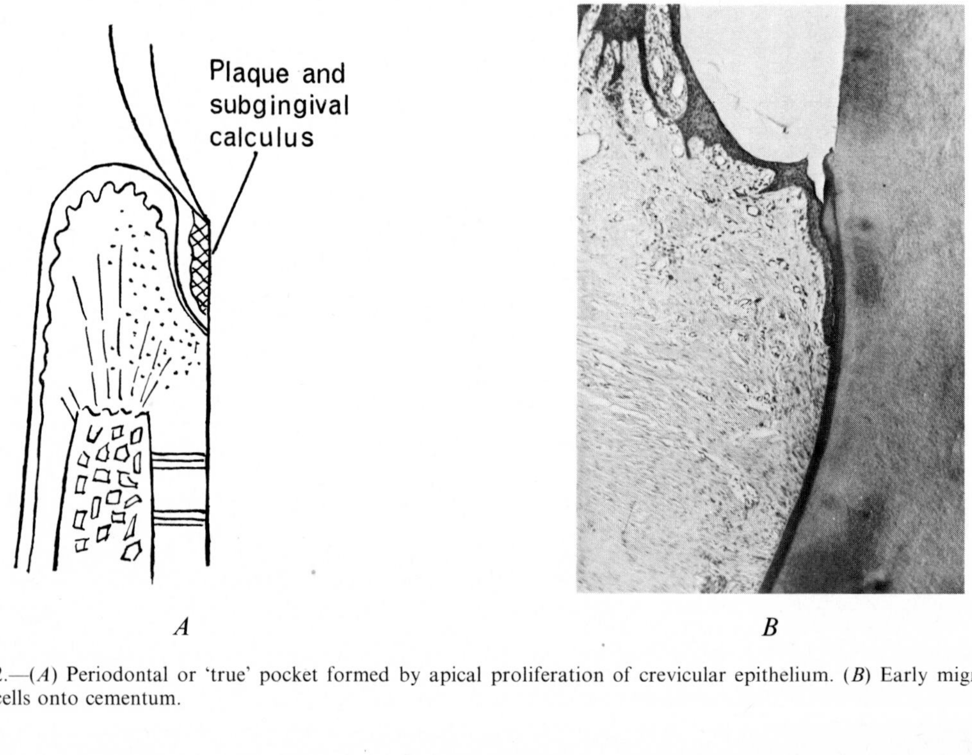

A *B*

FIG. 102.—(*A*) Periodontal or 'true' pocket formed by apical proliferation of crevicular epithelium. (*B*) Early migration of epithelial cells onto cementum.

pocket, plaque and subgingival calculus cannot be flushed away by the crevicular fluid exudate. Indeed the inflammatory exudate into the pocket is probably a factor in promoting the deposition of subgingival calculus and plaque.

The inflammatory process may be spread from the gingival margin along three paths (Fig. 103):

1. Through the attached gingiva.
2. Into the alveolar process.
3. Into the periodontal ligament.

The most common pathway appears to be through the alveolar bone. Inflammation extends via perivascular and perineural channels through the connective tissue into the alveolar crest, and then via trabecular spaces in the periodontal space and attached gingiva (Weinmann, 1941). It may also extend superficially from the gingival margin into the attached gingiva, and then through the bone into the periodontal ligament.

The periodontal ligament is the least vascular pathway; in addition the fibre bundles of the periodontal ligament are organized in layers perpendicular to the path of inflammation and therefore represent a relatively dense barrier.

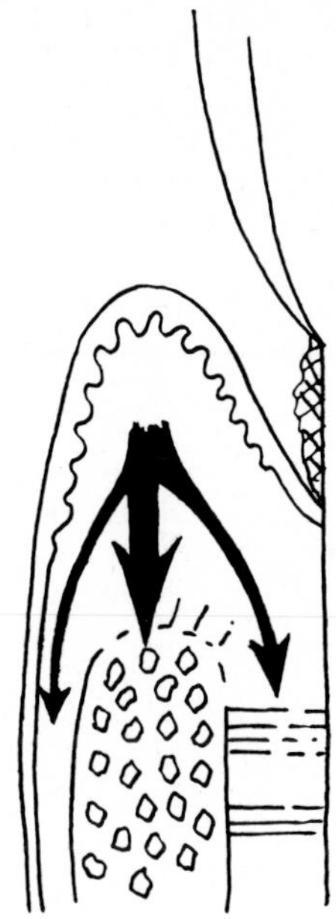

FIG. 103.—Inflammation may spread from the gingival margin along three pathways: (1) into the periodontal ligament; (2) into the alveolar bone, and (3) along the attached gingiva, and then through the bone.

Histology of the Pocket

Inflammatory changes in the gingival connective tissue appear to provoke epithelial changes and the epithelium of the pocket shows a proliferative and degenerative response. Projections of epithelium grow into the adjacent connective tissue. The epithelium becomes infiltrated with leucocytes and many cells undergo vacuolar degeneration. Progressive epithelial degeneration and necrosis can lead to ulceration of the pocket wall and exposure of the underlying connective tissue, but this is by no means a universal finding. In many sections the epithelial layer is intact (Fig. 104).

The connective tissue is oedematous and densely infiltrated with plasma cells and lymphocytes, some macrophages plus a few polymorphonuclear leucocytes (Fig. 104*C*). Vessels are dilated and increased in number. Some capillaries are thrombosed. There may be breakdown of vessel walls with haemorrhage into the surrounding tissue. The most evident feature is the loss of well-defined collagen bundles and in some areas there is degeneration of the connective tissue sometimes associated with patches of haemorrhage. This is in marked contrast to neighbouring areas where the organization of the periodontal fibres remains intact so that the periodontal lesion is well localized. The circumscribed nature of the periodontal lesion is one of its most obvious characteristics (Fig. 105). In some cases suppuration takes place and very large numbers of polymorphonuclear leucocytes are present.

Some areas of cementum undergo resorption with consequent exposure of dentine; even caries may result.

Extension of the inflammation into the alveolar process is marked by infiltration of the trabecular spaces by inflammatory cells, proliferating connective tissue cells and new capillaries. The bone surfaces become involved in resorption and the trabecular spaces increase in size. Endosteal surfaces are more reactive than periosteal surfaces and it is possible that alveolar bone loss is mainly brought about by increasing osteoporosis. At the same time interproximally the crestal surface undergoes resorption with the formation of an interdental crater (Fig. 106). The resorption process spreads laterally so that the entire crest becomes reduced.

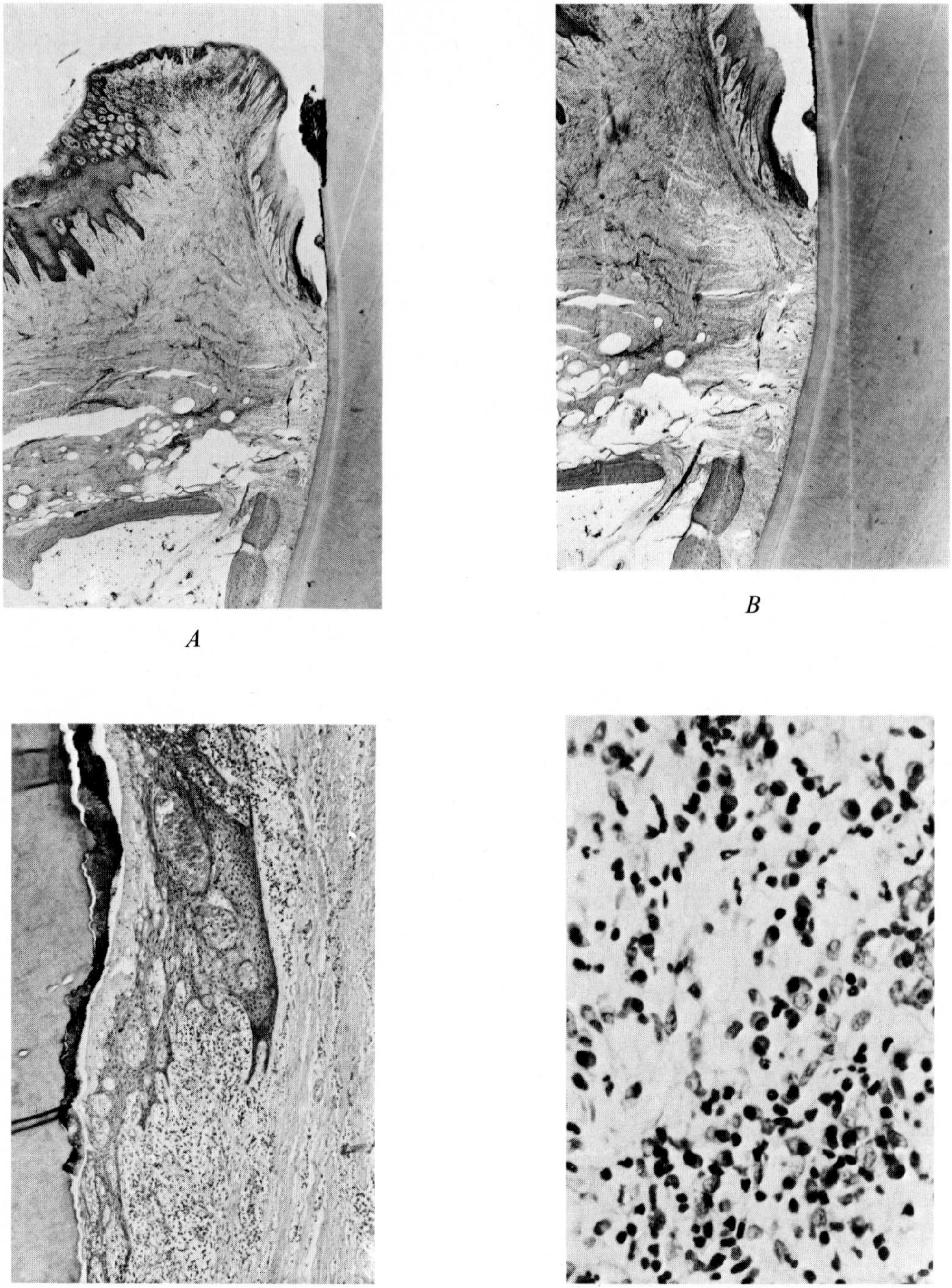

FIG. 104.—(*A*) Periodontal pocket with downgrowth of crevicular epithelium onto cementum. Note surface of epithelium conforms to shape of subgingival calculus. (*B*) Dilated vessels passing from inflammatory zone into the alveolar crest. (*C*) Higher power showing irregular proliferation of epithelium of pocket wall and inflammatory infiltrate in corium. (*D*) Dense infiltration of lymphocytes and plasma cells (which predominate) in pocket wall. (By courtesy of Professor I. R. H. Kramer.)

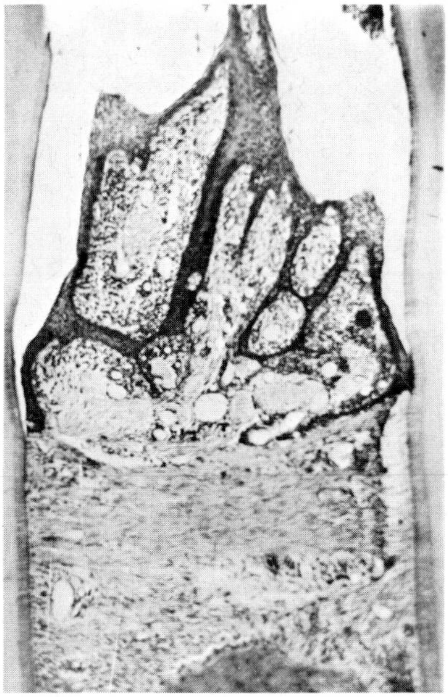

FIG. 105.—Inflammation well localized by reformation of transseptal fibres apical to periodontal pocket. (By courtesy of Professor B. Cohen.)

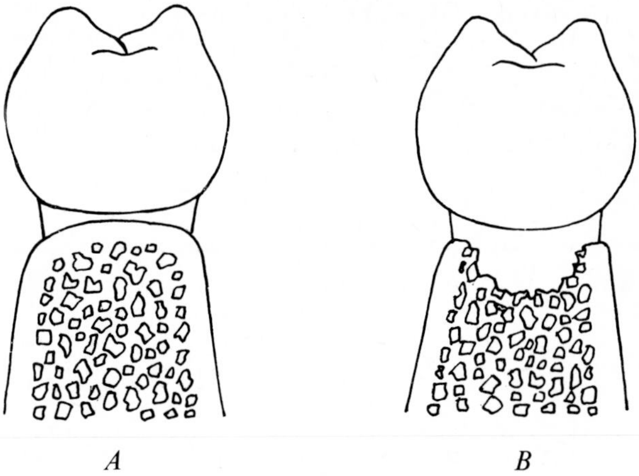

FIG. 106.—Variations in the pattern of alveolar bone contour. (*A*) Normal interdental bone contour. (*B*) Bone crater.

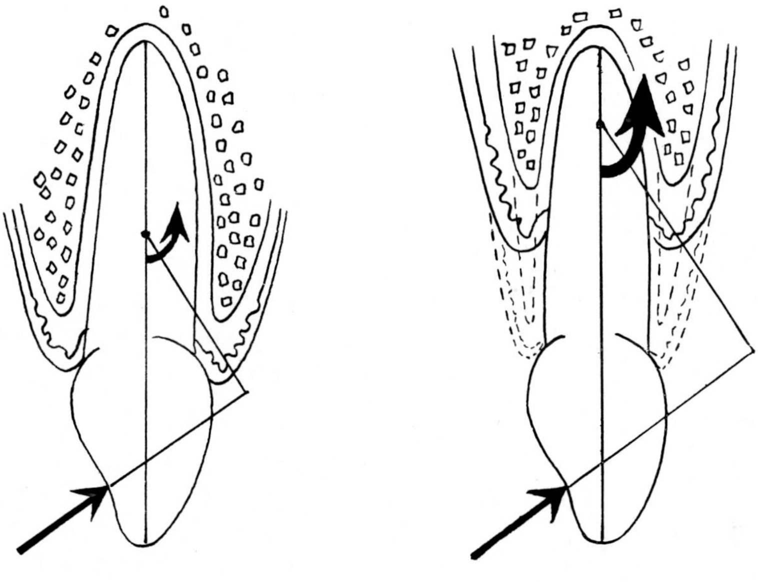

FIG. 107.—With progressive bone loss the crown-root ratio increases, therefore the moment of force on the remaining tissue also increases, and a vicious circle is established.

The process of bone loss is intermittent, periods of resorption alternate with periods of consolidation but the former is greater in the presence of inflammation and the aggregate result is loss of supporting tissue.

This process of tissue destruction may continue until the amount of supporting tissue can no longer absorb occlusal stresses and previously acceptable or physiological forces cause tissue damage (Fig. 107). This damage is called 'secondary occlusal trauma' (see Chapter 13).

From this point on the destructive process seems to accelerate until the tooth is shed or acute infection supervenes with the production of a periodontal abscess (Chapter 12).

OCCLUSAL TRAUMA

(see Chapters 13 and 14)

The periodontal tissues may be subject to two forms of irritation, gingival irritation and excessive occlusal stress, *i.e.* physical overloading of the tooth-supporting tissues by forces acting on the crown of the tooth. These two factors may occur alone but frequently occur together to produce respectively gingival inflammation and occlusal or periodontal trauma. Gingival inflammation and its sequelae have just been described. It is possible to study these tissue changes by biopsy of diseased gingivae from human patients, from tissue obtained at autopsy and from animal experiments. However, those tissue changes which result from excessive occlusal stress affect the deeper periodontal tissues which cannot be obtained for observation without tooth extraction and mutilation of the jaws. Therefore our knowledge of the changes which take place when the tooth-supporting tissues are exposed to excessive mechanical loads has been obtained from animal experiments. In the early experiments on rodents, dogs, even sheep, the occlusion was interfered with in a gross way and no attempt was made to simulate the conditions which actually occur in the human mouth. The experimental interference sometimes acted constantly and was in no way related to the stress system, quantitatively or qualitatively, which operates in the human mouth either in function or parafunction. Indeed in these experiments the animals were also rarely free of gingival inflammation.

Despite these limitations it has been assumed that the tissue changes described in these experiments demonstrate the kind of tissue changes produced by overloading of the human dentition. Under excessive loading the principal periodontal fibre bundles become disrupted and disorganised. Hyaline degeneration and necrosis takes place and the connective tissue may be replaced by granulation tissue. Vascular changes which take place include haemorrhage and thrombosis. There may be cementum resorption. The changes which take place in the bone depend on the direction and degree of force. On the tension side bone deposition is described, while on the pressure side the bone undergoes resorption. If pressure is not so great there is an increase in vascularity plus evident signs of osteoclasis. If pressure is great so that the tooth impinges on the bone and vascularity is severely interrupted, death of bone cells occurs in that area of bone next to the tooth, and undermining resorption takes place in the neighbouring trabecular spaces and the necrotic bone is removed. Tissue remodelling takes place so that new supporting tissue is formed with the tooth in its new position. The gingival fibres and the most coronal periodontal fibres are not disrupted, there is no apical migration of crevicular epithelium, and the whole phenomenon can be described as '*intra-alveolar*'. The tissues involved including bone have considerable reparative and remodelling powers and the periodontal changes produced by excessive occlusal forces are reversible when the forces are removed. It is fortunate that this is the case, otherwise orthodontics would be impossible.

The obvious criticism of most of this research work is that it does not simulate the stress system in the clinical situation. To overcome obvious differences, Wentz, Jarabak and Orban (1958) introduced a method of producing intermittent excessive loading through cuspal interference in the experimental animal. The periodontal damage produced by such forces could be reversed after three months but the periodontium did not return completely to normal. The periodontal fibre bundles appeared larger and the periodontal space stayed very much wider. However these changes remained *intra-alveolar* and were not those we identify with chronic periodontitis. The accumulated evidence of considerable experimentation is that whatever lesions may be produced by excessive occlusal stresses *alone* they are not the characteristic lesion of chronic periodontitis, the periodontal pocket.

The combined effects of gingival irritation and occlusal stress have been studied (Ewen and Stahl, 1962; Glickman and Smulow, 1962) and these studies indicate that the two factors enhance each other, *i.e.* there appears to be a more rapid spread of inflammation through tissue disrupted by excessive occlusal forces, and inflamed tissue disrupts more easily so that there is more rapid progression of the destruction of periodontal tissue than if each of the factors acted separately. Because of this Glickman (1971) has called inflammation and occlusal trauma 'co-destructive' factors.

This idea has general acceptance; a question still debated is whether occlusal stresses influence the actual shape of the bone lesion.

THE BONE LESION

As the periodontal lesion progresses bone resorption takes place as described. The resorption of the alveolar crest may take place evenly, *i.e.* 'horizontal' bone loss which proceeds at the same rate at the apical migration of the crevicular epithelium, in which case the soft tissue lesion remains coronal to the bone margin and is termed a 'suprabony' pocket. However in many cases bone resorption does not take place evenly. There may be considerable variation in the amount of bone resorption in different parts of the mouth and even on different aspects of the same tooth. The pattern of bone resorption and the form of the bone lesion demonstrates an almost infinite variety. There are three main groups of bone defects:

1. Intra-alveolar defects.
2. Marginal defects.
3. Perforations.

Intra-alveolar Defects

These are defects within the alveolar process. They are formed when periodontal fibres break down and epithelium migrates apically more rapidly than the bone of the alveolar margin is resorbed, so that the bottom of the pocket is apical to the bone crest (Fig. 108), *i.e.* bone

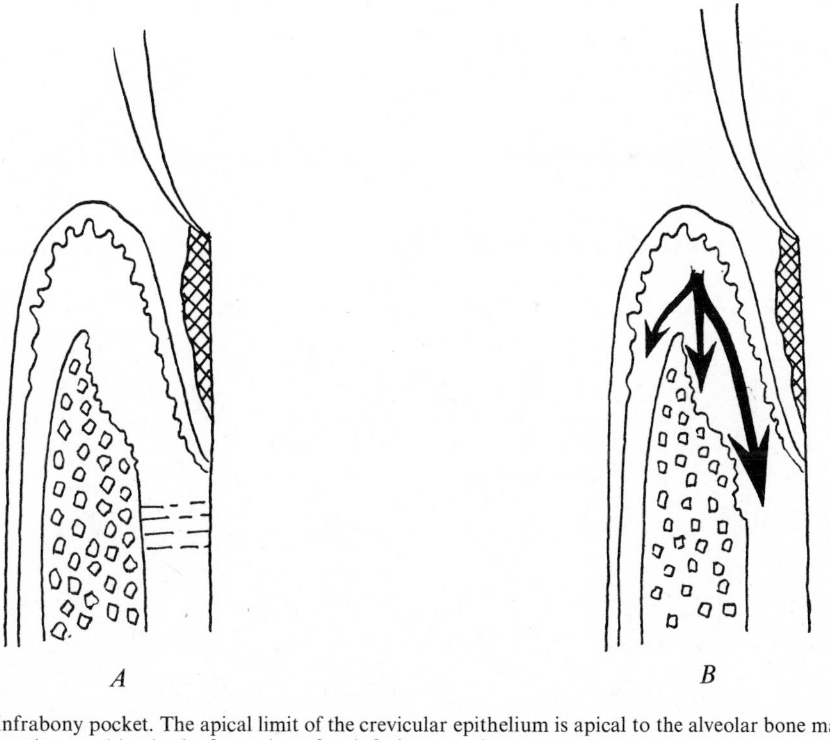

FIG. 108.—(*A*) Infrabony pocket. The apical limit of the crevicular epithelium is apical to the alveolar bone margin. (*B*) Altered pathway of inflammation resulting in the formation of an infrabony pocket.

resorption is *not horizontal*, it is uneven or oblique, or as it is loosely described, 'vertical'.

Intra-alveolar bone defects take up a multiplicity of shapes, and are designated according to their morphology and location.

(a) The interdental crater; concavities in the crest of the interdental septum confined within facial and lingual walls (Fig. 106*B*).

(b) The infrabony defect; areas of bone resorption alongside root surfaces and enclosed within one, two or three bony walls (Fig. 109).

(c) Hemisepta; where the mesial or distal portion of an interdental septum is resorbed leaving the other side of the septum more or less intact (Fig. 110).

Obviously bone defects do not always conform to the standard shapes under which they are classified and different parts of the same defect may be described as one-, two- or three-walled (Fig. 111). The base of a hemiseptum may have two or three walls; an interdental crater may be seen as a two-walled infrabony defect.

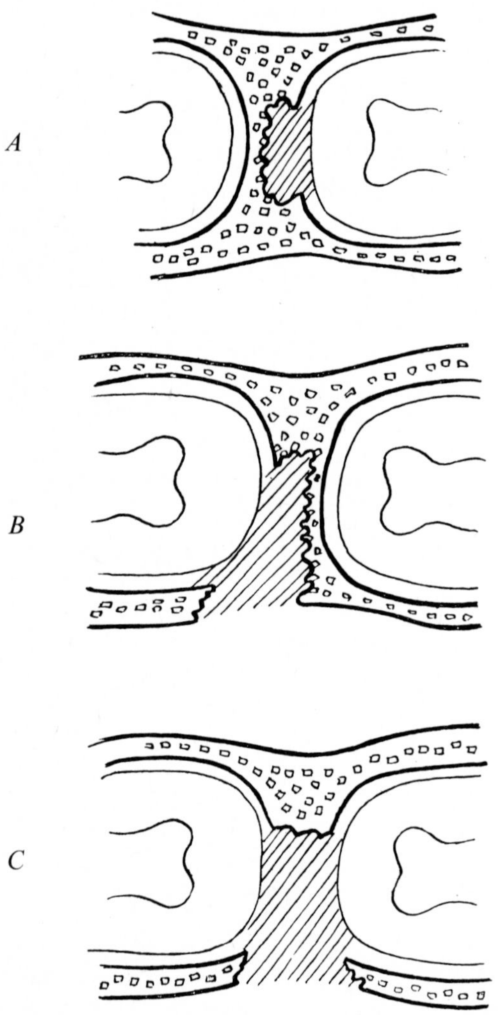

FIG. 109.—(*A*) Infrabony defect with three bone walls. (*B*) Infrabony defect with two bone walls. (*C*) Infrabony defect with one bone wall.

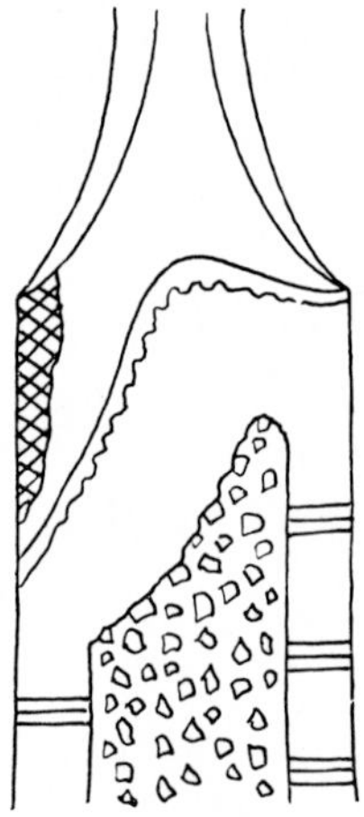

FIG. 110.—Infrabony pocket between teeth.

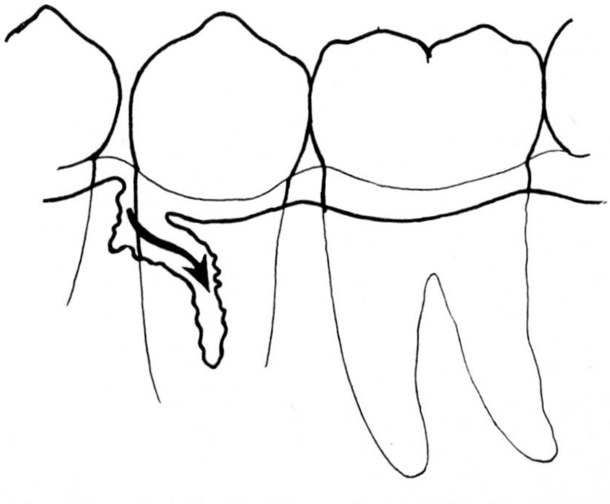

FIG. 111.—Spread of inflammation resulting in a tortuous bone defect.

Marginal Defects

The alveolar margin may become uneven because of irregular resorption or thickened by periosteal deposition (Fig. 112). It may also become remodelled by resorption of the bone surface next to the tooth and compensatory deposition on the periosteal surface to form a gutter. Marginal thickening appears to occur where tissue resistance is good and breakdown very slow, *i.e.* it is a typically chronic bone lesion.

Perforations

Perforation of the buccal or lingual alveolar plates may take place with or without involvement of the alveolar margin. A simple perforation is known as a 'fenestration' (Fig. 113). Where the perforation involves the alveolar margin the defect is known as a 'dehiscence'.

These perforations may be developmental but they may also be inflammatory induced resorptions through thin alveolar plates.

The Determinants of the Bone Defect

There are two general theories about the determinants of the site and morphology of bone defects:

1. The form of the defect is related to the occlusal stress on the related tooth or teeth (Glickman and Smulow, 1962).
2. The form of the defect is related to the original anatomy of the bone (Prichard, 1965), and therefore is influenced by tooth anatomy and position. Goldman and Cohen (1958) include the relationship of neighbouring marginal ridges, cemento-enamel junction and contact points. These writers also describe open contact points as leading to food impaction and accentuated interdental bone damage.

As described above many attempts have been made to replicate the conditions of the human mouth in animal experiments. It has been shown (Macapanpan and Weinmann, 1954) that occlusal loading can change the vascularity and therefore the main pathway of gingival inflammation into the deeper tissue from one which goes directly into the alveolar crest to one which goes primarily into the periodontal ligament (Fig. 108*B*).

Glickman and Smulow (1962) have shown in animals with gingival inflammation that excessive occlusal stresses produce angular bone defects and infrabony pockets. But these results have not been confirmed by other workers.

There is considerable variation in alveolar bone morphology, both in the form of cortical plates and trabecular pattern. The bone morphology is related to tooth position, tooth shape and tooth relationships. Cancellous bone is more vascular than cortical bone therefore inflammation, a vascular phenomenon, spreads more rapidly through cancellous than cortical bone. Where the cortex is thin or absent one would expect more rapid spread of inflammation than where the cortex is thick.

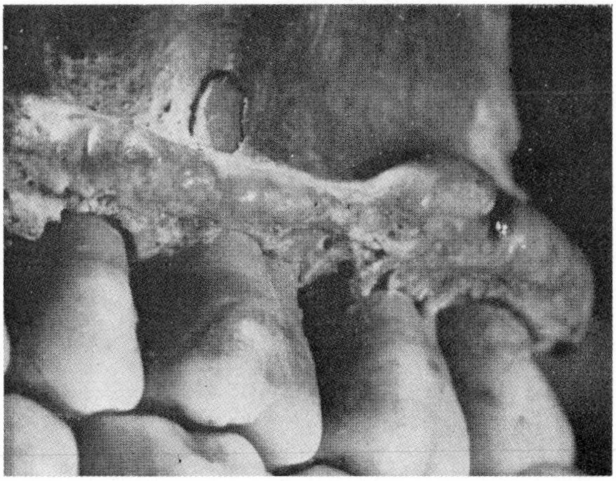

FIG. 112.—Thickening of the alveolar margin in response to low-grade irritation. (R.C.S. Odontological Museum Specimen No. 'A' 34.3.)

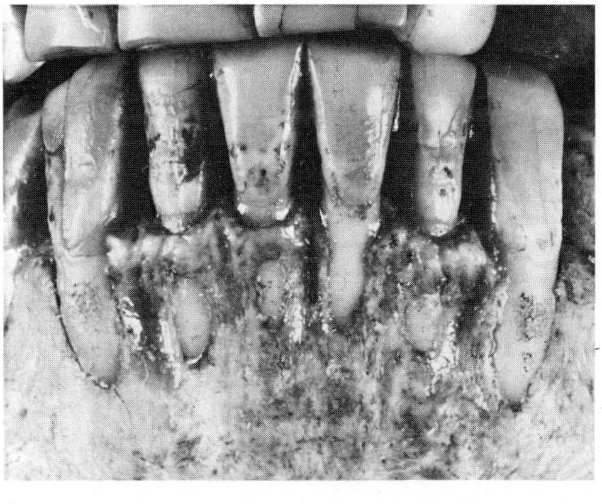

FIG. 113.—Dried skull of a young adult showing developmental faults in the alveolar bone.

A study of the distribution of bone defects does appear to support the idea that the primary determinant of the bone lesion is the original bone morphology (Manson and Nicholson, 1974).

The interdental crater is the commonest defect in the mandible and is found most frequently in the lower posterior segment. This would appear to be the result of an aggregate of factors:

1. The interdental area is very difficult to clean.
2. The epithelium of the col is thin and non-keratinized.
3. The normal bucco-lingual shape of the interdental septum between the lower molar is usually flat and occasionally concave. The centre of the crest of the septum is composed of cancellous trabeculation and there is a marked contrast between this and the cortical bone of the buccal and lingual plates.
4. Inflammation travels by vascular pathways and therefore most rapidly through cancellous bone.
5. Cancellous bone tends to have a higher turnover than cortical bone, *i.e.* it is more reactive.

Thus the most likely result of continuing plaque stagnation and inflammation in this area is an interdental crater.

Perforations, *i.e.* dehiscence and fenestrations, are found most commonly in the labial alveolar plate over the lower incisors. This plate is usually thin and where teeth are irregular bone defects of developmental origin are common. Inflammation will exaggerate the existing defect.

Infrabony defects, *i.e.* intra-alveolar defects apart from the interdental crater occur most commonly in the maxilla. The structure of the mandible and maxilla are quite different. The thick cortical plates of the major part of the mandible apart from the anterior segment are not present in the maxilla which consists of cancellous bone enclosed in thin cortical plates. The defects found in the maxilla demonstrate a much greater diversity of form than those found in the mandible and this can be explained by the complex pattern of the vascular cancellous bone which makes up the maxilla.

It is likely that the original alveolar morphology acts as a template on which such factors as food impaction and occlusal stresses can act to produce the rich diversity of forms in which the bone lesions are found.

CLINICAL FEATURES

In chronic periodontitis the clinical features of chronic gingivitis are present to some degree, associated with pocketing, and possibly tooth mobility, tooth migration and, occasionally, sensitivity to percussion.

As the site of active tissue destruction moves further away from the gingival margin, that is, as the pocket deepens, the overt manifestations of gingival inflammation may disappear almost completely. One of the intriguing features of periodontal disease is the apparent lack of correspondence between the degree of manifest inflammation and swelling of the gingivae and the amount of destruction of the deeper tissues. Frequently they appear to represent quite independent processes. The gingivae may be firm, pink and stippled, the contour may be almost normal and the patient may have no complaints of bleeding or discomfort; indeed he or she may be completely unaware that any disease is present. The disease can easily be overlooked unless a careful examination is carried out (Fig. 114).

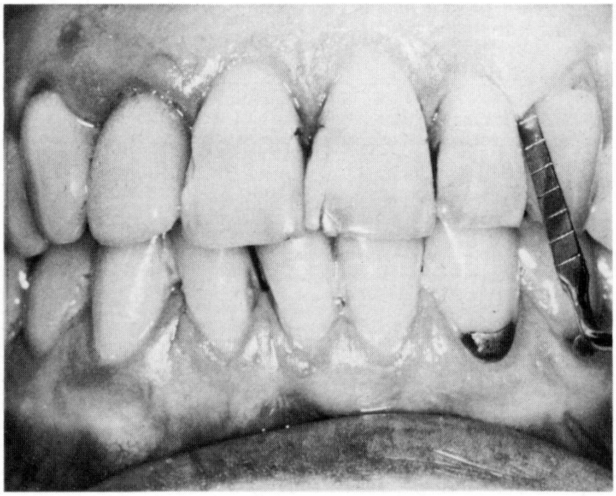

FIG. 114.—Generalized 4 mm pockets in a 40-year-old woman who had never known symptoms of gingival inflammation, and who refused to believe that pathology could be present.

Pocketing

If there is no gingival swelling, pockets of over 2 mm indicate apical migration of the crevicular epithelium and breakdown of periodontal fibres, *i.e.* periodontitis. In some cases gingival swelling may be considerable but it does not often account for more than another 2 mm of pocket depth, therefore a pocket of 4 mm almost always indicates breakdown of the periodontal ligament. If a patient has 4 mm pockets it is likely that he has an early chronic periodontitis.

Pockets are rarely of even depth all round the tooth. For several reasons they are usually deepest interproximally:

1. The interproximal area is the site of the most persistent stagnation.
2. The epithelium of the interdental col is not subject to functional stimulus and is therefore thin and non-keratinized.
3. The interproximal tissue is sheltered from the friction of toothbrushing and from the irritation of slightly abnormal function which causes atrophy and therefore recession of the buccal and lingual gingival margin.

In assessing the depth of a pocket the gingival crevice must be probed very gently with a fine but blunt-ended instrument, the pocket measuring probe (Fig. 115). The pocket wall may become quite firmly adapted to the root surface so that careful examination is essential to identify the pocket (Fig. 114). Even with care pocket measurement is a gross procedure in which many errors are possible. The deeper the pocket the greater the possible source of error. Coppes (1972) has demonstrated the diminishing reliability of pocket depth determinations at levels deeper than 3 mm. He shows that angulation of the probe, crown curvature, root angulation, morphology of the bone defect, cavities, restorations and subgingival calculus all conspire to invalidate the measurement (Fig. 116). Gentle probing should be painless, but the more sensitive patient may suffer slight discomfort. Excessive pain or bleeding is the result of careless examination.

Finger pressure over the pocket wall may cause exudation of materia alba or even pus. Retraction of the pocket wall often reveals subgingival calculus (Fig. 117).

Tooth Mobility

In health a just perceptible movement of teeth may be elicited in a labio-lingual direction. Excessive tooth mobility is the result of:

(a) Inflammation of the periodontal ligament in which the fibres become slack, disorientated or even broken. This is a reversible condition.

(b) Loss of supporting bone; this is irreversible.

These two features occur together in varying proportions and for this reason mobility alone is not a reliable index of tissue destruction. Mobility is elicited by finger or instrument pressure or by

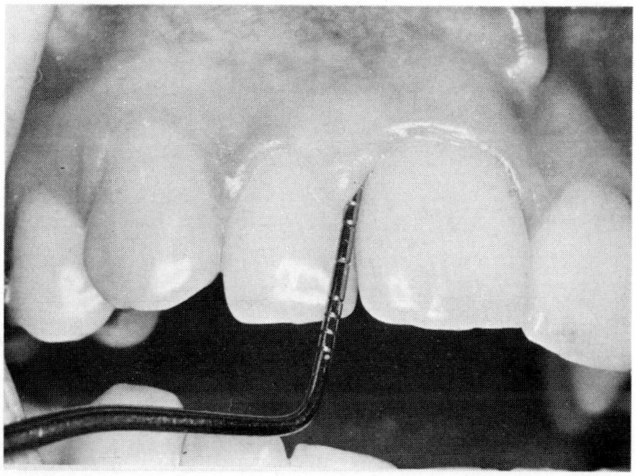

FIG. 115.—Pocket measuring probe (Williams) in shallow pocket.

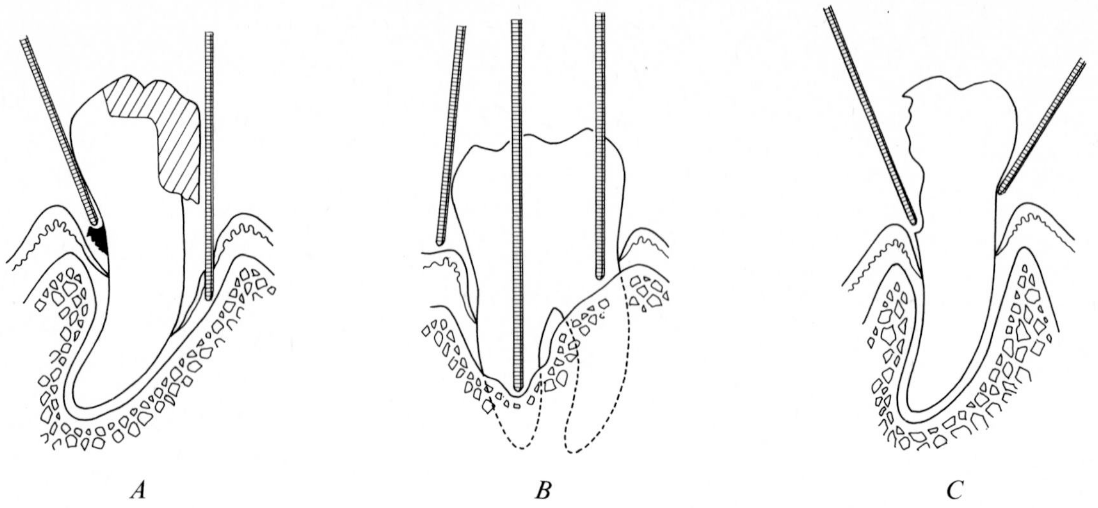

FIG. 116.—Diagrammatic illustration of the many factors which limit the accuracy of pocket measurements. (*A*) Subgingival calculus and overhanging restorations. (*B*) Irregular pocket depth and poor angulation of probe. (*C*) Cavity and crown contour. (By courtesy of Dr L. Coppes.)

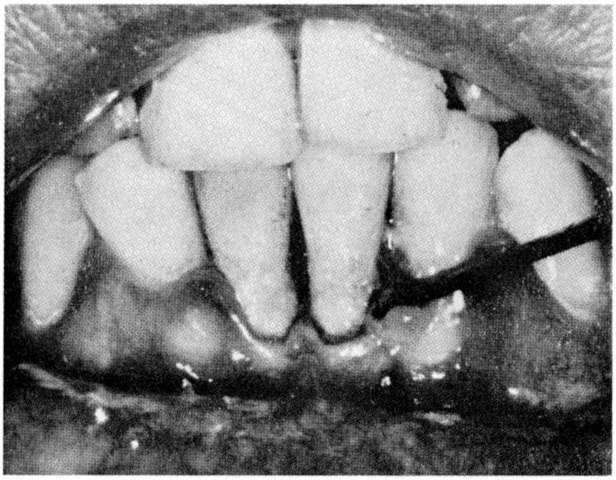

FIG. 117.—Retraction of the pocket wall reveals debris and subgingival calculus.

movement of the mandible with the teeth in contact. In assessing mobility by finger pressure it is important to grasp both the tooth under test and a neighbouring tooth. The latter is used as a fixed point so that the relative movement between the two teeth is felt and seen. Movement generally is labio-lingual, but with gross destruction a tooth may be movable up and down in an axial direction. The degree of mobility is usually indicated on an arbitrary scale from 0 to 3.

For purposes of description mobility is usually graded as follows:

Grade I – Just discernible.

Grade II – Obvious mobility but less than 1 mm of displacement.

Grade III – 1 mm or more labio-lingual displacement and including tooth movement up and down in an axial direction.

Although subjective this grading is extremely useful particularly for the operator's own records.

Tooth Migration

Pathologic migration of teeth is a common feature of periodontal disease. Frequently, the patient complains that the upper incisor teeth have moved, are now spaced and also appear longer (Fig. 118).

Tooth position is maintained by a balance of forces on the tooth and even in health a change in this balance may result in tooth movement. When the periodontal tissues are weakened by disease teeth can be moved by forces which are not great enough to move them in health. (This is discussed in more detail in Chapter 13.) The subsequent malposition of the tooth then becomes a factor causing further tissue destruction and further movement. Once a tooth moves a vicious circle is set up and tissue destruction accelerates.

The movement tends to occur in phases; periods of increased tooth mobility alternating with periods of repair during which the tooth becomes quite firm.

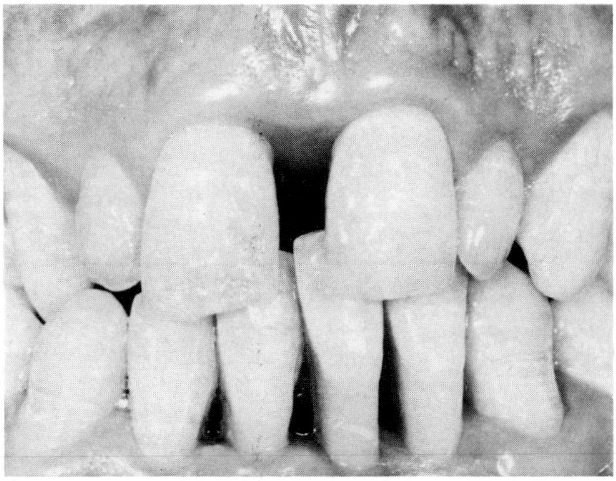

FIG. 118.—Migration and elongation of incisor teeth associated with advanced periodontal destruction (see Fig. 124A).

Sensitivity on Tooth Percussion

There may be considerable destruction of the supporting tissues without any discomfort on tooth percussion. Sensitivity or pain on percussion indicates inflammatory involvement of the periodontal tissues. When slight, the patient may feel the need to bite on the tooth to obtain relief, but when the inflammatory involvement is severe, for instance when an abscess develops, the tooth is exquisitely sensitive to touch.

In health a characteristic note is sounded on tooth percussion. With tissue destruction this sound becomes quite dull. Although a very gross test, a dull note indicates that further examination of that tooth is necessary.

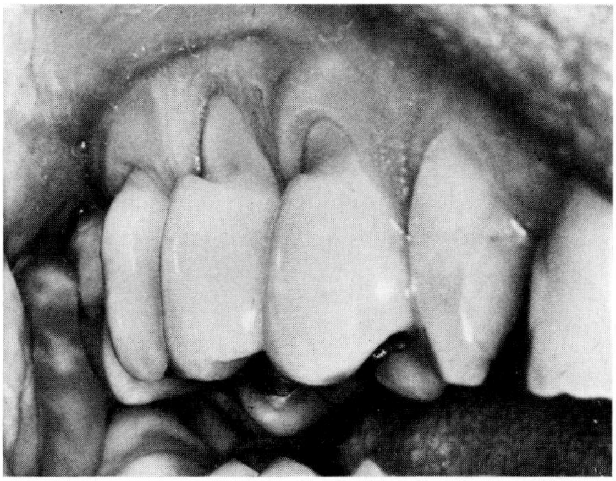

FIG. 119.—Toothbrush abrasion and gingival recession.

Gingival Recession

Healthy gingiva may atrophy under the stress of toothbrush abrasion (Fig. 119). In periodontal disease, as the pocket deepens the gingival margin may not remain at its original level in the region of the amelo-cemental junction. The marginal tissue may atrophy so that the depth of the pocket is less than the apical distance moved by the crevicular epithelium. The amount of recession may equal the distance moved by the crevicular epithelium so that although tissue is lost no pocket is formed (Fig. 120). This rarely happens in interdental areas where the gingiva is sheltered, but it is common in (a) areas subject to severe toothbrush abrasion, *e.g.* buccal surfaces of upper canines and premolars, and (b) where a root is so inclined that the plate of alveolar bone is thin or absent, *e.g.* palatal to the upper first molar, in which case moderate abrasion causes gingival atrophy and recession.

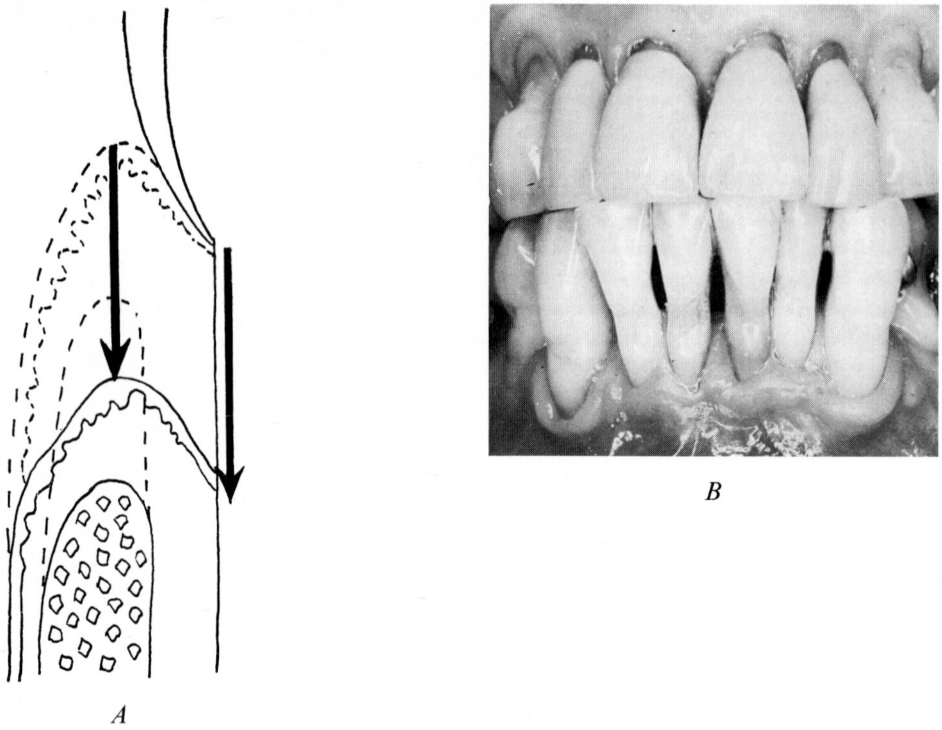

FIG. 120.—(*A*) Gingival atrophy proceeding at the same rate as apical migration of the crevicular epithelium. (*B*) Gingival recession without pocket formation in a 65-year-old woman.

Alveolar Bone Loss

The amount of bone destroyed and its rate of destruction varies considerably from one individual to another. As described above, in many cases the alveolar bone loss progresses evenly and at the same rate as the pocket deepens and the crest of the bone remains apical to the pocket, that is, the pocket is 'suprabony' (Fig. 121). Fairly even horizontal bone loss is characteristic of a 'marginal periodontitis'. One frequently encounters the disease in this form, but variations of this basic pattern occur just as frequently (Fig. 122).

It is imperative to define the degree and pattern of bone loss as accurately as possible. Pocket measurement can indicate the severity of tissue destruction but it is by no means an accurate or even reliable method of examination. It can never be a substitute for careful radiological examination.

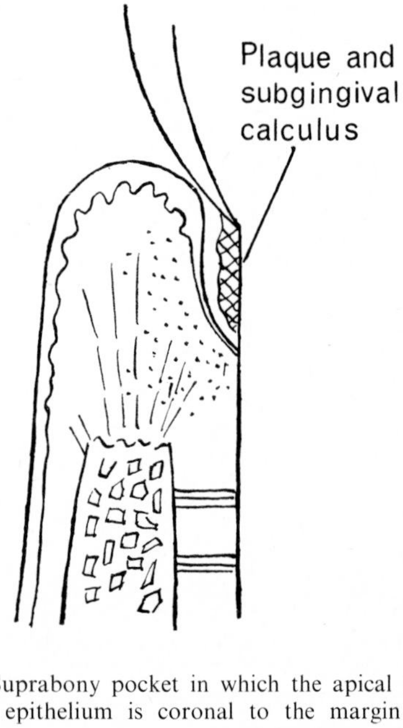

FIG. 121.—Suprabony pocket in which the apical limit of the crevicular epithelium is coronal to the margin of the alveolar bone.

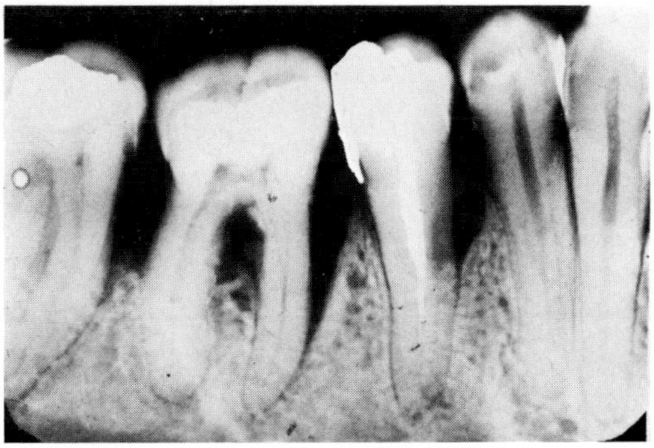

A

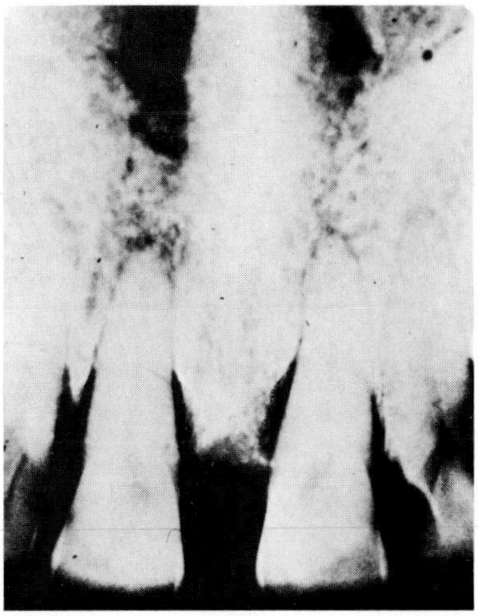

B

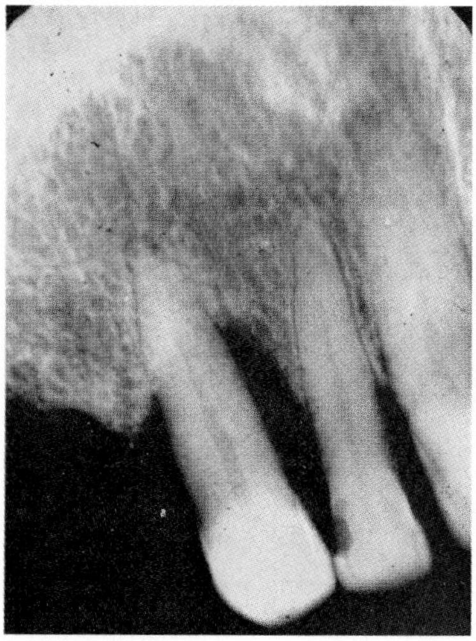

C

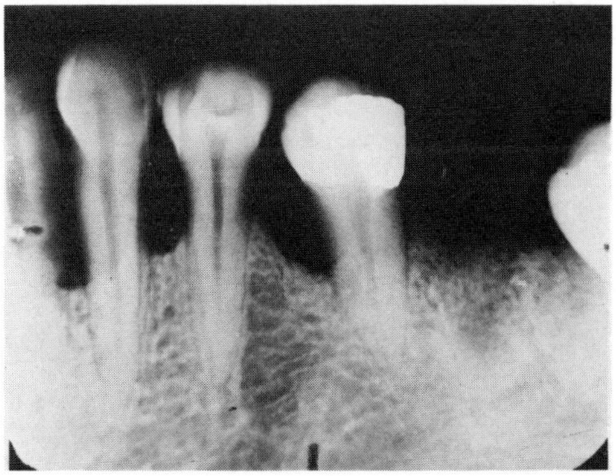

D

FIG. 122.—A variety of bone defects.

(*A*) Uneven pattern of bone destruction in a 33-year-old woman. (*B*) Crescentic bone loss around upper incisors usually said to be associated with excessive occlusal stress – actually poor X-ray angulation. (*C*) Typical bone destruction around an abutment tooth. (*D*) Uneven bone loss found in a 24-year-old woman. (*E*) Terminal bone loss. The clearly demarcated bone margin probably indicates the lingual aspect of the alveolar ridge. Careful examination of the radiograph reveals a shadow of some remaining buccal bone.

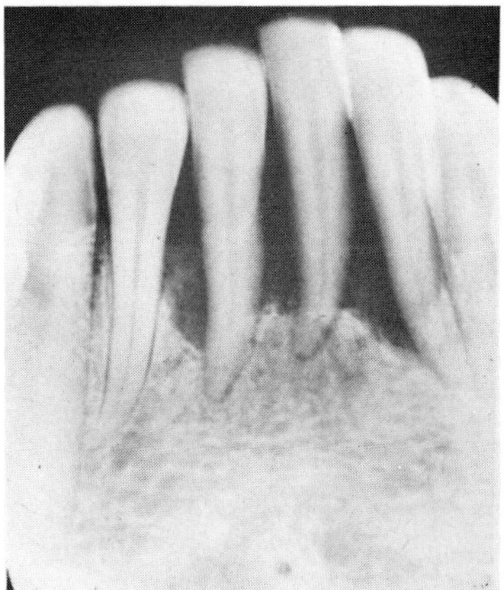

E

Radiographic Evidence

With certain reservations a properly taken radiograph will show the extent and pattern of bone loss. In a marginal periodontitis bone destruction is indicated first by the loss of the dense margin which delineates the alveolar process in health. As bone density decreases the bone margin becomes radiolucent and indistinct (Fig. 123). With continuing bone resorption the height of the alveolar bone is reduced (Fig. 124).

Even when correctly oriented in one plane the X-ray may not reveal a bone defect in another plane. This is particularly so in the case of interdental craters and the infrabony pocket. Defects may go undetected if radiographs are taken only from one angle; if the direction of the beam is altered the defect is usually revealed (Figs. 125 and 126). Where there is uneven loss of either the buccal or lingual plates of bone it is often difficult to say which of the two plates is involved without careful examination of the lesion, and in many cases the true situation is not revealed until the soft tissue is laid back and the bone exposed.

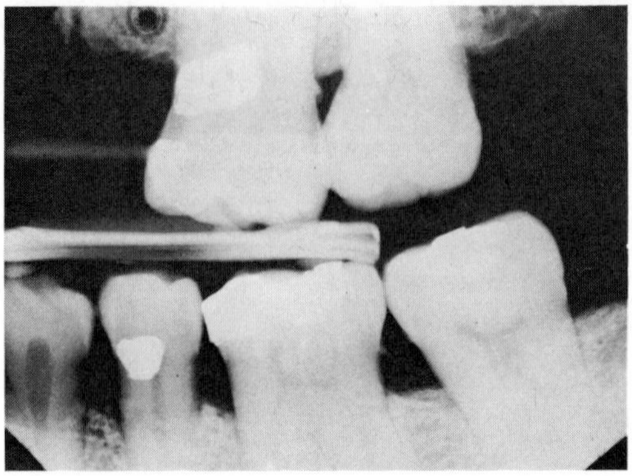

FIG. 123.—Marginal periodontitis with diminished radiodensity of alveolar margin.

Loss of bone in the bifurcation may be obscured by the presence of one intact bone plate. On the other hand, some radiolucency in the bifurcation area does not always indicate that bone is absent from this site; when initially affected by the inflammatory process bone trabeculae may become thinned (osteoporosis). This is a reversible change, but one which may be seen on the radiograph as an area of radiolucency and interpreted as an area of bone loss, *i.e.* as an irreversible condition.

Treatment often depends upon radiographic interpretation. Radiographs must be examined critically and interpreted with caution. While it is sometimes possible to devise a treatment plan on the basis of a radiographic examination alone this is never wise. The radiograph should be used as a tool along with all the other methods of clinical examination.

TREATMENT OF CHRONIC PERIODONTITIS

The lesion of chronic periodontitis is progressive, and although this progress may be very slow with a natural history of the order of thirty or forty years in some individuals, there is no evidence that unlike say the tubercle, the disease ever comes to a spontaneous halt. Nor is there any evidence that suffering the disease confers any immunity which prevents occurrence after the disease is eliminated. Indeed all the evidence available (*i.e.* clinical impression) on the subject of recurrence suggests that susceptibility persists and that recurrence is virtually inevitable if plaque control is inadequate.

Therefore treatment has always two major objectives, the elimination of the progressive lesion and the prevention of its recurrence. There is little advantage in attempting to achieve the first objective unless the second is assured.

As described the periodontal lesion can occur in a variety of forms. The pocket may be shallow or deep; it may be of regular depth around the tooth or it may vary considerably from one aspect of the tooth to another. The bone margin may be resorbed evenly or very irregularly. Pockets may be completely enclosed by soft tissue or involve bone deformities. There may be associated soft tissue problems such as muscle attachments, a narrow width of attached gingiva or a shallow vestibule. In attempting to achieve the above objectives each case must be examined with care so that all aetiological factors are defined and a complete assessment of the problems specific to that case is made. Only then should treatment be initiated.

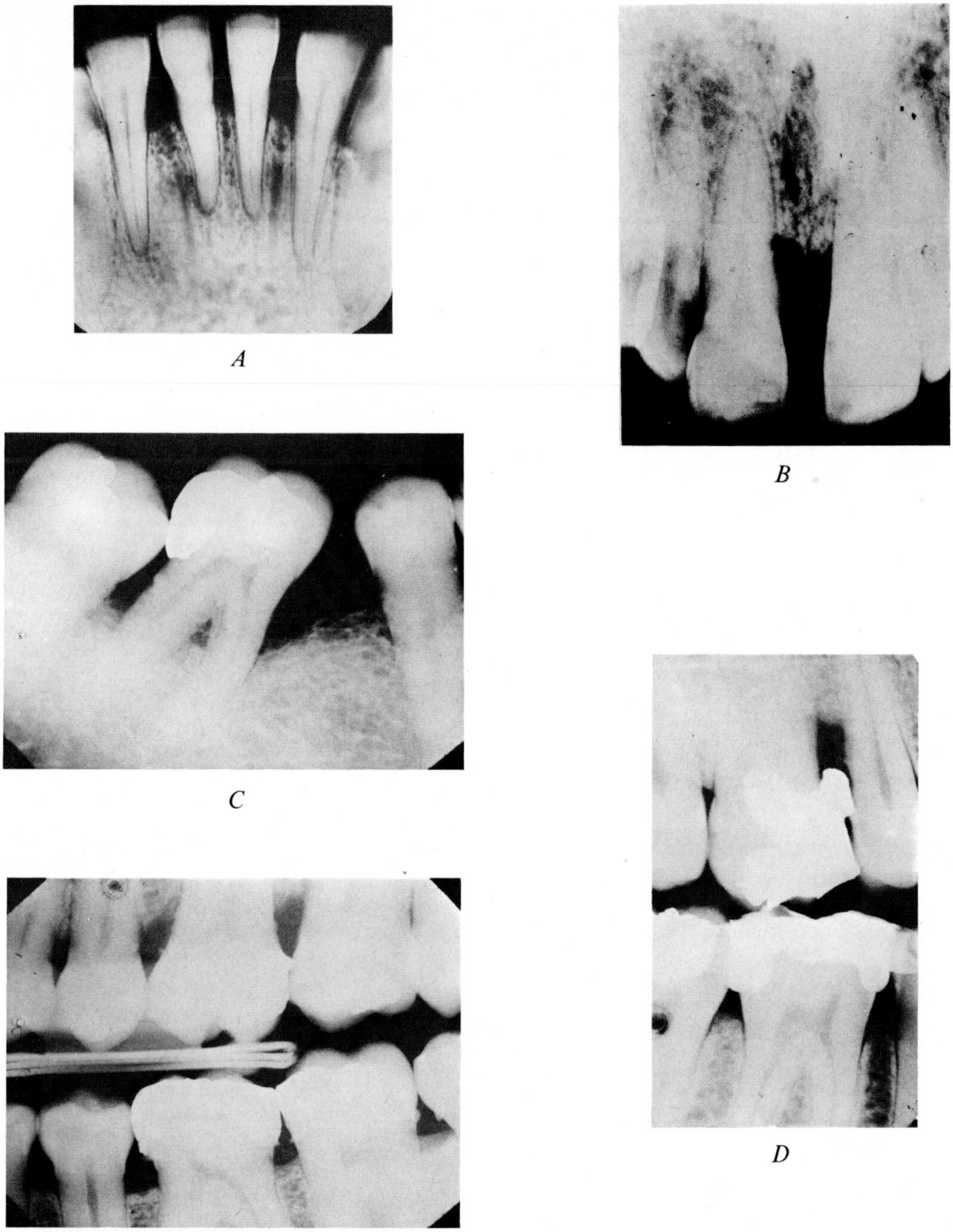

A *B* *C* *D* *E*

FIG. 124.—(*A*) Marginal bone loss around lower incisors. Widened periodontal space indicates excessive occlusal stress. (*B*) Bone loss around teeth shown in Fig. 94. (*C*) Bone loss involving the bifurcation of a lower molar. (*D*) Bone loss in relation to an overhanging edge of amalgam. (*E*) Common finding. Healthy alveolar margin in lower posterior region plus bone loss about upper molars in relation to calculus deposits.

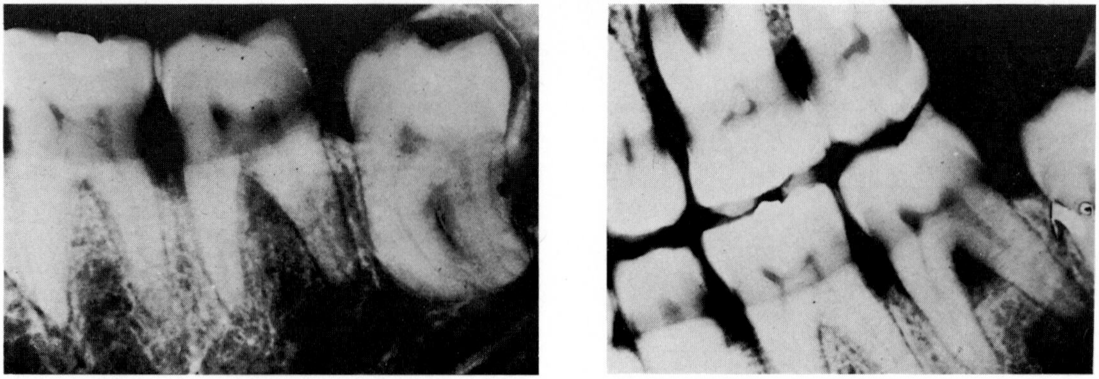

A *B*

FIG. 125.—(*A*) Standard periapical view of lower second molar indicates only marginal bone loss. (*B*) Bitewing radiograph demonstrates bone loss in bifurcation.

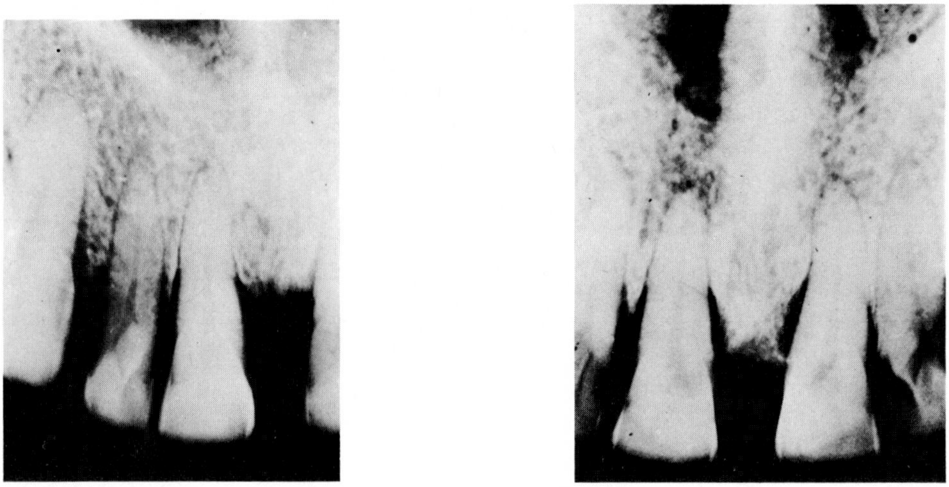

A *B*

FIG. 126.—(*A*) Radiograph indicates horizontal bone loss around central incisors. (*B*) Alteration of beam angle demonstrates crescentic bone loss.

We can list the aims of treatment as follows:

1. To remove the immediate cause of disease, *i.e.* plaque and calculus.
2. To gain the patient's co-operation so that recurrence is avoided.
3. To eliminate the lesion, *i.e.* the periodontal pocket.
4. To achieve a tissue morphology conducive to the maintenance of good oral hygiene.
5. To correct predisposing factors as in the treatment of chronic gingivitis, *e.g.* badly contoured fillings, 'gum-stripping' dentures, etc.
6. To correct the occlusion if it is thought that occlusal stresses may be a contributing factor to the progress of the disease (Chapter 14).

Three general forms of treatment are used to obtain these ends. These are:

1. Oral hygiene control, *i.e.* scaling and patient instruction in plaque control.
2. Surgical techniques.
3. Occlusal analysis and adjustment.

In some cases all three forms of treatment may be needed, in others only two but in *all cases oral hygiene control is essential*, and more advanced treatment is not undertaken unless the patient is able and willing to control plaque deposition.

Scaling and instruction in plaque control can be the definitive treatment for chronic periodontitis. It is not essential to resort to surgical techniques merely because there is pocketing and alveolar bone loss. If pockets are no deeper than 4 mm it may be possible for the experienced operator to remove all the calculus present by careful scaling, but subgingival scaling is a blind procedure and it is possible for even the most experienced and skilful operator to leave calculus behind.

Where some inflammatory swelling is present even a less than perfect scaling may help to reduce inflammation and therefore reduce pocket depth from 4 mm to 3 mm or even 2 mm so that any calculus or plaque still present in the depths of the pocket becomes accessible to further scaling. Where inflammation is minimal and the tissue is fibrous, a reduction in pocket depth may not take place even after the most thorough scaling. Therefore more radical techniques, *i.e.* surgical procedures, must be used whereby all calculus can be removed and the periodontal lesion eradicated. However, surgery should not be resorted to unless scaling has been carried out carefully and plaque control measures instituted with the full co-operation of the patient, and still pathology persists.

There are basically only three types of surgical situation involving the periodontal lesion. These are:

1. Where the lesion is confined within the soft tissue, *i.e.* the suprabony lesion.
2. Where an alveolar bone lesion is involved, *e.g.* the infrabony pocket.
3. Where the periodontal lesion is associated with a muco-gingival problem.

The problems involved in dealing with these three situations are discussed in the following chapters.

REFERENCES

COPPES, L. (1972). Routine-Sulcus-Dieptemetingen in de Parodontologie: het belang-de betrouwbaarheid-de toe passing. Thesis. Amsterdam University.

EWEN, S. J. and STAHL, S. S. (1962). The response of the periodontium to chronic gingival irritation and long-term tilting forces in adult dogs. *Oral Surg.*, **15**, 1426.

GLICKMAN, I. (1971). Role of occlusion in the etiology and treatment in periodontal disease. *J. dent. Res.*, **50**, Suppl. to No. 2, p. 199.

GLICKMAN, I. and SMULOW, J. B. (1962). Alterations in the pathway of gingival inflammation into the underlying tissues induced by excessive occlusal forces. *J. Peridont.*, **33**, 7.

GOLDMAN, H. M. (1942). Relationship of the gingival crevice and the alveolar crest. *J. dent. Res.*, **21**, 561.

GOLDMAN, H. M. and COHEN, D. W. (1958). Infrabony pocket: classification and treatment. *J. Periodont.*, **29**, 272.

MACAPANPAN, L. C. and WEINMANN, J. P. (1954). The influence of injury to the periodontal membrane on the spread of gingival inflammation. *J. dent. Res.*, **33**, 263.

MANSON, J. D. and NICHOLSON, K. (1974). The distribution of bone defects in chronic periodontitis. *J. Periodont.*, **45**, 88.

PRICHARD, J. F. (1965). Advanced Periodontal Disease: Surgical and Prosthetic Management. Saunders, Philadelphia.

WEINMANN, J. P. (1941). Progress of gingival inflammation into the supporting structures of the teeth. *J. Periodont.*, **12**, 71.

WENTZ, F. M., JARABAK, J. and ORBAN, B. (1958). Experimental occlusal trauma imitating cuspal interferences. *J. Periodont.*, **29**, 117.

9. Surgical Treatment of the Simple Suprabony Pocket

The objectives of surgical treatment, as of all treatment, should be two-fold: (1) to remove disease, and (2) to prevent its recurrence. Therefore the aims of surgical treatment of the simple suprabony pocket, *i.e.* the periodontal lesion which is entirely enclosed within soft tissues are:

1. To eradicate the lesion by removing its soft tissue wall and all subgingival plaque and calculus.
2. To improve the tissue contour so that plaque control procedures are facilitated and recurrence of disease prevented.

In attempting to achieve these aims several surgical techniques have been developed. These may be summarized under four headings:

1. Gingivectomy (Fig. 127*A*).
2. Inverse bevel gingivectomy (Fig. 127*B*).
3. Apically repositioned flap (Fig. 127*C*).
4. Subgingival curettage (Fig. 127*D*).

Whichever of these techniques is employed pre-operative scaling and instruction in plaque control techniques is essential and should achieve:

1. A cleaner field in which to operate.
2. Some reduction in inflammation which will
   (a) help reduce operative bleeding and thus improve working conditions.
   (b) improve the quality of the tissue and facilitate its surgical manipulation.
3. A better understanding of the patient's attitude to dental health. If pre-operative co-operation is unsatisfactory it is unlikely to improve after surgery. No surgery should be carried out until the oral hygiene improves.

Contra-indications to Surgery

1. Where patient co-operation is doubtful. If the patient is not prepared to spend time and effort keeping his mouth clean then surgery may be a waste of time.
2. Where complete eradication of pockets would result in the exposure of so much tooth that the patient would be unhappy about the post-operative appearance.
3. Where so much bone has been destroyed that tooth loss is inevitable.
4. Where the patient is of advanced age and it is likely that the teeth will be retained without radical treatment for several years. Despite this limitation the mouth should be rendered as clean and free from infection as possible.
5. Where the presence of some systemic disease such as anaemia or heart disease contra-indicates surgery. In case of doubt the patient's physician must be consulted (see Chapter 17).
6. Where acute gingival disease, such as acute ulcerative gingivitis, is present.

Management of Surgery

If full-mouth surgery is necessary it may be carried out in one stage or in several stages with sections of the mouth being treated at separate visits. The schedules shown in Table I may be followed, taking into account:

1. The patient's wishes. He may not have time to pay many visits; may wish to have treatment carried out in as short a time as possible; may be afraid of surgery and prefer to have the operation carried out in one visit under sedation and local anaesthesia, or under general anaesthesia in a hospital.
2. An assessment of operative and post-operative problems. The patient may report that he bleeds copiously or heals slowly, in which case it may be advisable to observe the healing of one segment before extending the treatment to other areas.

Anaesthesia

Where surgery is to be carried out in several stages local anaesthesia is almost always preferred to general anaesthesia for the following reasons:

1. Adequate anaesthesia of the area is easily obtained.
2. A reduction of bleeding results from capillary contraction.
3. It allows sufficient time for a careful operative technique.
4. The patient can co-operate fully and is completely ambulatory.
5. Multiple general anaesthetics are avoided.

However where full mouth surgery is required

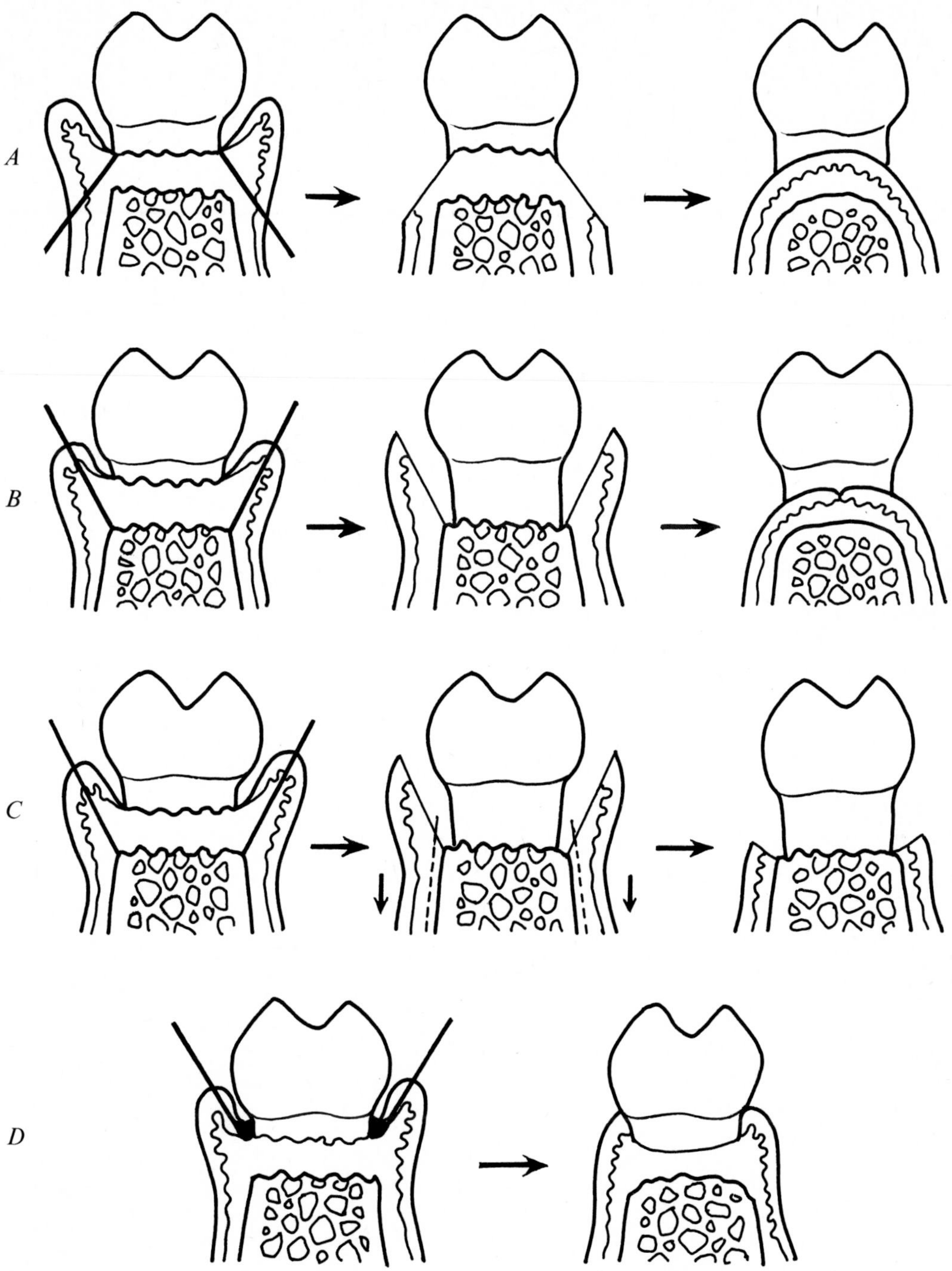

FIG. 127.—Diagrams to show various methods of elimination of the simple suprabony pocket. (*A*) Gingivectomy: radical removal of tissue and healing by secondary intention. (*B*) Inverse bevel gingivectomy: retention of tissue to effect closure of wound. (*C*) Apically repositioned flap: retention of tissue and apical movement so that bone margin is exposed to heal by secondary intention. (*D*) Subgingival curettage: blind removal of pocket contents and crevicular epithelium.

	First Visit	Second Visit	Third Visit	Fourth Visit
Plan I	Gingivectomy quadrant A	Remove periodontal dressing quadrant A	Gingivectomy quadrant B; inspect quadrant A	Remove dressing quadrant B; inspect quadrant A
Plan II	Gingivectomy quadrant A	Gingivectomy quadrant B; remove dressing quadrant A	Gingivectomy quadrant C; remove dressing quadrant B; inspect quadrant A	Gingivectomy quadrant D; remove dressing quadrant C; inspect A and B
	Fifth Visit	**Sixth Visit**	**Seventh Visit**	**Eighth Visit**
Plan I	Gingivectomy quadrant C; inspect quadrants A and B	Remove dressing quadrant C; inspect A and B	Gingivectomy quadrant D; inspect B and C	Remove dressing quadrant D; inspect B and C
Plan II	Remove dressing quadrant D; inspect quadrant C	Inspect complete mouth	Inspection (after further one week)	Inspection (after further four weeks)

Table I. Schedule of Weekly Visits.

there are several advantages to the use of general anaesthesia. These are:

1. It allows a one-stage procedure. Multiple procedures are avoided. This has a considerable psychological advantage.
2. The patient is unconscious and the operator can proceed at his own speed unencumbered by any patient personality problems.
3. The total time taken to complete full mouth surgery is less than the sum of multiple smaller procedures.
4. Because all the surgery is completed in one stage the total period of periodontal therapy is reduced.
5. There appears to be less pain after surgery under general anaesthesia than when carried out under local anaesthesia.

Disadvantages of general anaesthesia are as follows:

1. General medical disadvantages of general anaesthesia especially as anaesthesia for periodontal surgery may be lengthy.
2. Hospitalization is necessary. Although the procedure can be carried out in the dental surgery, supervision during the recovery period is more efficient in hospital.
3. Full-mouth surgery can be demanding on the operator, particularly when inexperienced.
4. Access and visibility to the lingual surface of the lower molar region can be poor unless the anaesthetist understands the problem and arranges the throat packing to suit the operator's requirements. With good tongue relaxation and unimpeded movement access to lingual surfaces may even be easier than under local anaesthesia. It is essential that operator and anaesthetist work out an acceptable technique together.
5. Bleeding tends to be more profuse under general anaesthesia.
6. Post-operatively, eating is drastically interfered with while the dressings are in place.

GINGIVECTOMY

Gingivectomy, the complete removal of the gingiva forming the wall of the suprabony pocket, is the most radical of the soft tissue surgery techniques. It immediately removes the lesion and makes the subgingival deposits visible and accessible. Gingivoplasty (as described in Chapter 7) indicates the surgical reshaping of the gingiva, an end *automatically produced by correct gingivectomy procedure* (see Goldman, 1951).

The indications for gingivectomy are:

1. The presence of suprabony pockets 4 mm and deeper, which persist despite thorough cleaning.
2. The presence of persistent gingival enlargement.
3. Furcation involvement.
4. The suprabony or gingival abscess.
5. The pericoronal flap.

N.B. An important condition applies in these situations, that is that an adequate zone of attached gingiva shall remain after gingivectomy.

Local Anaesthesia

As root surfaces are to be planed it is advisable to obtain anaesthesia of the teeth as well as of the soft tissues. In the lower posterior regions a regional block plus local infiltration is necessary; in other regions buccal and lingual infiltration is normally sufficient. The region of anaesthesia must be at least one tooth on either side wider than the field of operation. Several injections are required for even a very localized gingivectomy, and in order to minimize the discomfort of multiple injections it is recommended that after the first injection is made the needle is moved more or less horizontally under the mucosa, the anaesthetic solution being deposited as the needle is moved along.

Pocket-marking

The apical limit of the pocket must be marked so that an accurate incision can be made. An examination of the bone margin on the radiograph is a useful guide but there are occasions on which the radiograph is misleading. The bottom of the pocket may also be indicated by a line on the gingiva defining the apical limit of the loose pocket wall and the beginning of tightly bound-down soft tissue. The experienced operator may well need no other guides to pocket depth, but it is generally advisable to mark out the pockets with a special pocket-marking instrument (Fig. 128). This is inserted into the pocket parallel to the axis of the tooth. The blades are pressed together so that the gingiva is perforated opposite the

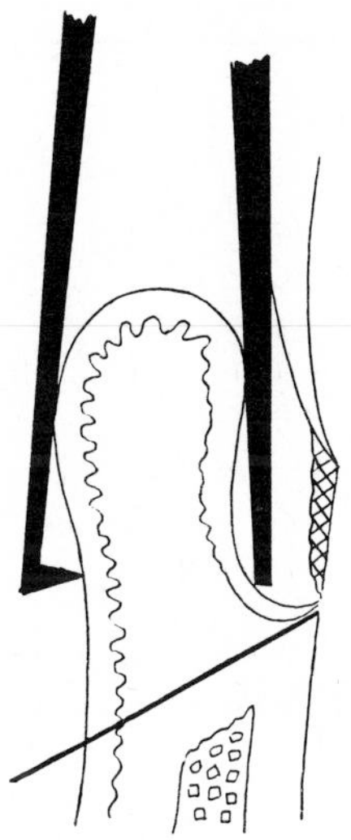

FIG. 128.—Pocket marking forceps in relation to the incision, which is made at 45° in such a position that the instrument contacts tooth at the bottom of the pocket.

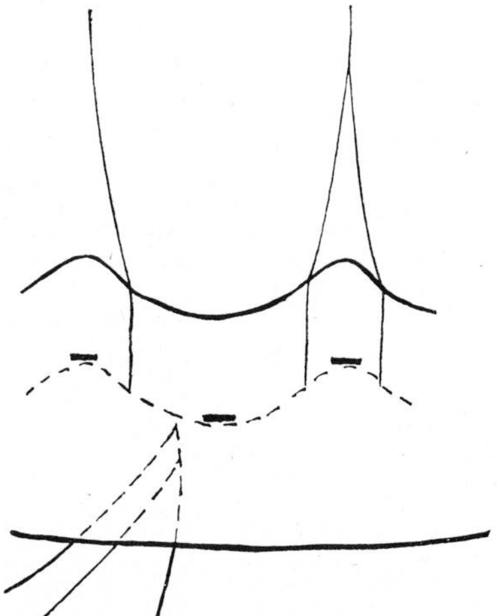

FIG. 129.—The relationship of bleeding points to the incision.

bottom of the pocket, which is then defined by a bleeding point. Markings are made on both labial and lingual surfaces, interdentally, and opposite the midline of the tooth (Fig. 129). Markings may also be made with a pocket measuring probe.

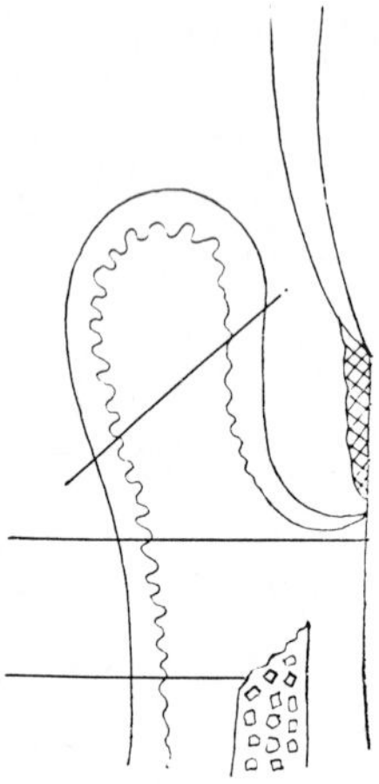

FIG. 130.—Incorrect position for incision.

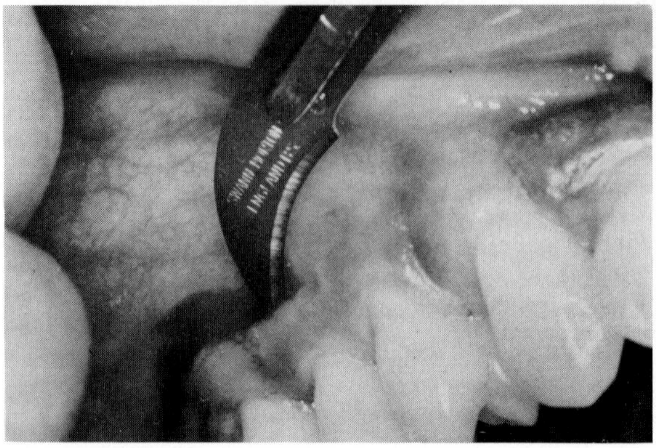

A

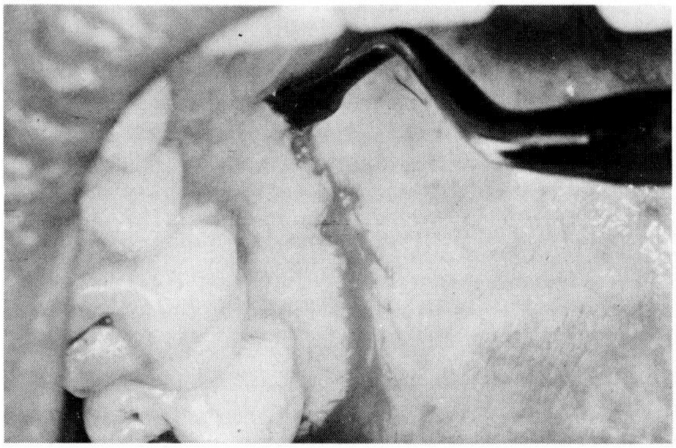

B

Incision

The row of bleeding points left by the pocket marker is a guide to the line of incision, but it is NOT the line of incision. If the incision is made on this line the pocket will not be completely removed and the resulting gingival contour will be poor. The incision must be planned so that the pocket is eliminated and a good contour produced by the one incision. With the blade held at approximately 45° the incision is made apical to the line of bleeding points in such a position that the blade contacts tooth at the bottom of the pocket (Figs. 128–130). When the gingivectomy is being carried out in segments the incision should start and end at the mid-point of the buccal or lingual surface of a tooth, not in an interdental papilla. A continuous straight line incision is made (Fig. 131). It is difficult to obtain an acceptable gingival contour with a discontinuous scalloped incision.

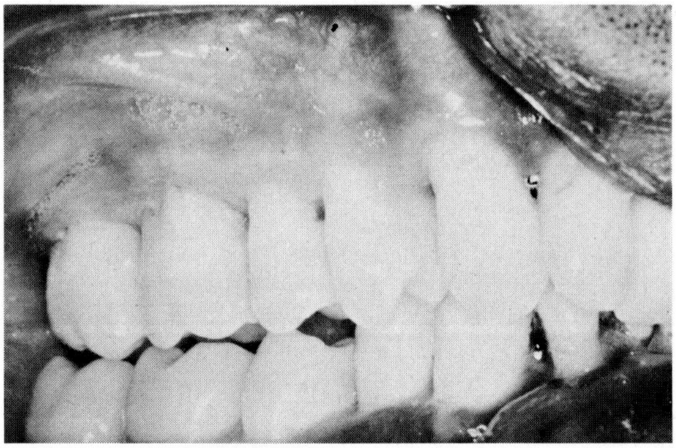

C

FIG. 131.—(*A*) Gingivectomy incision being made in buccal gingiva. Note apical position of incision and angulation of blade. (*B*) Gingivectomy incision in palate with Kirkland knife. (*C*) Two-weeks post-gingivectomy. Note final contour resulting from incision shown in (*A*).

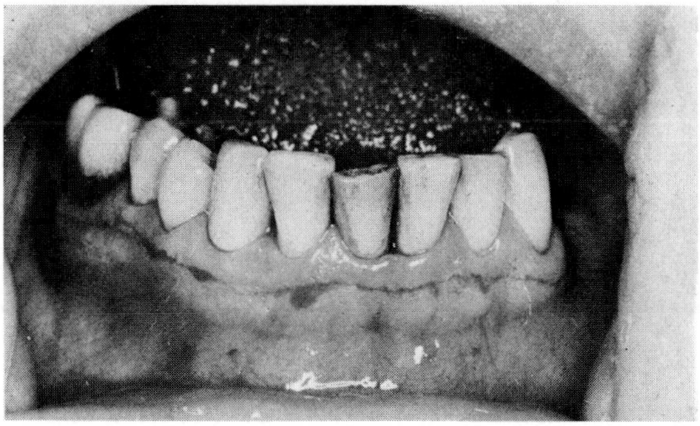

A

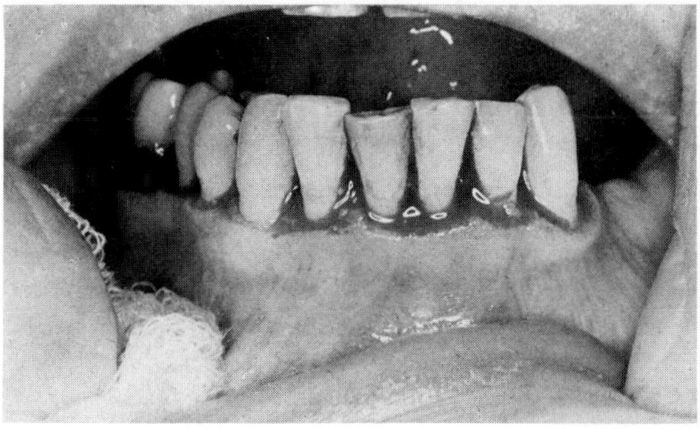

B

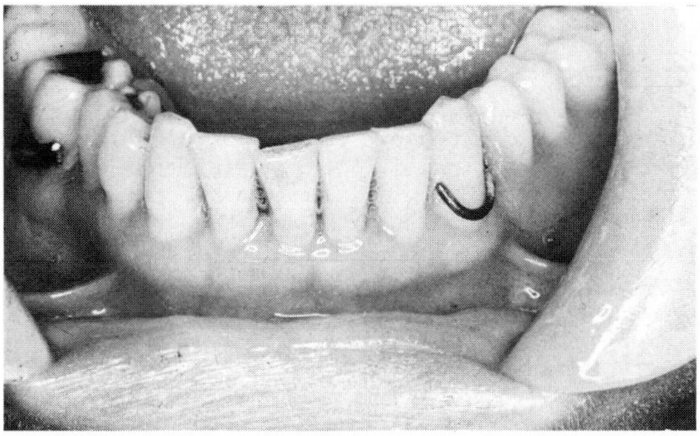

C

FIG. 132.—(*A*) Continuous gingivectomy incision following the line of the bottom of the pockets. (*B*) Gingivectomy wound with pocket wall removed. (*C*) Post-operative appearance.

The blade should make contact with tooth substance throughout the incision so that the tissue is completely and neatly incised. Care must be taken to follow the path indicated by the pocket-marker. The contour of the bottom of the pockets may be very irregular and this irregularity must be followed (Fig. 132). It is extremely easy, particularly on the lingual aspect of lower posterior teeth, to lose sight of the markings and to remove too little tissue so that the pocket remains.

The Incision in Special Situations

1. In linking up with a previous gingivectomy a good contour is produced by overlapping the limits of the incision.
2. Where an edentulous area is involved in the field of operation it is advisable to extend the incision completely through the edentulous ridge so that an acceptable contour is achieved (Fig. 133).
3. Distal to third molars there may be a considerable thickness of soft tissue, and gingivectomy can produce a large heavily bleeding wound.

Conservative elimination of the pocket will result in recurrence of the pocket. In these sites it is important to remove sufficient tissue to produce a self-cleansing area, and this may well mean removing a soft-tissue tuberosity completely (Fig. 134). Where the pocket is deep there is sometimes the risk of incising a palatal vessel unless due care is taken. Obviously, if such a risk seems to be present, the incision must not be so radical. The bulk of tissue behind a third molar can also be reduced by cutting out a wedge of tissue and undermining the edges of the wound before suturing them together. This technique obviates the risk of haemorrhage and allows healing by primary intention (see page 113).

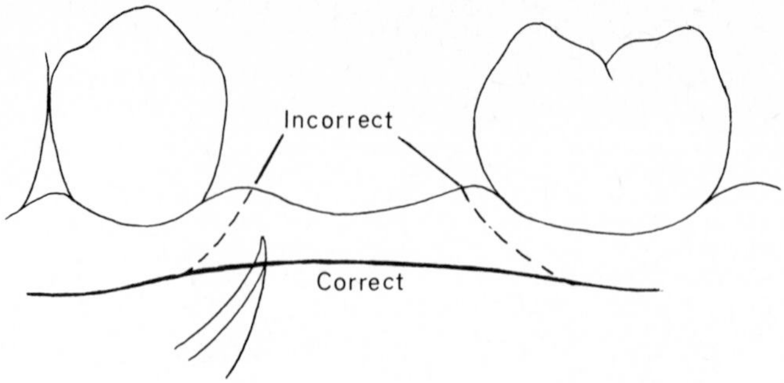

FIG. 133.—Incision through edentulous area to produce an acceptable contour.

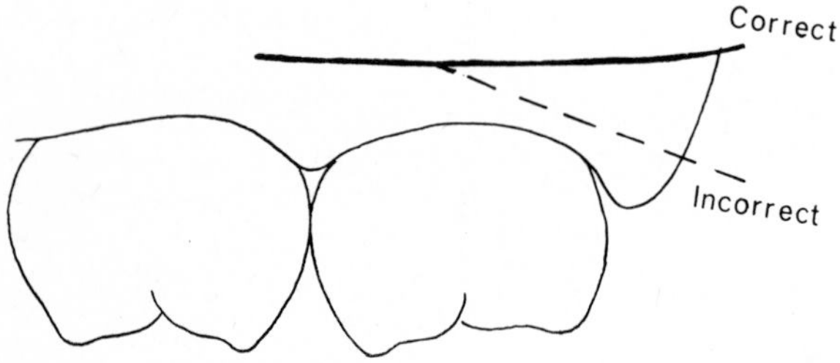

FIG. 134.—The incision through the tuberosity should produce a self-cleansing area.

Tissue Removal

When both labial and lingual incisions have been completed the loose tissue is detached with a suitable scaler or curette. Any remaining attachment is severed carefully with the scalpel or pointed scissors; the tissue must not be torn away. After the tissue is removed swabs are pressed over the wound to control haemorrhage. At this stage bleeding remnants of inflamed connective tissue or granulation tissue are usually present, particularly in the interdental spaces. These must be thoroughly removed with sharp curettes; after their removal haemorrhage diminishes considerably, and any calculus present can be clearly seen. It is essential to have teeth clean before the dressing is applied. The practice of delaying the scaling until some healing has taken place is to be condemned; only a poor surgeon would leave dirt near a wound! If all loose tags of tissue have been removed haemorrhage is usually not excessive, and the efficient use of an aspirator should make a thorough scaling possible. All calculus must be removed, but root planing must be carried out with discretion or very sensitive dentine will be exposed, and even a pulpitis may result. At the same time rough cervical margins of fillings should be smoothed.

When all calculus and tissue tags are removed absolutely clean teeth should stand surrounded by a firm, well contoured, gingival wound (Fig. 132). Should improvement of the contour be required, it can be completed with scalpel, diamond stone, or electrocautery as described for gingivoplasty. Tissue which does not feel firm and which is obviously not well tied down to the underlying bone should be trimmed.

When the operator is satisfied that the pockets are completely eliminated and that the contour is as good as can be achieved, swabs are pressed over the wound to control haemorrhage while the periodontal dressing is being prepared.

Bleeding from the gingivectomy wound can be vigorous (Berdon, 1965) but excessive bleeding after gingivectomy is uncommon. Pressure may be applied with dry swabs, or swabs soaked in fairly hot saline or epinephrine (1:25,000) solution. Persistent bleeding is a rare occurrence after gingivectomy: if it occurs it may be controlled by suturing or by the topical application of Epsilon Aminocaproic acid (Epsikapron).

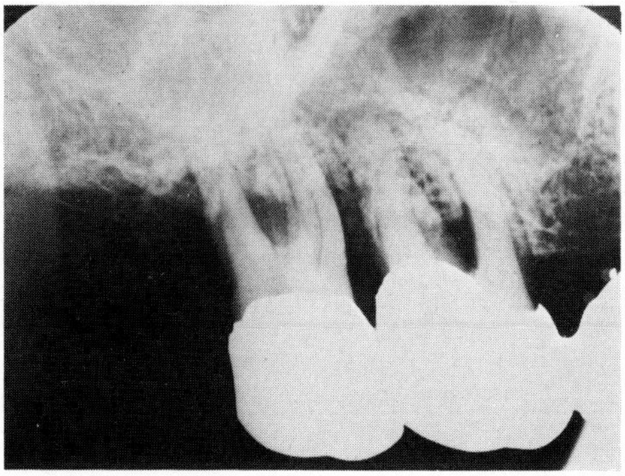

FIG. 135.—Molars with gross bone loss used as twin abutments for a bridge. The bridge was in use for ten years before further bone loss.

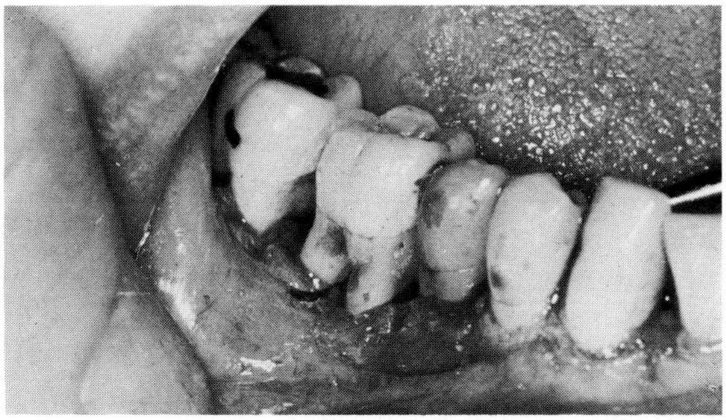

FIG. 136.—Bifurcation exposed completely so that the area can be curetted thoroughly. Note curette passing between roots.

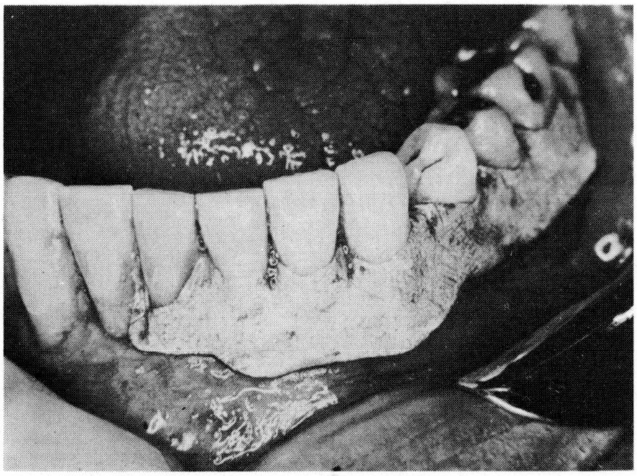

FIG. 137.—Asbestos resin periodontal dressing in place.

Trifurcation and Bifurcation Involvement

The extension of the periodontal pocket into the area between molar roots is often regarded as justification for extraction. In fact, because of the divergent roots, many molars with bone loss from the interradicular septum are firmly embedded, and may even be used as abutment teeth for bridges (Fig. 135). In treating bifurcation and trifurcation areas it is essential to remove the pocket and its contents thoroughly and to expose the area completely down to and including the bone margin (Fig. 136). Failure to remove the pocket wall completely or to leave calculus or necrotic cementum in place will not only lead to treatment failure but may result in the formation of a periodontal abscess.

Application of the Dressing

When bleeding has stopped the periodontal dressing is applied. It should be placed so that it covers the wound and fills the interdental spaces completely (Fig. 137). The presence of dead space may allow granulation tissue to proliferate, which if epithelialized could form a recurrent pocket. Linking the facial and lingual dressings through the interdental space pegs them into position. Where a dressing is placed around an isolated tooth it can be kept in place by first tying a cotton or wire ligature around the tooth as an anchor for the dressing.

The dressing is usually kept in place for one week, after which it is removed and the wound is irrigated and inspected. Frequently the wound is sufficiently well epithelialized by this time to obviate the need for further dressing, but if this is not so and the wound is still raw and sensitive the dressing must be re-applied for a further week (see post-operative care).

Instruction to Patient

It is mandatory to give comprehensive instruction to the patient and to ensure that all eventualities are dealt with. Although it is possible to do this by giving the patient a printed sheet this must be reinforced by verbal instruction. The following advice should be given:

1. Avoid eating or drinking for one hour.
2. Avoid eating very hard, sharp or sticky food, *e.g.* toast, toffee.
3. Use the toothbrush with care in other regions of the mouth.
4. Use copious amounts of a warm water

mouth-wash to keep the mouth clean; at least one tumblerful four times a day.
5. Return immediately if the dressing is dislodged.
6. If there is some haemorrhage, exert pressure on the dressing over the site for 15 minutes; do not rinse; return to the surgery if it does not stop.
7. Take a suitable analgesic, *e.g.* aspirin, paracetamol, or any other analgesic preferred if there is pain when the anaesthetic wears off.
8. Return in 5–7 days for removal of the dressing.

Post-operative Care

The dressing should be removed 5–7 days after operation. If part of the dressing dislodges before this time it is advisable to renew it completely. All debris, stain or calculus must be carefully removed with scalers and curettes and the area thoroughly irrigated with warm water, or, if very dirty, with warm water and hydrogen peroxide. Retention of any irritant will stimulate the production of granulation tissue which is difficult to control.

There is considerable individual variation in gingival healing. In some patients the tissue heals and epithelializes rapidly and no further dressing is needed; in others epithelialization is slow and the wound needs to be covered for a further week or, rarely, a further two weeks.

If granulations are present this may be a sign that some calculus has been overlooked in that area. It is often possible to remove small beads of granulation tissue with a curette without causing any pain. After drying the area and compressing it gently to arrest bleeding, any calculus present is revealed and can be removed. Some patients seem to form considerable amounts of granulation tissue in response to the slightest gingival irritation. A loose or dirty dressing will produce exuberant granulations over a great part of the wound surface. If these are not completely removed the tissue organizes and becomes covered in epithelium with the result that the final gingival contour is as bad as the original contour. Very careful application of a drop of pure phenol or 30 per cent trichloracetic acid should control isolated areas of granulations. If granulations are extensive or healing is progressing slowly a second dressing should be placed firmly so that no movement of the dressing on the wound is possible. Before the dressing is placed the area must be dried and a topical anaesthetic applied. If granulations persist when this second dressing is removed after 5–7 days, it may be necessary to anaesthetize and remove the granulations with electrocautery, after which another dressing must be placed.

Patient Care

At the time of removing the periodontal dressing it is advisable to reinforce the instruction of oral hygiene technique which should have been thoroughly discussed at the time of scaling. The patient must be informed that the future health of the gingivae depends on him. Without adequate home care the original condition will recur.

When the dressing is removed the wound is sensitive and even a soft toothbrush is uncomfortable to use; despite this the patient must prevent food debris from collecting about the gingival margin, therefore frequent and vigorous mouthwashing is essential. A tumblerful of warm salt water used 5–6 times a day is recommended. After 24 hours a soft toothbrush used gently but thoroughly can be tolerated; as the wound heals the toothbrush can be used more vigorously each day and a medium brush can often be used within one week of removing the dressing. The patient is seen again a week after the dressing is removed and the mouth is inspected for debris, granulations and inflammation. Disclosing solution should be used and if the mouth is not perfectly clean any debris must be shown to the patient before it is removed. Thus he is made aware of areas where extra attention is required. One week later (three weeks post-operative) the procedure is repeated.

Four weeks later the mouth is further inspected and if healing is satisfactory and the patient is keeping his mouth clean, he can be dismissed for three months (Figs. 138–140).

Post-operative use of the Dental Woodstick

Woodsticks are often routinely recommended after gingivectomy and gingivoplasty to stimulate keratinization. Very often after gingivoplasty healthy interdental papillae fill the spaces between the teeth so that there is no room for the insertion of a woodstick. It may still be possible to use the stick gently on the gingival margin but its use is limited and may have no advantage over the

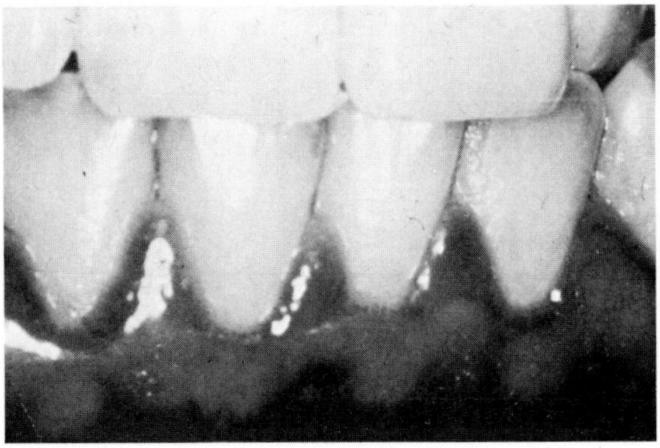

A

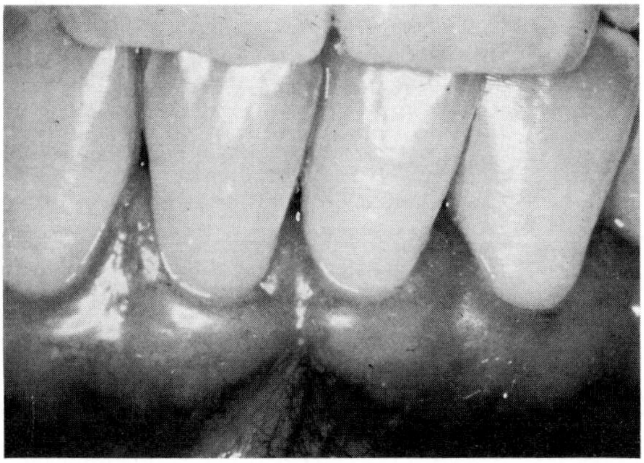

B

FIG. 138.—(*A*) Pre-operative appearance. (*B*) Two months post-operative.

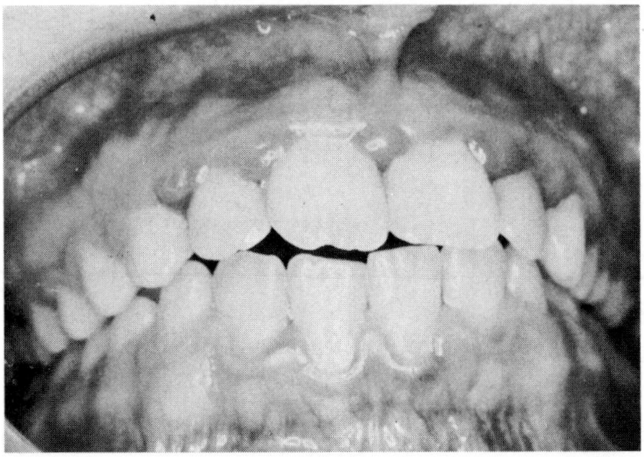

A

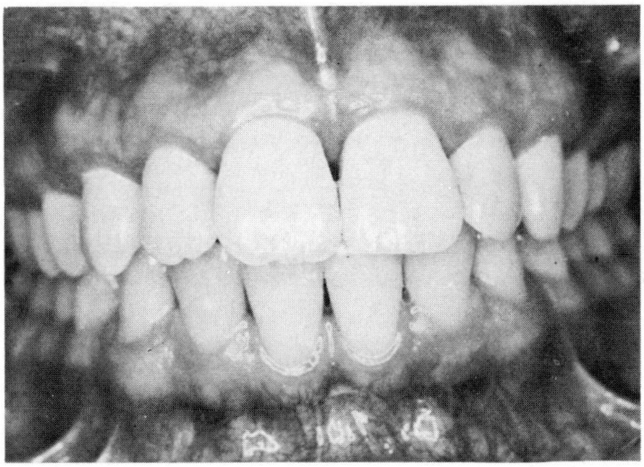

B

FIG. 139.—(*A*) Pre-operative appearance of a 23-year-old woman with chronic periodontitis on which a Vincent's disease had been superimposed in the lower incisor region. (*B*) After gingivectomy and frenectomy of upper labial frenum.

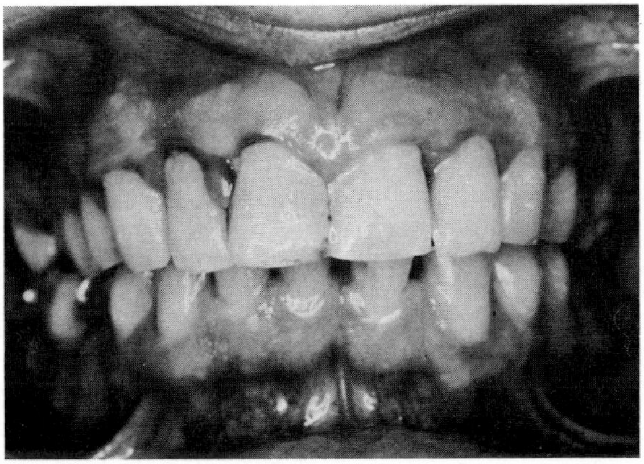

A

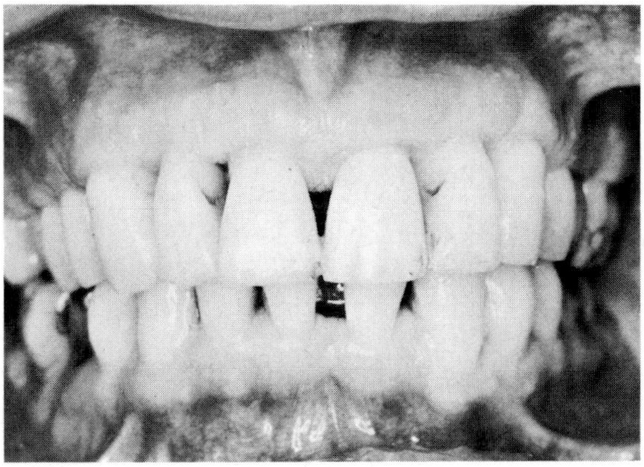

B

FIG. 140.—(*A*) Pre-operative appearance. (*B*) Post-operative appearance. Dental woodsticks are very useful in this case.

proper use of the toothbrush.

The criterion to use when advising any adjunct to toothbrushing, *e.g.* pipecleaners for bifurcation areas, is whether or not it can help to keep the area about the gingival margin clean. If it can without in any way damaging the tissues, then it is valuable. If it is potentially harmful to the gingiva, but is a great deal more effective in certain areas than the toothbrush, then it can be used with caution. The dental woodstick can, if used carelessly, damage the gingiva but it can also clean areas not easily cleaned by a toothbrush, therefore its careful use in selected cases is advised. Thus the cases illustrated in Figs. 139 and 140 are suitable, but the case shown in Fig. 138 is not. The use of the woodstick has also been discussed in Chapter 6.

Sensitive Root

After gingivectomy, any exposed root surface may be extremely sensitive to sweet foods and to changes in temperature. In some individuals sensitivity is slight and transient, in others it is severe and persistent so that eating and even breathing cold air causes distress. Nevertheless, even when severe the sensitivity gradually decreases without treatment. When sensitivity persists for more than a week after gingivectomy the use of some desensitizing agent is indicated. One of the most effective is sodium fluoride. This may be conveniently used as a paste as, for example, Lukomsky's paste (equal parts by weight of sodium fluoride, kaolin and glycerine) or fluoride-containing proprietory products for this purpose. Another effective remedy is topical application of 1% hydrocortisone solution to the dried root surface.

To treat sensitive root the tooth is first dried thoroughly, and the medicament is rubbed firmly over the surface to be desensitized. This procedure may be painful, but after a few seconds the initial pain gradually subsides. The paste should be left in position for 2–3 minutes before the patient is allowed to rinse out. If the root surface is not too sensitive the paste may be applied on a rubber cup rotated against the tooth surface.

Two or three applications of desensitizing paste at intervals of two or three days will reduce sensitivity considerably. The patient is advised to use one of the toothpastes containing desensitizing agents (Emoform, Sensodyne). This procedure is generally effective in completely eliminating sensitivity. If sensitivity recurs in any area sodium fluoride paste can be applied again.

Limitations of Gingivectomy

1. The conventional gingivectomy removes a great deal of tissue and creates an open wound which must heal by secondary intention. Therefore post-operative discomfort is almost inevitable and the healing period is prolonged. It can be several weeks before the wound has healed and is covered by a layer of mature epithelium.
2. Tissue is sacrificed which could be used to close the wound so that healing by primary intention could be obtained.
3. The alveolar margin is not exposed so that bone defects are revealed. The radiographic appearance of the alveolar margin can be misleading about the presence and form of bone lesions, particularly those on buccal and lingual surfaces, and they may be missed at gingivectomy. If bone defects are to be treated adequately they must be fully exposed.
4. If the zone of attached gingivae is narrow it may be reduced or even eliminated by gingivectomy so that the gingival margin is made close to or actually composed of alveolar mucosa, a non-functional tissue. The depth of the vestibule may also be reduced so that cleaning the gingival margin becomes difficult (Fig. 141).

Therefore gingivectomy should be used only where careful pocket-measuring and X-ray examination indicate that bone defects are unlikely to be present, and where there is a wide zone of attached gingivae so that after gingivectomy 2–3 mm of attached gingivae remains.

Because of these limitations other techniques have been devised for the elimination of the periodontal lesion.

INVERSE BEVEL GINGIVECTOMY

The inverse bevel incision allows tissue to be conserved and used to cover the wound so that no connective tissue is left exposed and healing by primary intention might take place (see Morris, 1965).

Procedure

1. The scalpel blade (No. 11 Bard-Parker) is

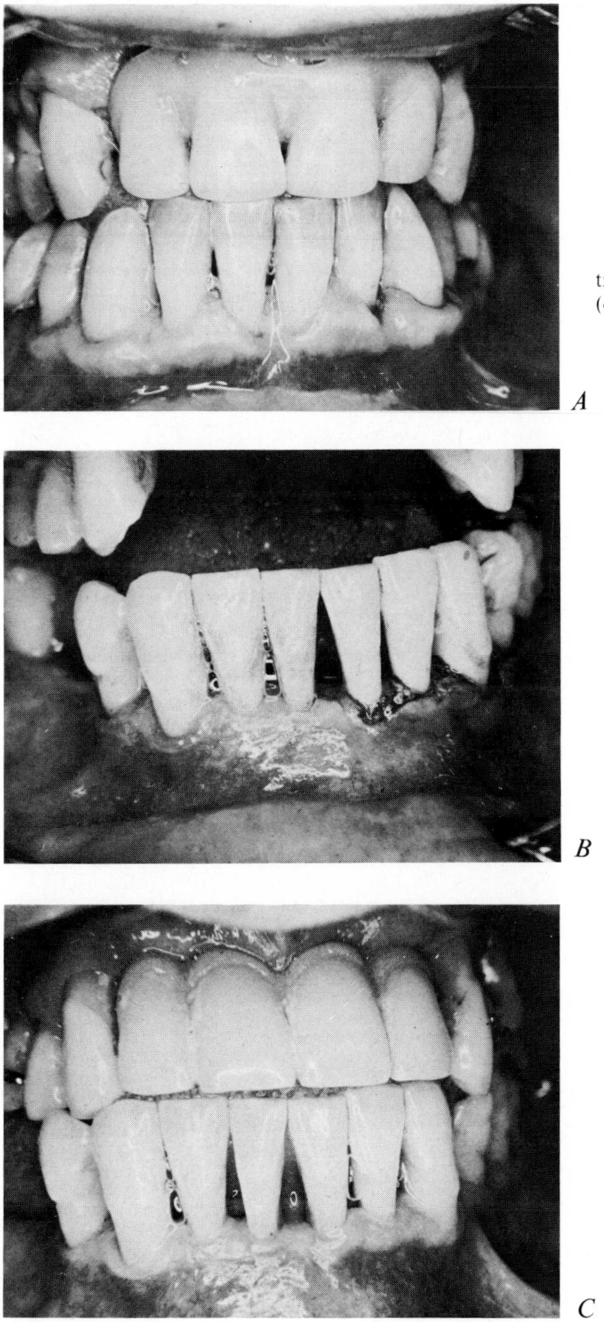

FIG. 141.—(*A*) Pre-operative appearance of gingivae in a 50-year-old man. Generalized 4–5 mm pockets in lower anterior region. (*B*) Gingivectomy wound on left side demonstrating the production of a well contoured wound with teeth completely free of calculus and debris. The right side had been operated on 3 weeks earlier. (*C*) Post-operative appearance. Firm, well contoured gingival margin which the patient is keeping clean.

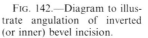

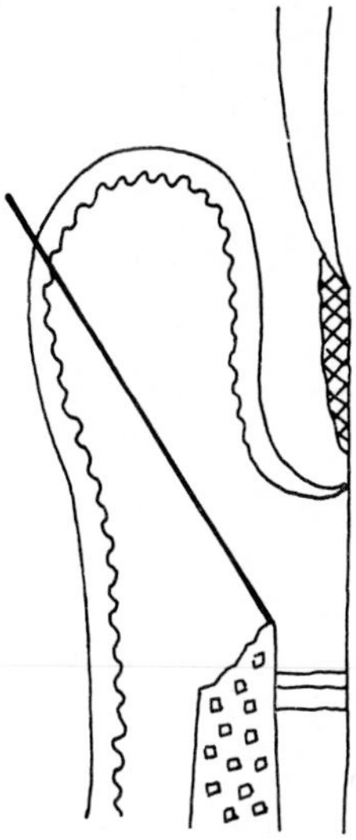

FIG. 142.—Diagram to illustrate angulation of inverted (or inner) bevel incision.

held pointing apically at the bone margin and the incision is made into the gingiva so that the crevicular epithelium is separated from the rest of the tissue (Figs. 142 and 143). The angle of the incision is approximately 45° but this varies with the depth of the pocket and thickness of the gingiva. A scalloped incision is made through both facial and lingual gingivae.

2. Using a periosteal elevator the gingival margins are raised so that the alveolar margin, root surface and calculus are exposed (Fig. 143*C*).
3. The collar of gingival tissue plus all granulation tissue and calculus is curetted away. One considerable advantage of the technique is that any bone defect present but not identified by X-ray examination is revealed, and can be treated (Figs. 143*D* and *E*).
4. The flaps are replaced and an attempt is made to close the interdental wound tightly with interrupted sutures so that pocketing is eliminated and a good contour achieved (Fig. 143*F*).

To this end it is sometimes necessary to trim the margins of the flaps so that the concavity of the bevel is deep enough to allow the interdental tissue to be approximated.

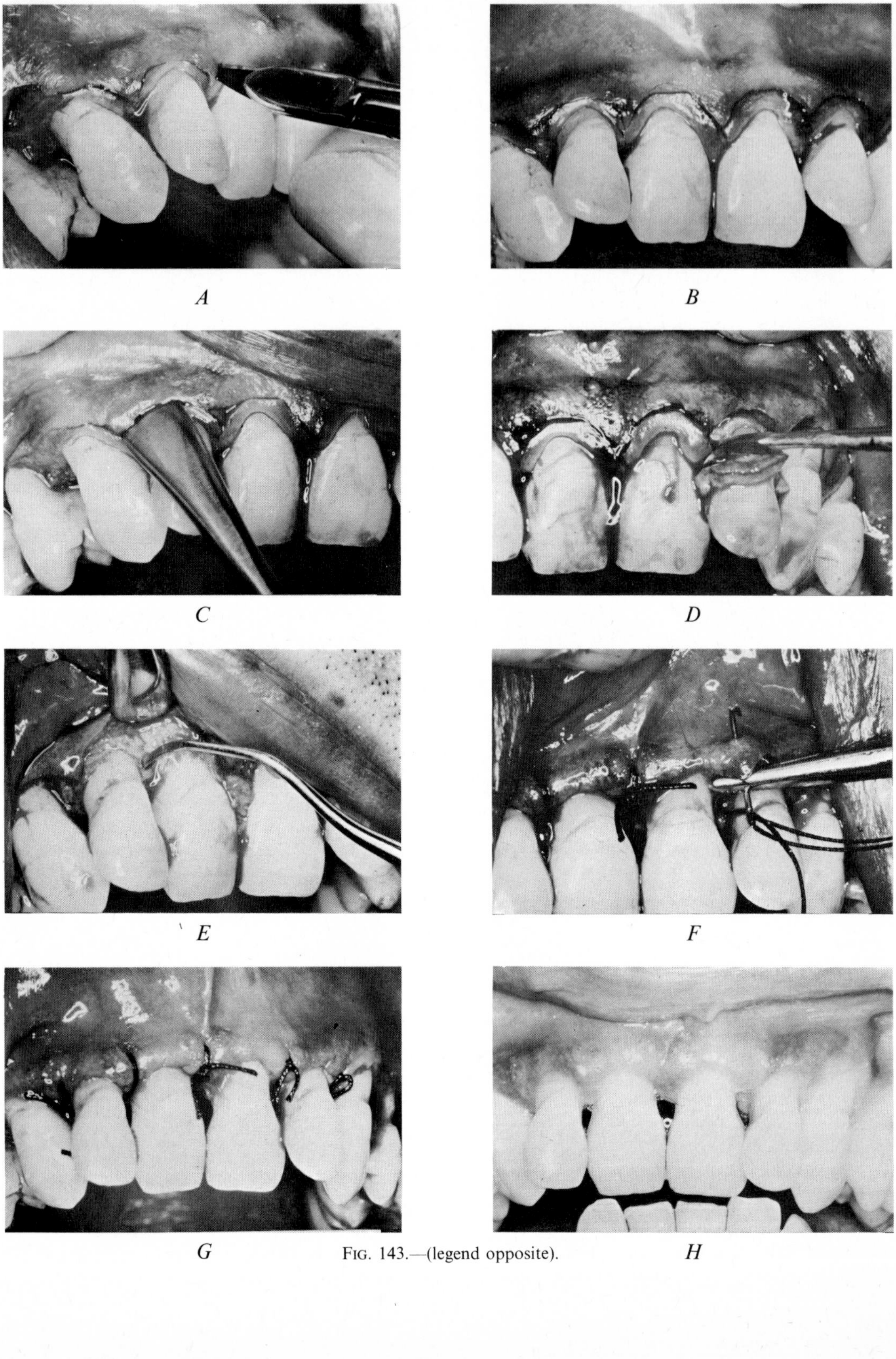

A B C D E F G H

FIG. 143.—(legend opposite).

FIG. 143.—Stages of inverted bevel gingivectomy. (*A*) Incision being made. (*B*) Scalloped pattern of incision. (*C*) Flap being raised. (*D*) Marginal and crevicular tissue being removed. (*E*) Granulation tissue being curetted. (*F*) Palatal and labial flaps sutured together. (*G*) Sutures in place. (*H*) Two-weeks post-operation.

5. A periodontal dressing is placed over the wound.
6. The dressing can be removed after 5–7 days. Post-operative care follows the pattern described for gingivectomy.

This is a more sophisticated technique than the classical gingivectomy but it requires more skill to achieve pocket elimination and a good tissue contour. Theoretically it should replace gingivectomy but from a practical point of view gingivectomy remains the simplest and the most definitive method of pocket elimination where there are no intrabony defects and where there is an adequate width of attached gingiva.

The Edentulous Ridge

An edentulous area may lie between teeth involved in surgery and frequently the alveolar ridge is covered by hyperplastic tissue which has to be reduced. This situation can be managed by making an incision along the crest of the ridge linking the incisions about the related teeth so that facial and lingual flaps can be raised (Fig. 144). When the flaps are replaced those over the edentulous ridge are trimmed until they just meet over the ridge.

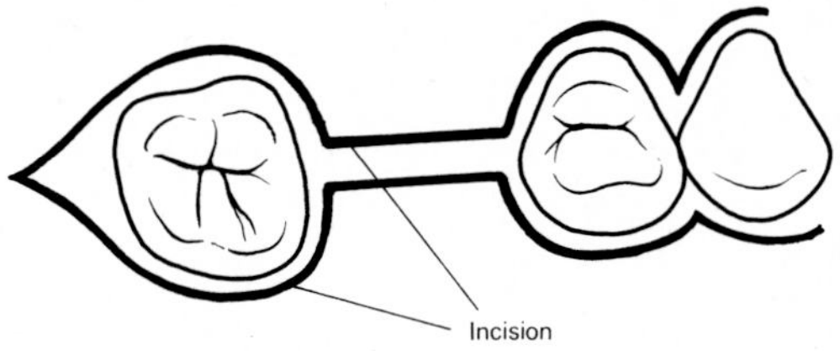

FIG. 144.—Incisions used where edentulous ridge is involved in flap procedure.

The Tuberosity and Retromolar Pad (Distal Wedge)

In some cases the tuberosity is very bulbous or the retromolar pad a flabby mass of tissue distal to a deep pocket. Both situations are dealt with using the 'distal wedge' procedure (Robinson, 1966). The facial and lingual incisions are made (No. 12 Swann-Morton blade) to extend through the tuberosity or retromolar pad to form a triangular wedge (Fig. 145). The incisions are deepened to dissect the wedge from the underlying bone. Loose tags of tissue are curetted and the distal surface of the adjacent tooth is scaled, then the facial and lingual margins of the wound are sutured.

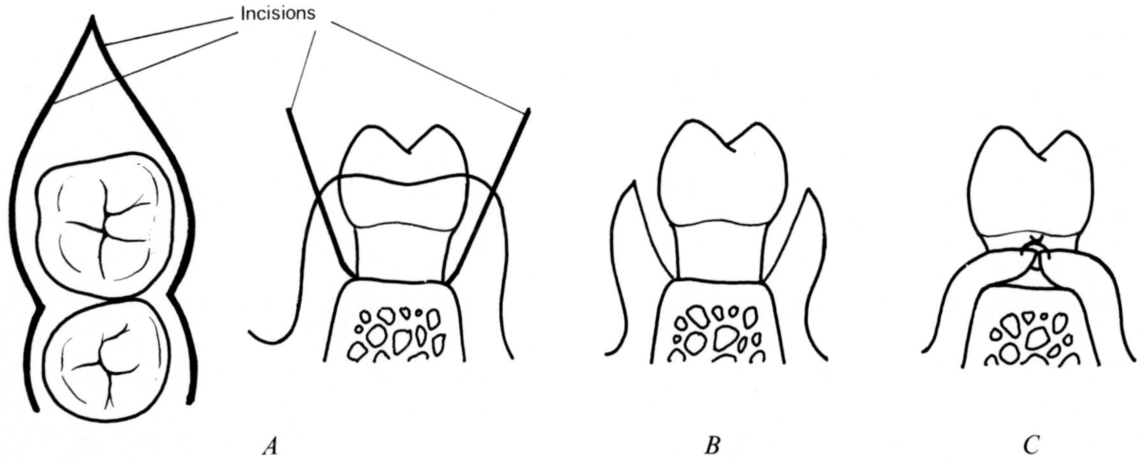

FIG. 145.—Distal wedge procedure for the elimination of a deep retromolar pocket.
(*A*) Diagram to show incision lines. (*B*) Distal wedge of tissue removed. (*C*) Distal tissue sutured.

THE APICALLY REPOSITIONED FLAP

(see also p. 133)

It is obviously possible to create a new pocket when replacing a flap. If the mucosa is not held firmly down against the alveolar crest such an error can occur. Where pocketing is deep this possibility becomes greater, therefore unless pocketing is fairly shallow it is advisable to reposition the flaps in an apical position. This procedure was introduced primarily to increase the width of the attached gingiva and deepen the vestibule (Nabers, 1954; Friedman, 1962).

The procedure is identical to that just described for the inverse bevel gingivectomy except that the flaps are dissected back further to increase their mobility. Mobility can be further improved by releasing incisions made at either end of the flaps. When the wound is closed the flap is moved apically until its edge just covers the bone margin. It can be held in this position by sutures across the releasing incisions after which interdental sutures are placed, care being taken that the flaps are not pulled in a coronal direction (Fig. 146). The periodontal dressing also helps to keep the flaps well adapted to the underlying bone.

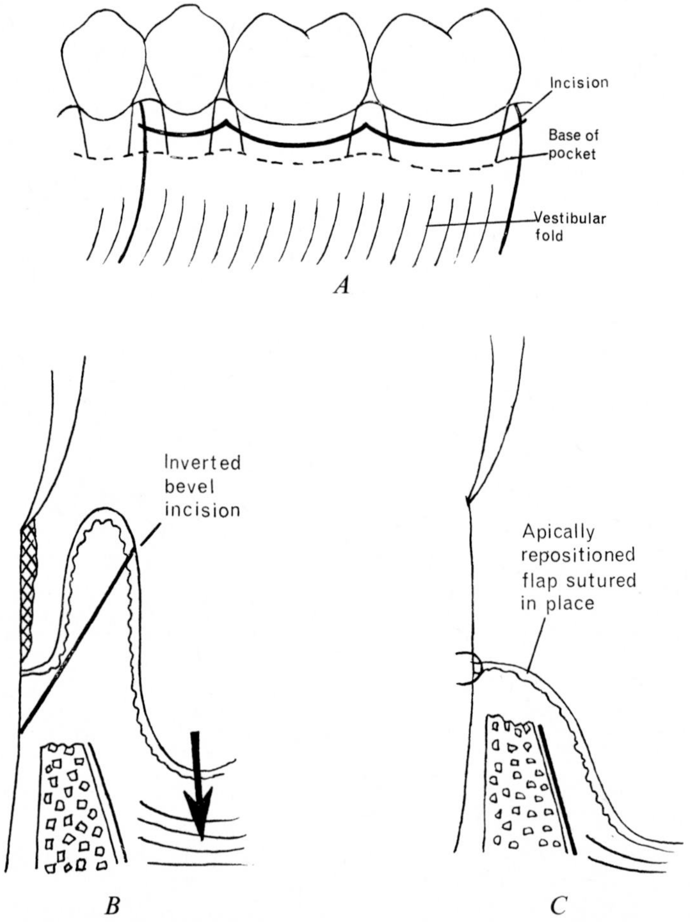

FIG. 146.—The apically repositioned flap technique.
(*A*) Three incisions are made so that a full flap can be raised. (*B*) Gingival tissue is conserved and the pocket wall is separated by using an inverted bevel when making the horizontal incision. After freeing the flap from its attachment to the periosteum it is repositioned deeper in the vestibule. (*C*) After removing all calculus and granulation tissue the flap can be sutured over the wound.

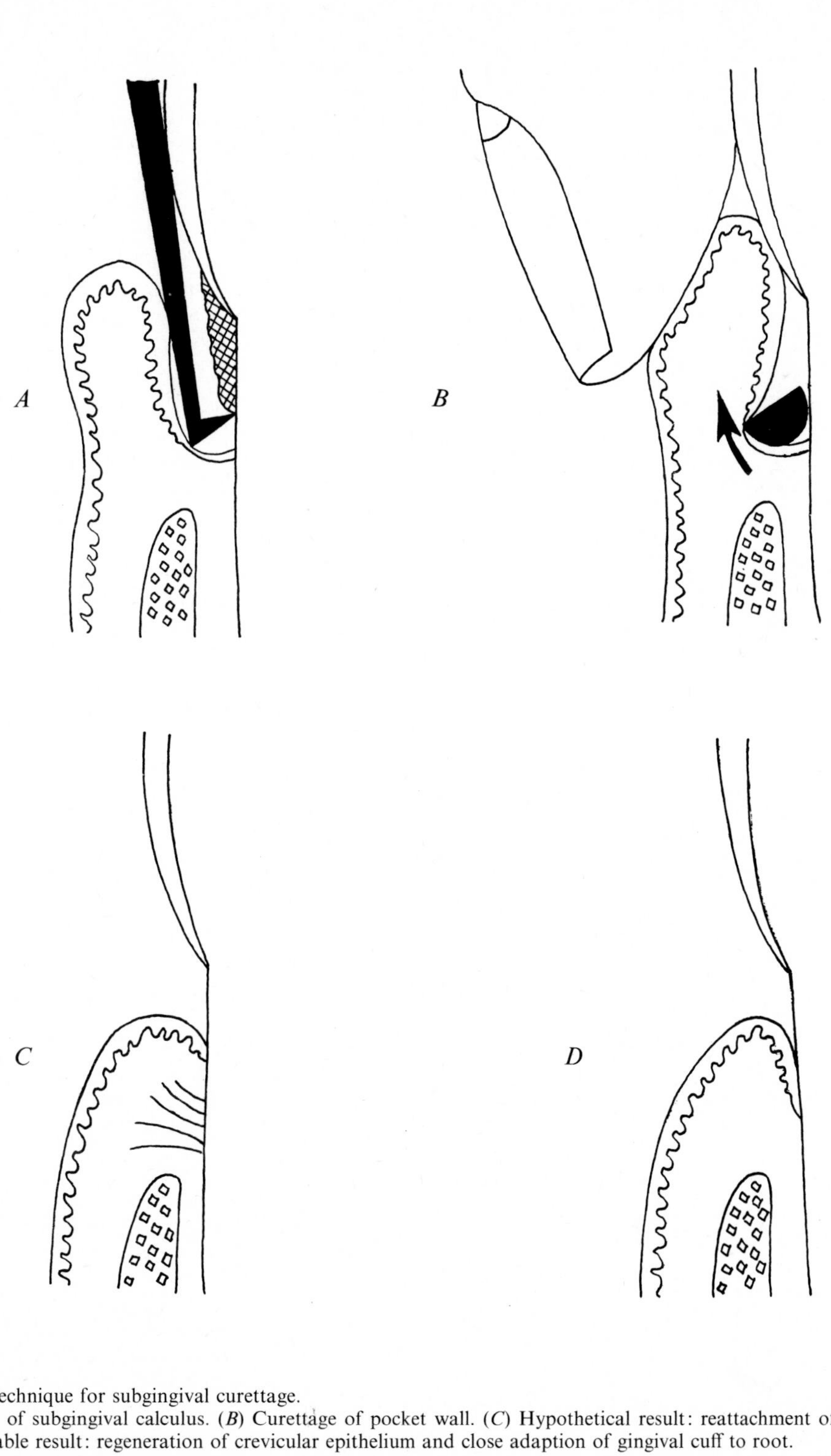

FIG. 147.—Technique for subgingival curettage.

(*A*) Removal of subgingival calculus. (*B*) Curettage of pocket wall. (*C*) Hypothetical result: reattachment of pocket wall to root. (*D*) Probable result: regeneration of crevicular epithelium and close adaption of gingival cuff to root.

SUBGINGIVAL CURETTAGE

Whilst scaling is the most conservative and gingivectomy the radical technique for treating periodontal pockets, subgingival curettage, is a compromise between the two (see Chaikin, 1954; Ramfjord *et al.*, 1968).

The aim of the technique is to remove all subgingival calculus, necrotic cementum and crevicular epithelium without excising gingival tissue.

At one time it was thought that this might result in some fibrous re-attachment of the pocket wall to the tooth, but it seems unlikely that this end is ever achieved (Fig. 147). Nevertheless, the complete removal of irritants and the bleeding of the tissues must result in some resolution of the inflammation, a decrease in pocket depth, and some organization of the periodontal fibres of the gingival margin so that a comparatively tight and healthy gingival cuff is produced (Fig. 147*D*).

The major drawback of the technique is that it is blind, therefore it is impossible to be sure that all calculus, necrotic cementum and crevicular epithelium have been removed. Also there is the danger that an assidiously applied curette will tear into the bottom of the pocket and deepen it. Indeed, it is likely that the tissue changes that take place after subgingival curettage are very little different from the tissue changes after an efficient scaling.

Indications

1. Where 3–4 mm pockets are present and the patient is reluctant to undergo gingivectomy.
2. Where 3–4 mm pockets are present about upper anterior teeth and gingivectomy will produce an objectionable appearance. A common situation is where the upper incisors are crowned and the exposed margins would be unsightly (Moral: carry out periodontal treatment prior to restorative work!)
3. Where for systemic reasons gingivectomy is contra-indicated.

Procedure

1. Management and anaesthesia is as for gingivectomy.
2. A subgingival scaling is carried out as thoroughly as possible. The hoes or other subgingival scalers are used firmly so that any necrotic cementum will be removed at the same time as the calculus (Fig. 147*A*).
3. The correct curette, *i.e.* one which fits the curvature of the tooth surface, is gently inserted into the pocket. The ultrasonic curette is a useful instrument in this procedure. A finger is pressed on to the gingiva over the curette so that as it is withdrawn from the pocket the crevicular epithelium is removed (Fig. 147*B*).

   This procedure is repeated on all surfaces of the teeth in the area, great care being taken that correctly angulated curettes are used. If the wrong curette is used the tissue may be perforated.
4. A periodontal dressing is applied as in gingivoplasty and, although there is very little danger of bleeding and of post-operative pain, instructions as after gingivectomy are given to the patient. The dressing is removed after 5–7 days. If it falls off before this time there is usually no need to apply a second dressing providing the patient uses frequent warm water mouthwashes to keep the area clean. Patient care follows the same pattern as for gingivectomy.

CAUSES OF RECURRENCE OF PERIODONTAL DISEASE
(see Wade, 1954)

1. Poor patient selection

It is the patient's co-operation which determines long-term success or failure. In no other form of dental treatment is patient co-operation so important. Observing the patient's response to scaling and instruction in oral hygiene techniques prior to gingivectomy is a useful guide to the selection of patients for further periodontal treatment.

2. Failure to instruct the patient adequately

The patient's understanding of his periodontal problem is essential to complete co-operation. An unco-operative patient is often one who does not understand why he needs periodontal treatment. The dentist must be prepared to spend time in informing and instructing the patient.

3. Incomplete removal of the pocket

The neophyte is usually too conservative. Failure to remove the entire pocket wall not only preserves the lesion but makes it impossible to remove all subgingival debris. Very often following inadequate surgery inflammation subsides, the gingival margin becomes firm and pink and, initially, both patient and dentist may be deceived into believing that the disease has been eliminated. But continuation of pocket deepening is inevitable and this soon becomes obvious. (Enthusiastic use of the dental woodstick will not compensate for poor surgical technique.)

4. **Failure to produce a tissue contour conducive to efficient food-shedding**

In gingivectomy this may result from making the incision at too shallow an angle, or from failure to take into account the morphology of the underlying bone, or complicating soft tissue factors. (These factors are discussed more fully in the next sections.)

5. **Incomplete scaling**

If subgingival calculus is left in place it may act as an irritant to the healing gingiva so that exuberant granulation tissue is produced. This may be epithelialized and subsequently organized in mature connective tissue and thus constitute the beginning of a new pocket wall. Also plaque, calculus, or any rough surface will act as a focus for the further deposition of calculus.

6. **An ineffective periodontal dressing**

If the dressing is chemically irritant, or does not cover the wound completely, or is not well retained so that it moves or is dislodged completely, or if it breaks, or its surface is rough or dirty the tissues will be irritated, healing will be retarded, granulation tissue will proliferate and the subsequent contour may be poor.

7. **Failure to recognize and eliminate predisposing factors**

The retention of badly contoured fillings with overhanging margins, or 'gum-stripping' dentures, and the failure to correct other predisposing factors must lead to gingival irritation and recurrence of disease. Correction of these factors implies their recognition in the first place. Many failures after surgery stem from incomplete examination of the mouth.

N.B. Eliminating pockets is a comparatively simple technical matter. Making certain that they do not recur requires skill, understanding and patience.

THE PERIODONTAL DRESSING

The purpose of the dressing is:

1. To protect the healing wound from saliva, food stagnation and trauma, therefore making the post-operative period comfortable and healing more rapid.
2. To prevent the proliferation of granulation tissue by filling 'dead' spaces, primarily the interdental space.
3. To control haemorrhage.

Requirements of a Periodontal Dressing

1. It should be non-irritant to the tissues.
2. Before setting it must be sufficiently plastic to be moulded by gentle pressure around the teeth and into the interdental areas so that no dead spaces are left.
3. It should set slowly enough to allow careful manipulation.
4. Its surface should be dense and smooth so that the mucosa is not irritated and the dressing remains clean.
5. It should not induce allergic reactions.
6. It should inhibit bacterial growth on its surface.
7. It must be sufficiently firm when set to resist displacement or distortion by cheeks, lips and tongue. Once in place the dressing must not move.
8. It must be sufficiently strong and coherent to withstand the stresses to which it will be exposed without being bulky, so that there is minimum interference with function.
9. Its taste must be acceptable.

Several types of periodontal dressings are available. The two described below are representative and meet most of these requirements.

The Asbestos-Resin Dressing

Several asbestos-resin dressings are available. Two typical formulae are:

1. *Powder*	*gm*	*Liquid*	*cc*
Zinc oxide	60	Eugenol	80
Resin	30	Olive oil	20
Asbestos-fibre	5		
Zinc acetate	2		

2. *Powder*	%	*Liquid*	%
Zinc oxide	45	Eugenol	98
Powdered resin	38	Thymol	2
Tannic acid	10		

Shredded asbestos	7
Kaolin	2

The powder and liquid are mixed on a paper pad to a thick putty consistency. After initial mixing with a wooden spatula it is helpful to complete the mix by kneading it with the fingers well coated in the powder. In this way a firm, easily-manipulated mix is obtained which can be rolled out into a long thin roll. Small pieces are cut off and pressed firmly between the teeth with a flat plastic instrument. The rest of the dressing is applied in one piece to the labial and lingual surfaces, pressed into place and muscle-trimmed. Where interdental spaces are small there is no need to place the small interdental pieces separately. If there are no interdental spaces retention of this type of dressing is poor and may be improved by threading strands of cotton-wool, ligature, or even short pieces of barbed broach between the teeth before applying the asbestos-resin mix. Generally, because more tissue has been removed in gingivectomy than in gingivoplasty, the interdental spaces are larger, giving better retention of the dressing. Any edentulous areas involved in the operation must be covered, and the asbestos resin dressing is particularly useful in these cases. It is retained effectively around a lone standing tooth if a cotton or wire ligature is tied around the tooth before the dressing is applied. When in place it must be muscle-trimmed and checked for any interference with the occlusion.

Eugenol-free Dressings

There is some evidence that eugenol is irritant to the tissues and may in fact retard the healing process. Many patients find its all-pervading taste objectionable and some complain of a burning sensation.

Several dressings without eugenol have been devised. One of these (Coe-pak) has proved to be very successful in use. It is supplied as two pastes which are mixed together four minutes before application. One paste consists of zinc oxide, magnesium oxide, calcium hydroxide and hexachlorophene; the other is a hydrogenated resin with chlorothymol and benzyl alcohol. The pastes are easy to mix (on paperpad) and to apply once the required consistency is attained. The dressing is smooth-textured, cohesive and plastic, and when set has a very dense smooth surface which is well tolerated by the tissues. The main retention is effected by pressing the dressing through the interproximal spaces. If used after gingivoplasty where little or no interproximal space is present the dressing may not be well retained without the added retention of cotton loops. The bacteriostatic and germicidal qualities of the chlorothymol are better than those of eugenol, and it is also fungicidal. There is no evidence that this pack produces a sensitization reaction. It remains cleaner in the mouth than the asbestos-resin dressings, has no unpleasant taste and is well accepted by the patient.

Cyanoacrylate Dressings

The conventional periodontal dressing is bulky and causes some inconvenience. During the past decade new adhesives with a capacity to adhere to tissue have been developed. The higher homologues of the cyanoacrylates have been shown to be safe to apply to human tissue, and Bhaskar *et al.* (1966) have tested these materials as periodontal dressings. They claim the following advantages:

1. The material is easy to apply.
2. It is not bulky.
3. It is haemostatic.
4. It helps reduce post-operative pain.
5. It prevents the formation of excess granulation tissue and therefore helps healing.

Butyl cyanoacrylate has been found to be the most suitable homologue and is used either as a liquid or as an anhydride powder (Cyanodont) which is mixed with a liquid monomer to form a jelly.

The preparation is run onto the wound with an applicator, and with rapid evaporation of the stabilizing sulphurous anhydride, it polymerizes and adheres to the wound surface.

In practice application of the dressing to form a smooth covering can be difficult and there is a tendency for the surface to become rough. These drawbacks are most noticeable where a large wound surface has to be covered; however, where the wound area is small as in the free gingival graft, particularly in the donor site, the cyanoacrylate dressing is easy to use and well tolerated by the patient.

REFERENCES

BERDON, J. K. (1965). Blood loss during gingival surgery. *J. Periodont.*, **36**, 102.

BHASKAR, S. N., JACOWAY, J. R., MARGETIS, P. M., LEONARD, F. and PANI, K. C. (1966). Oral tissue responses to chemical adhesives (cyanoacrylates). *Oral Surg.*, **22**, 394.

CHAIKIN, B. S. (1954). Subgingival curettage. *J. Periodont.*, **45**, 240.

FRIEDMAN, N. (1962). Muco-gingival surgery: the apically repositioned flap. *J. Periodont.*, **33**, 328.

GOLDMAN, H. M. (1951). Gingivectomy. *Oral Surg.*, **4**, 1136.

MORRIS, M. L. (1965). The unrepositioned muco-periosteal flap. *Periodontics*, **3**, 147.

NABERS, C. L. (1954). Repositioning of the attached gingiva. *J. Periodont.*, **25**, 38.

RAMFJORD, S. P., NISSLE, R. R., SCHICK, R. A. and COOPER, H. (1968). Subgingival curettage versus surgical elimination of periodontal pockets. *J. Periodont.*, **39**, 167.

ROBINSON, R. E. (1966). The distal wedge operation. *Periodontics*, **4**, 256.

WADE, A. B. (1954). Where gingivectomy fails. *J. Periodont.*, **25**, 189.

10. Treatment of Alveolar Bone Defects

As described in Chapter 8 the bone changes associated with periodontal disease are either (a) productive, or (b) destructive.

(a) Where pocket deepening is very slow, reduction in the height of the alveolar process may be accompanied by a thickening of the bone margin, which prevents simple gingivoplasty from achieving a good tissue contour. The thickened margin interferes with food shedding, and the retention of plaque on the flat interdental table maintains irritation and therefore periodontal disease. This bone thickening is found most often on the buccal aspect of the upper molar teeth, and in bifurcation and trifurcation areas (Fig. 148).

(b) As periodontal disease progresses the margin of the alveolar bone may be reduced unevenly so that bone defects of various shapes may occur on all aspects of the teeth (Fig. 149). This change in bone contour may take place with or without gingival recession. If loss of bone and atrophy of the soft tissues progress at about the same rate, the deformities in the bone are apparent on visual examination of the mouth. If, as is more commonly the case, little gingival recession takes place the bone lesions are apparent only on critical radiographic examination. Some bone defects, including the interdental bone crater, may not be disclosed even then (Fig. 150).

The presence of a bone deformity may make elimination of the periodontal pocket impossible by soft tissue surgery alone, and even where this can be achieved, will predispose to plaque retention in the mis-shaped areas and cause rapid recurrence of periodontal disease.

The objectives in the treatment of bone defects are those of all periodontal surgery:

1. To eliminate pathology.
2. To achieve a tissue architecture which is conducive to the maintenance of health by judicious bone shaping or grafting.

A variety of techniques have been used to deal with bone problems, including 'open' and 'closed' procedures. It is now recommended that all bone defects be treated by the 'open' approach. This allows complete visualization of the defect and a more reliable appraisal of the problems to be overcome, with therefore a greater chance of success.

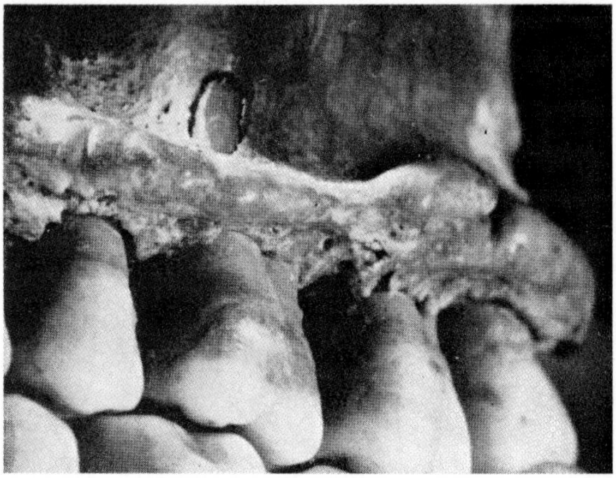

FIG. 148.—Thickening of alveolar margin about upper molars. (R.C.S. Odontological Museum specimen No. 'A' 34.3.)

The procedure must produce a bone shape, and therefore gingival contour which allows food shedding to take place and cleansing techniques to be effective, without at the same time reducing the bone support of the teeth (Fig. 151) (see Ochsenbein, 1958; Ochsenbein and Ross, 1969). In altering the shape of the alveolar bone it has to be remembered that irritation to the bone is likely to stimulate bone resorption and it is possible that some bone remodelling takes place even when a mucoperiosteal flap is raised, therefore, over-enthusiastic reshaping of bone can result in loss of support for the teeth.

It should also be recognized that the interdental bone margin between molars is usually flat, but may be either slightly convex or concave. These variations may be within normal limits and the reshaping of interdental bone in an attempt to conform to some stereotype is quite unjustified.

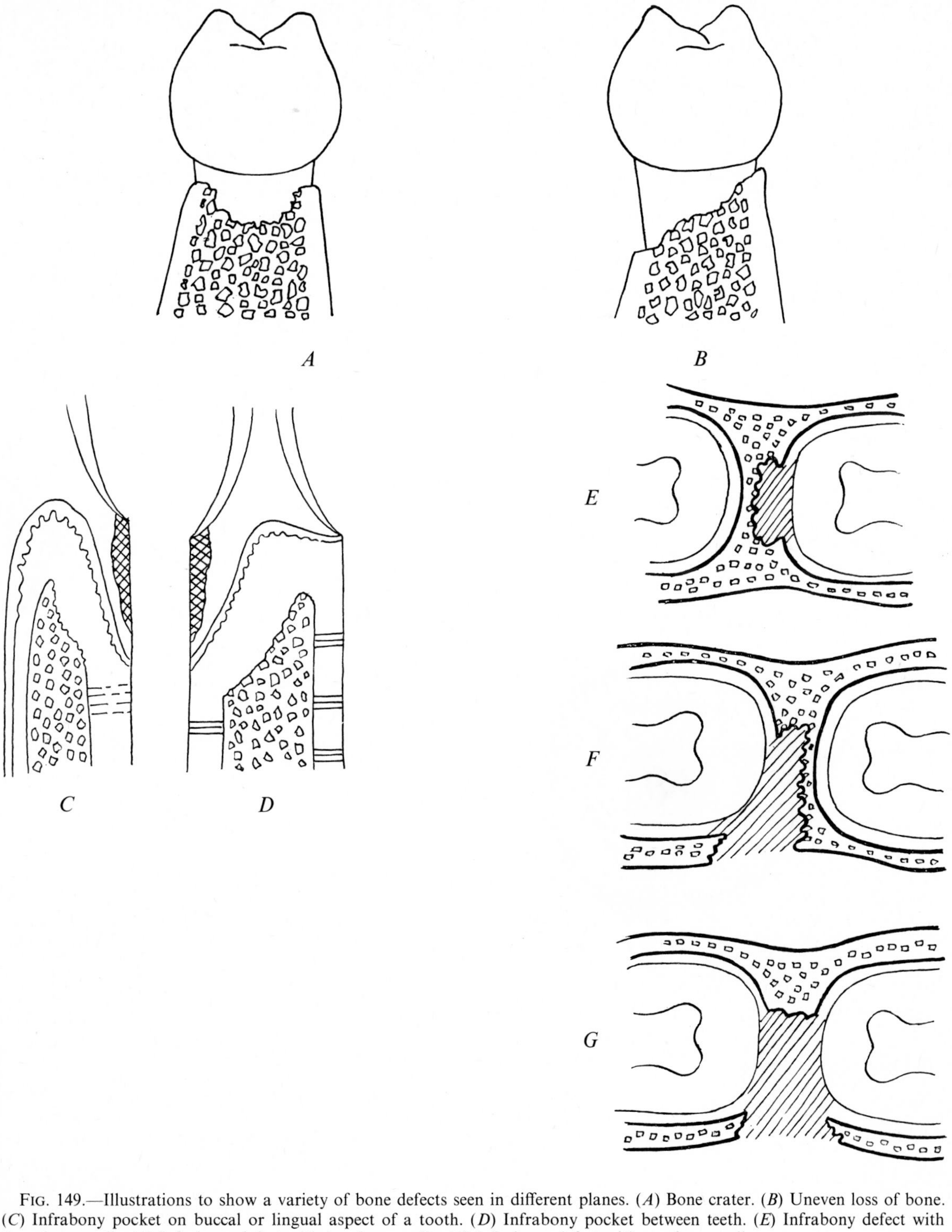

FIG. 149.—Illustrations to show a variety of bone defects seen in different planes. (*A*) Bone crater. (*B*) Uneven loss of bone. (*C*) Infrabony pocket on buccal or lingual aspect of a tooth. (*D*) Infrabony pocket between teeth. (*E*) Infrabony defect with three bone walls. (*F*) Infrabony defect with two bone walls. (*G*) Infrabony defect with one bone wall.

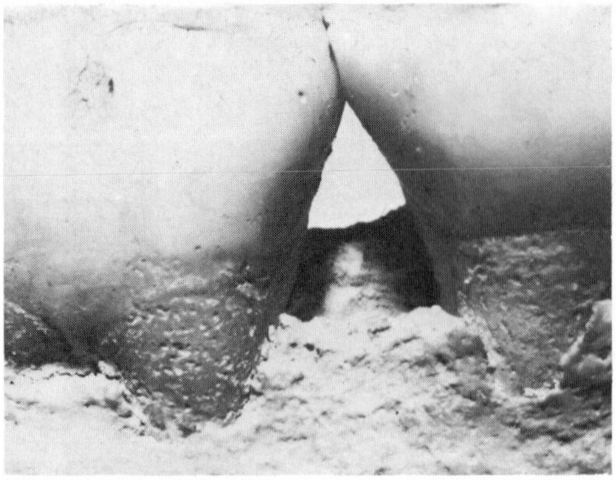

A

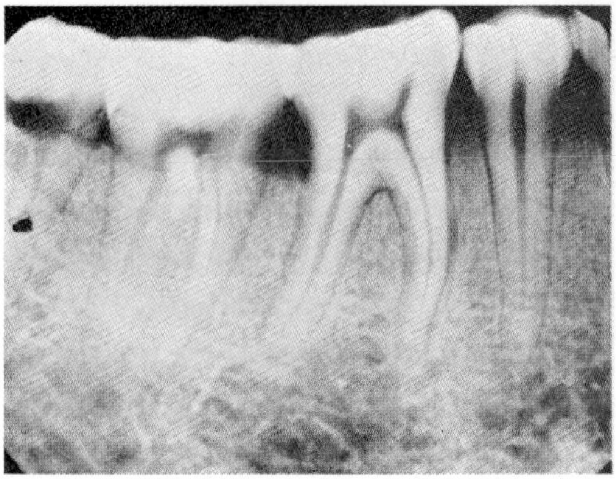

B

FIG. 150.—(*A*) Artificial dental crater in a dry skull. (*B*) Radiograph of this shows no obvious bone defect.

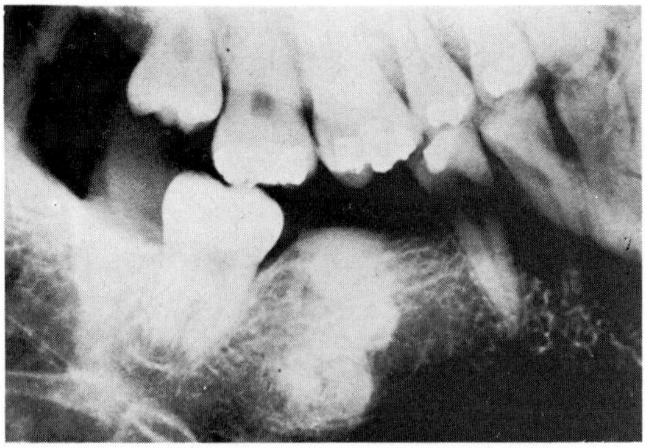

A

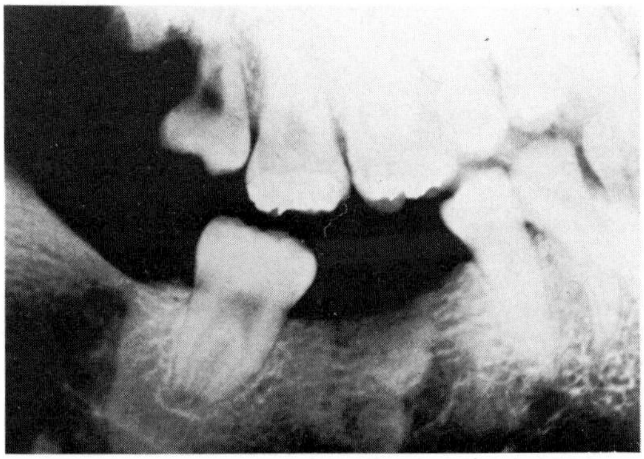

B

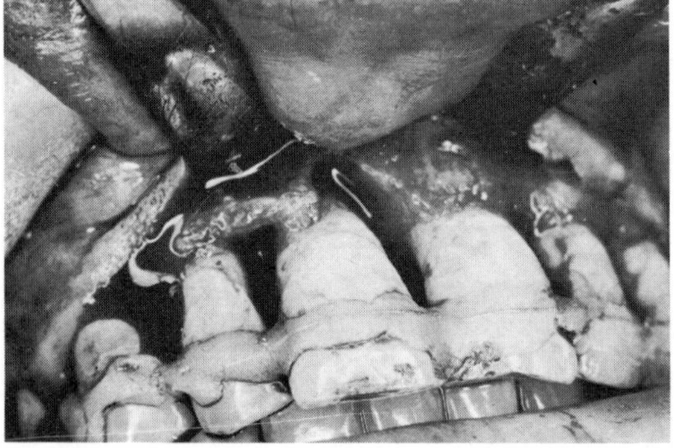

C

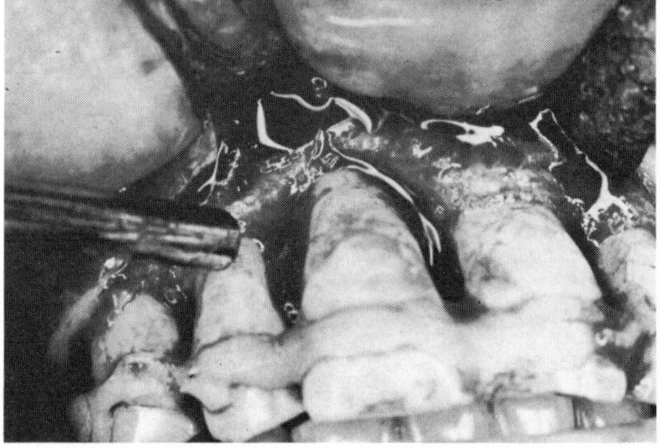

D

FIG. 151.—Bone reshaping carried out to bring partially erupted tooth into function. (*A*) Pre-operative radiograph. (*B*) Post-operative radiograph. (*C*) Labial margin defect. (*D*) Defect reshaped retaining as much marginal bone as possible.

Bone surgery should not be undertaken without careful consideration.

Open surgical techniques are used routinely for the treatment of soft tissue lesions, *e.g.* inverted bevel gingivectomy, and the treatment of bone defects can be readily undertaken at the same time. Indeed the separation of the treatment of soft and hard tissues is quite artificial and only justified for descriptive purposes. Perhaps the main interest in the treatment of bone defects is that some situations offer the opportunity for achieving that 'holy grail' of periodontics, the formation of a new attachment between bone and tooth (Fig. 152). Such repair must involve:

1. The formation of a healthy blood clot.
2. Organization of the clot.

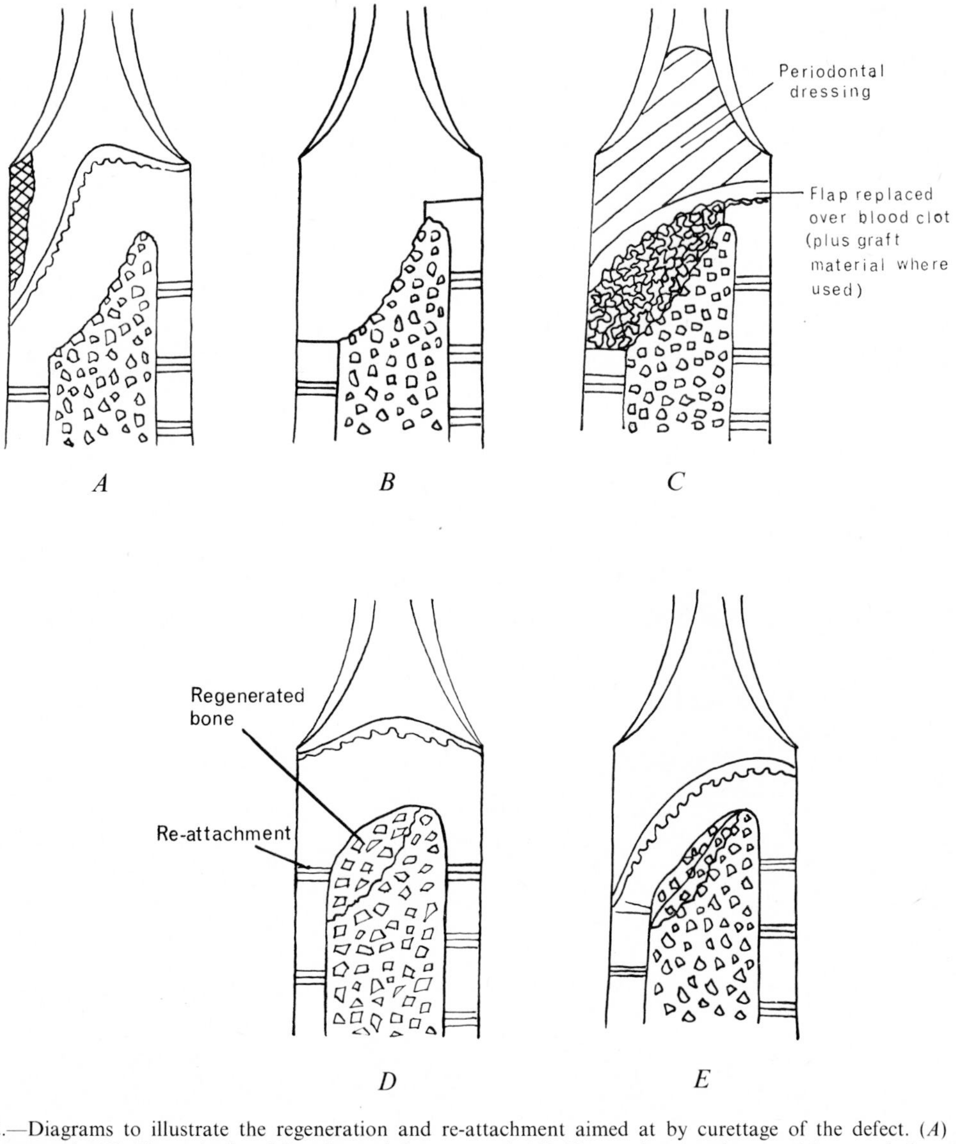

FIG. 152.—Diagrams to illustrate the regeneration and re-attachment aimed at by curettage of the defect. (*A*) Intrabony defect between teeth. (*B*) Flap raised and intrabony defect curetted. (*C*) Flap replaced and covered by a periodontal dressing. (*D*) Ideal result; regeneration of bone and fibrous tissue re-attachment to the root. (*E*) Usual result; regeneration by secondary intention produces an improved contour.

3. Deposition of new bone in the alveolar defect.
4. Deposition of cementum on the root surface.
5. The organization of mature periodontal fibres linking bone to cementum.

So that this sequence of events may take place certain conditions are essential:

1. The defect must be exposed completely.
2. All plaque, calculus, infected tissue and necrotic cementum must be removed.
3. The blood clot and surrounding tissue must be protected from infection.
4. The gingival epithelium must be prevented from proliferating into the defect.
5. The tooth must be held in a stable relationship with surrounding tissues; excessive movement is bound to interfere with healing.
6. Cells capable of forming the new tissues must be present in the area, and conditions must be such as to allow their activity.

The chances of obtaining re-attachment depend to a large extent on the morphology of the lesion. An intrabony defect with three bone walls must offer better chances of re-attachment than one with two bone walls. A deep, narrow lesion is more likely to be bridged by connective tissue than a shallower, but wider one.

In deciding on the definitive treatment of an individual bone defect one must ask:

1. What are the chances of re-attachment?
2. If the chances of re-attachment are poor because the defect is wide or has only two (or even one) bone walls, will bone reshaping result in (a) weakening of tooth support? (b) a poor appearance? (c) a self-cleansing area?

Therefore one must take into consideration:

1. The exact morphology of the pocket. Radiographs from two slightly different angles and taken with some radiopaque pocket marking device (gutta percha point, Hirshfeld point) in place are helpful (Fig. 153). Careful examination with a probe is essential.
2. The total amount of bone loss about the tooth and, if it can be determined, the rapidity of that loss. A tooth which is firmly supported obviously has a better prognosis than one with considerable bone loss.
3. The age of the patient. It is generally assumed that tissues in the young have the greatest regenerative power. On the other hand an intrabony defect in a young individual may well indicate the presence of some factor which might interfere with tissue repair; therefore it is imperative to define as well as possible all factors which are involved in the aetiology of the infrabony pocket before treatment.
4. The position of the defect in the mouth. If the infrabony pocket is in the front of the mouth conservative methods of treatment are obviously to be preferred, particularly if it is deep and localized. In the posterior region of the mouth it is often better to eliminate the pocket and bone lesion radically by bone reshaping and produce a predictable result than take a chance on obtaining re-attachment.

Thus the ideal case for attempting to obtain re-attachment is one in which a single narrow three bone-walled defect is present on an anterior tooth which is otherwise well supported by bone.

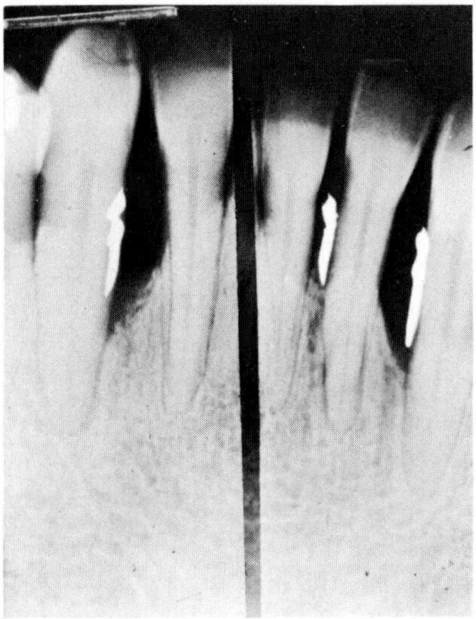

A *B*

FIG. 153.—(*A*) Infrabony defect mesial to molar. The apical limit of the defect is not defined. (*B*) Hirschfeld point in place defines depth of defect.

Procedure

1. Anaethesia is given as for other surgery.
2. Inverted bevel scalloped incisions are made in the margin of the facial and lingual gingivae. Releasing incisions are made where

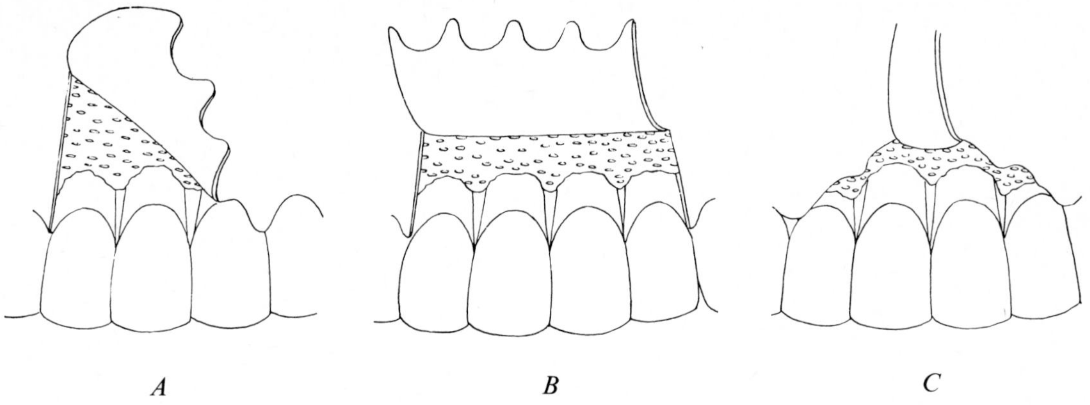

FIG. 154.—(*A*) Triangular flap; two incisions are made. (*B*) Full flap made with three incisions. (*C*) Modified flap; only the gingival margin is incised.

required to obtain exposure of the alveolar process. The design of the flap depends upon the extent of the area to be worked on and the size of the defect (Fig. 154).

3. Flaps are lifted using a periosteal elevator and scalpel dissection where the muco-periosteum is tightly bound down by fibrous tissue. This is frequently the case over bone lesions on the facial or lingual surfaces where scar tissue is formed.
4. All tissue tags and granulations are curetted so that the shape of the bone defect can be seen.
5. Root surfaces are planed free of subgingival calculus and necrotic cementum.
6. The bone defect is carefully examined and an assessment of any necessary modifications is made. At this time a decision about the possibility of 'fill-in' has to be made. A narrow defect offers a greater chance of re-attachment than a wide defect: a three-walled defect has more chance than a two- or one-wall defect. Where re-attachment does not seem possible the edges of the defect have to be trimmed to provide a shape which when covered by gingiva will allow some food shedding and the opportunity for good home care. Bone edges may be trimmed with a well-cooled airotor-driven diamond fissure bur or better, with a chisel, which is less traumatic and allows the fragments to be pushed into the defect (Figs. 155, 156). An old Kirkland knife which has been reduced in size by repeated sharpening provides a perfect tool for whittling down bone margins.

Interdental craters may be treated by fracturing one or two bone walls and pressing them together to form a new interdental septum – so called 'ramping'. This is carried out with chisels or forceps.

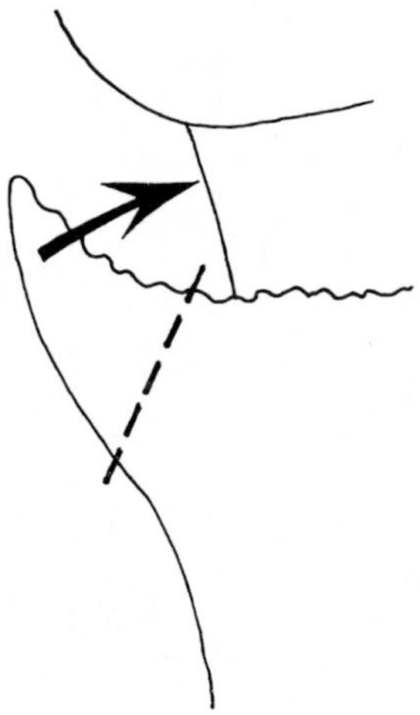

FIG. 155.—The edge of a bone defect can be trimmed and the fragments placed in the defect.

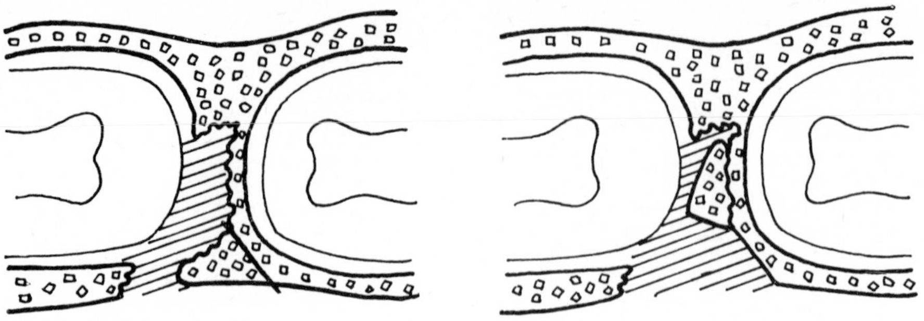

FIG. 156.—Illustration to show the way in which a bone edge which does not support bone can be used to help fill in a two-walled bone defect and produce a better morphology.

7. Interdental sutures are then placed so that the bone defects are well covered. If possible the facial and lingual flaps are brought into contact by carefully placed and tight suturing (Fig. 157). In order to produce a good soft tissue contour the margin of the flap may need trimming with scissors.
8. A periodontal dressing is then placed securely over the wound. If an interdental defect needs extra protection this can be provided by suitably shaped pieces of metal foil placed over the interdental area prior to the application of the dressing.

Post-operative Instructions

These follow the same pattern as those given after soft tissue surgery. Care must be taken not to disturb the wound, and at the same time the mouth must be kept clean. Frequent warm water mouthwashes are essential.

The main post-operative complication after treatment of the bone defect is infection. Drainage is poor, therefore if infection of the wound occurs a periodontal abscess may develop. Some operators routinely provide antibiotic cover for this procedure, but while this seems to be justified in many cases especially where the bone defect is

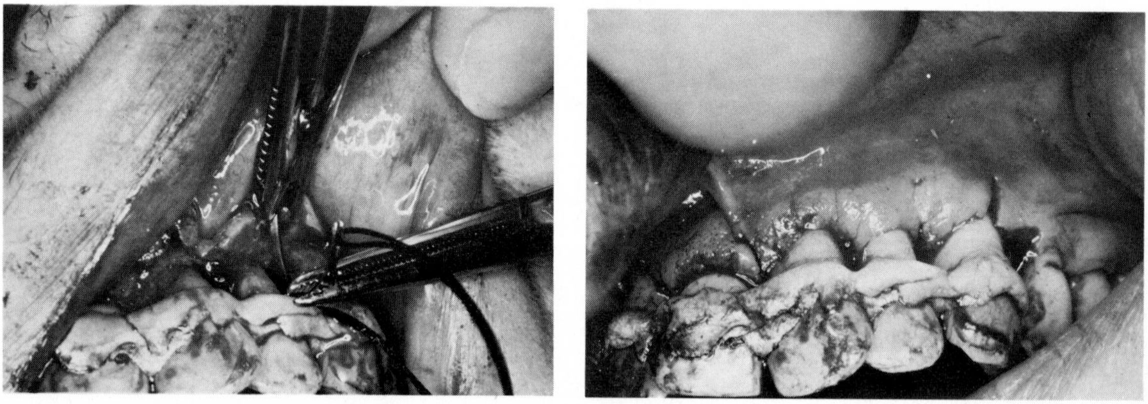

A *B*

FIG. 157.—(*A*) Suture needle being placed through papilla in labial flap held firm by special split-beak forceps. (*B*) Sutures in place pulling flap tight around the teeth.

deep, its use is empirical and it is also essential to use sound surgical techniques and to maintain as high a degree of surgical sterility as possible in the mouth. If no antibiotic has been given and post-operative infection supervenes, antibiotics should be prescribed (Caps. penicillin V or Caps. erythromycin; dose, 250 mg four times a day for five days). Penicillin is contra-indicated where allergic symptoms have followed its previous administration, and in individuals suffering from asthma, hay-fever or eczema. Sometimes pain and swelling immediately post-operative indicate that antibiotics are necessary, and their prompt use may abort the infection, but it is more than likely that if a patient suffers from marked post-operative symptoms irreversible damage to the wound has already taken place. In this case antibiotics are prescribed to prevent increased destruction of the periodontal tissues and spread of infection. Hot salt-water mouthwashes used every two or three hours help to establish and maintain drainage.

When the infection is under control it may be possible to repeat the flap operation but it is advisable to wait for at least two weeks so that any bone changes due to the infection are evident on radiographs. At that time it may be seen that bone loss is too extensive to make hopes of re-attachment justified, in which case an alternative form of treatment, even extraction, must be considered.

If the immediate post-operative period is uneventful the dressing and sutures are removed after one week. The area is gently but thoroughly cleaned and the patient is instructed to use the toothbrush and mouthwashes.

One week later (two post-operative) the healing wound is inspected. Sometimes after a flap operation, the gingival contour is poor. It is not necessary to recontour the tissues immediately because given time the tissues can remodel and the contour improves considerably. Where a wire and acrylic splint is in place this should be removed six weeks after surgery. Retaining a splint longer will serve no purpose; if re-attachment has not taken place within six weeks it is definitely not going to take place in a longer period. The splint also interferes with the maintenance of good oral hygiene. After the splint has been removed it is possible for the patient to keep the area clean.

After three months radiographs of the treated infrabony lesion should be taken to determine whether bone deposition has taken place (Fig. 158). The interpretation of these radiographs presents real problems. Ideally pre- and post-operative X-rays should be taken with identical orientation of the beam and placement of the film, but this precaution involves the use of special equipment which the practitioner may not possess. Therefore, in taking radiographs of periodontal lesions, some attempt must be made to standardize the procedure. Two radiographs taken from slightly different angles provide more reliable information than can be obtained from one radiograph, and comparisons of two pre-operative and two post-operative radiographs will provide more valid information about bone changes than a comparison of single radiographs. But estimations of the success or failure of the treatment should not be made on radiographic evidence alone. Tooth mobility and pocket depth provide equally valuable information about the results of treatment.

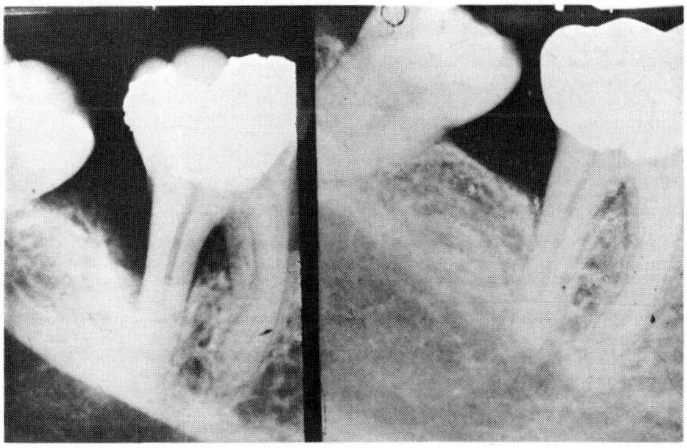

FIG. 158.—Radiographs showing pre- and post-operative bone contour where crest of bone between molars was used to fill intrabony defect.

After removing the splint and completing all the gingival treatment it is essential to check the occlusion before dismissing the patient. Tissue changes take place in healing which result in tooth movement. A tooth which was in good occlusion before surgery may be in traumatic occlusion after surgery. Failure to check the occlusion after treatment of the infrabony defect may result in the failure of otherwise successful treatment. The maintenance of good oral hygiene is essential.

BONE GRAFTS

A variety of graft materials have been used in attempts to obtain filling-in of the bone defect. These include treated ox-bone, calf-bone, cartilage, cementum and dentine fragments, even Plaster of Paris.

The heterografts provide occasional but unpredictable success. All antigenic properties must be destroyed; ox-bone treated with ethylene diamine produces an anorganic graft which can be used with occasional success (Cross, 1960) (Figs. 159 and 160). The best hope lies in the use of autogenous bone, that is bone from the patient himself. Autogenous transplants are obtained from the different parts of the jaw (Nabers and O'Leary, 1965) usually a neighbouring area, an edentulous ridge or the tuberosity (Fig. 161). Cancellous bone which is highly cellular and has a vast surface area which is exposed to the host tissue fluids and cells, is a more useful graft material than fragments of cortical bone. Hip

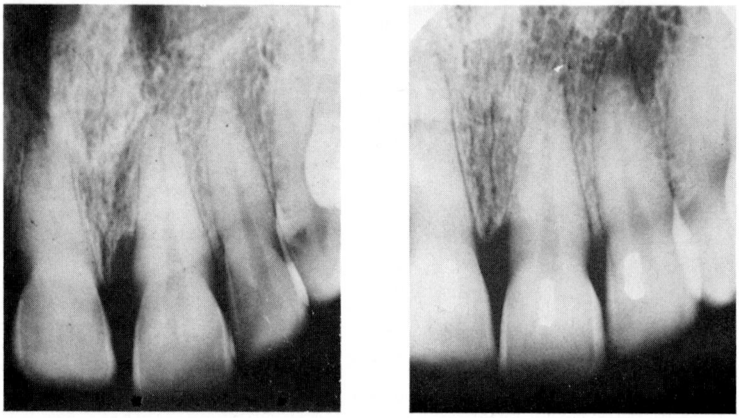

A *B*

FIG. 159.—(*A*) Two-walled infrabony defect in a 26-year-old woman. (*B*) One year after curettage at open operation when a graft of anorganic bone was inserted.

Radio-opaque areas in teeth are thimbles for Weissenfluh splint.

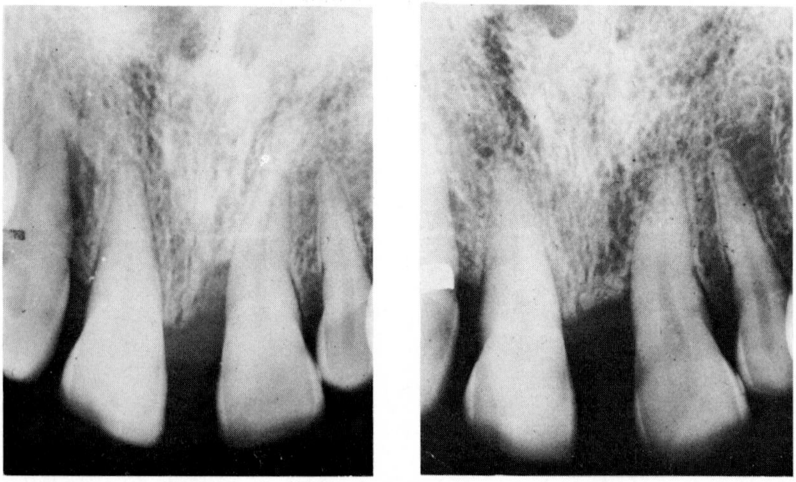

A *B*

FIG. 160.—(*A*) Two-walled infrabony defect in a 52-year-old woman. (*B*) Three years after curettage at open operation. Anorganic bone was also placed in this case.

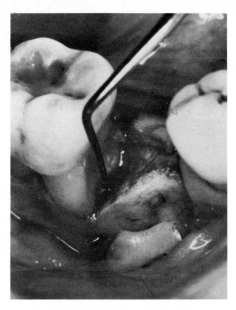

A

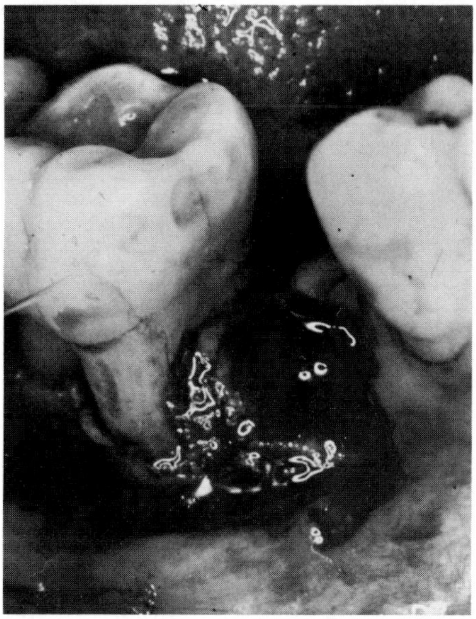

B

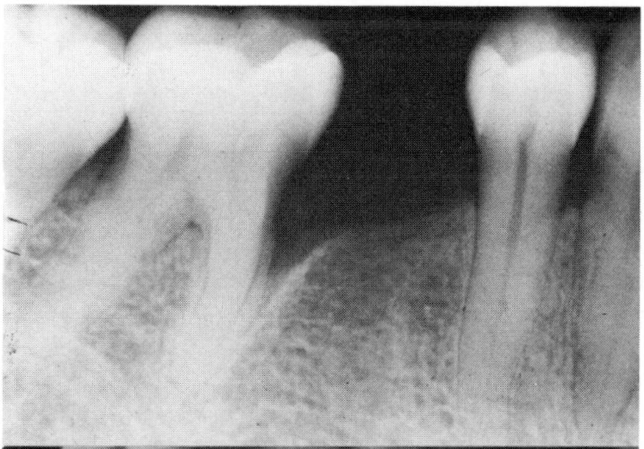

C

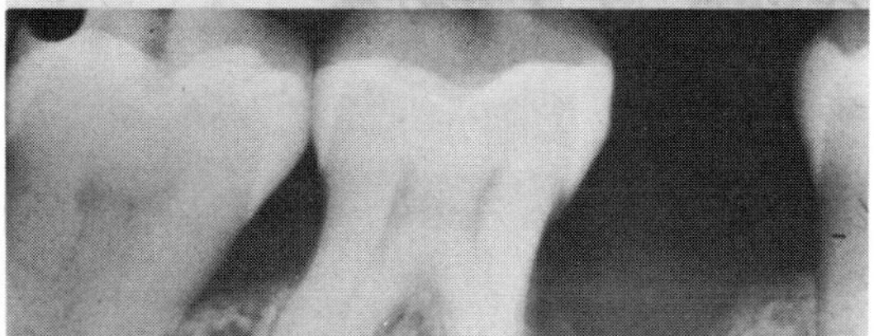

D

FIG. 161.—Autogenous graft. (*A*) One-wall defect next to edentulous area. (*B*) Fragments of bone from edentulous ridge filling defect prior to replacement of mucoperiosteal flap over bone. (*C*) Pre-operative radiograph. (*D*) Post-operative radiograph showing signs of filling-in of defect.

bone marrow has been found to be an effective transplant (Schallhorn, Hiatt and Boyce, 1970).

The way in which these graft materials are used by the host tissues is not yet known but several mechanisms are possible:

1. Bone cells in the graft may stay alive, particularly when the graft is moved expeditiously from donor to recipient sites.
2. Chemical inductors in the graft may stimulate differentiation of osteoblasts from precursor cells in the host.
3. The graft may provide a calcific framework for host cell activity.

Heterografts such as anorganic bone may provide a calcific honeycomb framework which at the least reduces the amount of blood clot present.

Whichever implant is used the evidence suggests that some of the graft is resorbed and the rest acts as a nucleus for the deposition of bone by the host.

REFERENCES

CROSS, W. G. (1960). The use of bone implants in the treatment of periodontal pockets. *Dent. Clin, N. Amer.*, March, p. 107.

NABERS, C. L. and O'LEARY, T. J. (1965). Autogenous bone transplants in the treatment of osseous defects. *J. Periodont.*, **36**, 5.

OCHSENBEIN, C. (1958). Osseous resection in periodontal surgery. *J. Periodont.*, **29**, 15.

OCHSENBEIN, C. and ROSS, S. (1969). A reevaluation of osseous surgery. *Dent. Clin. N. Amer.*, **13**, 87.

SCHALLHORN, R. G., HIATT, W. H. and BOYCE, W. (1970). Iliac transplants in periodontal therapy. *J. Periodont.*, **41**, 566.

11. Mucogingival Surgery

Treatment of the periodontal pocket is often complicated by (a) the proximity of a frenum or other prominent muscle attachment; or (b) loss of gingival tissue resulting in reduction of the width of attached gingivae with proximity of the base of the pocket to the mucogingival junction and reduction in the depth of the vestibule. These complicating factors often occur together.

The depth of the oral vestibule is not as important for gingival health as is the width of the attached gingiva (Bowers, 1963). The vestibule should be deep enough to allow efficient food shedding away from the gingival margin and manipulation of the toothbrush (Bergenholtz and Hugoson, 1967). A minimum width of attached gingiva appears to be essential to stability of the gingival fibres and therefore to the dento-gingival relationship. If tension on the lips or cheeks is transmitted to the gingival margin the attached gingiva is certainly not wide enough.

A frenum is sometimes abnormally placed and inserted close to the gingival margin. This may interfere with the use of the toothbrush so that neighbouring teeth are not thoroughly cleaned and a gingivitis ensues, but this is not always the case (Fig. 162). If a pocket forms, the frenum may be attached to its wall so that movement of the lip opens the pocket, allowing access to food debris. With gingival recession a normally placed frenum or muscle attachment sometimes becomes involved in the marginal tissue (Gottsegen, 1954) (Fig. 163).

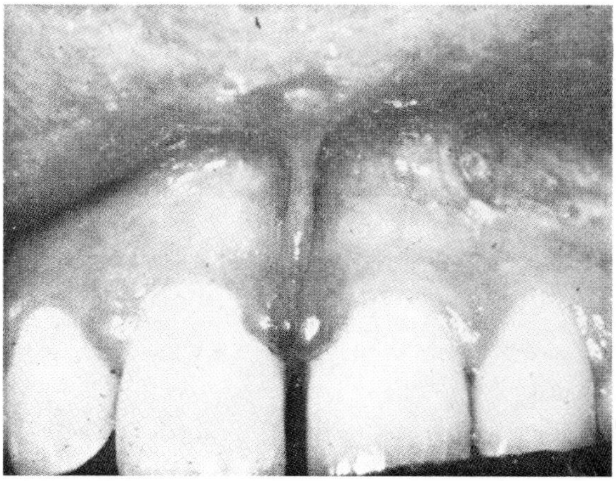

A

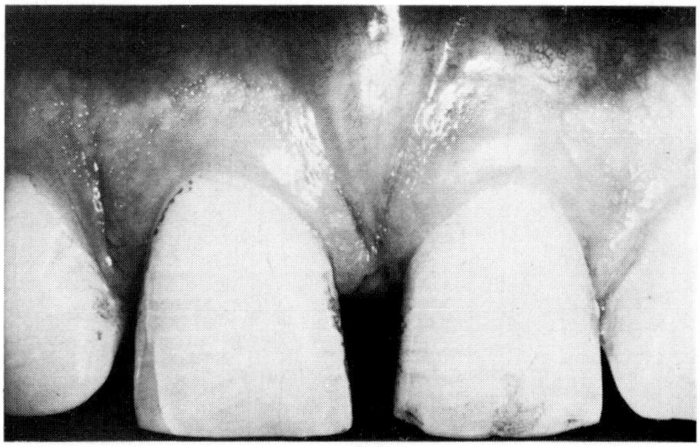

B

FIG. 162.—(*A*) Labial frenum which interferes with toothbrushing and so maintains a marginal gingivitis. (*B*) Pronounced labial frenum without any associated gingival disease in a 40-year-old man.

When gingival recession occurs the band of attached gingiva becomes narrower, and a periodontal lesion may extend into alveolar mucosa (Fig. 164). This is particularly common in the lower posterior region where the attached gingiva is very narrow in health. Removal of the lesion by simple gingivectomy would result in:

(a) a reduction in the depth of the vestibule so that the gingival margin area is extremely difficult to keep clean.

(b) the creation of a gingival margin from alveolar mucosa. Alveolar mucosa is normally not well keratinized, is comparatively fragile, and is loosely bound down to the underlying periosteum. Although changes must take place in the new marginal tissue after gingivectomy in response to change in function, it is unlikely that this tissue will form a hardy and streamlined gingival margin capable of withstanding the stresses to which the region is subject.

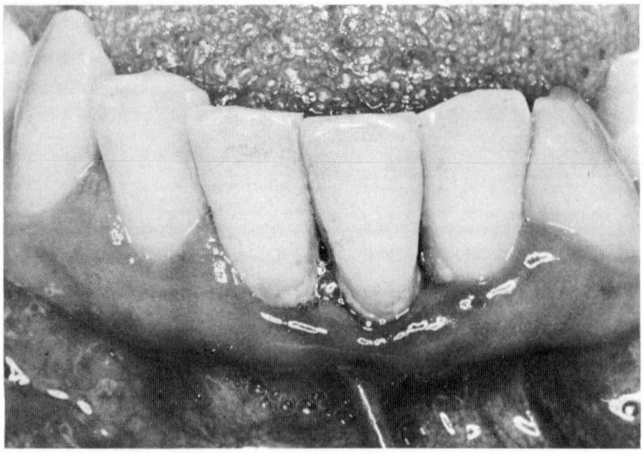

FIG. 163.—Normally placed frenum attached to marginal tissue after recession has taken place. Retraction of the lip opens the pockets.

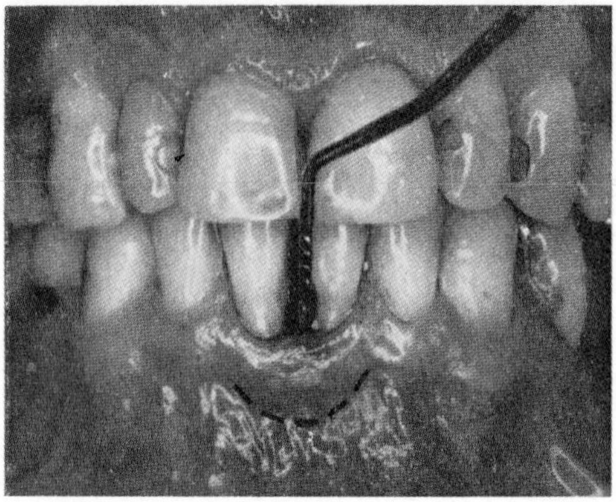

FIG. 164.—Pocketing extends into area of alveolar mucosa in a 44-year-old man. The apical limit of the pocket is marked by the black line.

A number of techniques have been devised to solve mucogingival problems; to remove frena and muscle attachments, to deepen the vestibule, and most important to produce a broader zone of attached gingiva.
These are:
1. Frenectomy.
2. Apically repositioned flap.
3. Apically displaced flap.
4. The Edlan technique.
5. Laterally repositioned flap.
6. Free gingival graft.

FRENECTOMY

Frenectomy is indicated where an abnormally large frenum, usually upper labial, interferes with the use of the toothbrush and is responsible for the persistence of gingival inflammation (Fig. 162*A*).

A frenum frequently regenerates following even radical excision but, as the aim of the operation may be limited to repositioning the frenum to a more apical position where it will no longer interfere with toothbrushing, the following simple technique is recommended.

Procedure

1. After inducing anaesthesia the lip is extended and the frenum gripped with mosquito forceps. Incisions are made on either side of the instrument (Fig. 165*A*), the incision on the alveolar side being made close to the alveolar process, and the triangle of frenum tissue is removed (Fig. 165*B*).
2. If the edges of the wound can be approximated without creating tension these are undermined slightly and sutured together (Fig. 165*C*). Frequently this cannot be done, and it may be necessary to widen the wound slightly with lateral incisions so that the edges of the wound can lay smoothly in the vestibule (Fig. 165*D*).
3. Swabs are pressed over the wound to control bleeding, and a firm periodontal dressing is then placed and moulded into the vestibule (Fig. 165*C*). If there are no interdental spaces the dressing is retained by wire or cotton loops tied around the teeth. The patient is not dismissed until the dressing has set and is seen to be securely placed in the vestibule.
4. After one week the dressing and any sutures are removed. Usually healing is rapid and there is rarely need for further dressing.

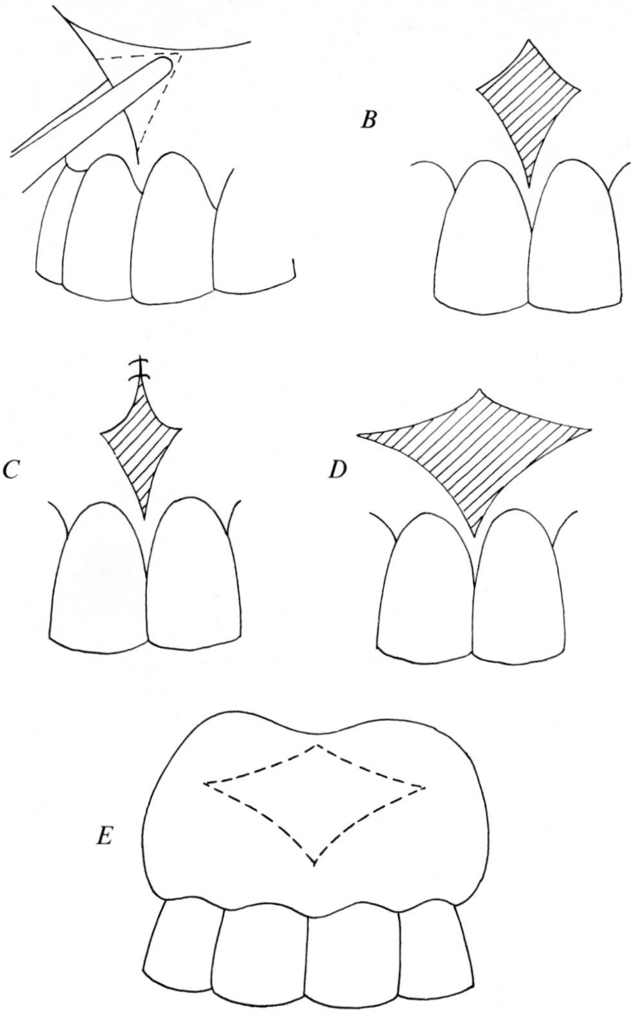

FIG. 165.—Stages in frenectomy procedure.
(*A*) Incision. (*B*) Diamond-shaped wound after frenum tissue is removed. (*C*) Suturing lip wound; it is not often possible to suture the alveolar side of wound. (*D*) Wound widened to allow edges to lie smoothly in vestibule. (*E*) Dressing in place.

THE APICALLY REPOSITIONED FLAP

The early techniques of vestibular deepening had very real disadvantages. Extensive open wounds were made, which healed by secondary intention with consequent prolonged healing time and discomfort. Also the tendency to fibrous tissue contraction was so marked that an initial gain in vestibule depth could be more than lost after several months (Bohannan, 1962a, 1962b, 1963).

The technique of repositioning a mucous membrane flap as described on page 114 represents one of the most useful advances in periodontal surgery (Friedman, 1962). At one operation pockets are eliminated, bone defects exposed for modification, muscle attachments repositioned, the vestibule deepened and a zone of attached gingiva produced. Also if there is sufficient mucosa available the wound is closed so that healing by primary intention can take place. This is without doubt a sound surgical technique; some shrinkage of the vestibule may take place, but this should not be significant.

Procedure

1. A localized flap is made with three incisions. Releasing incisions are extended from the gingival margin across attached gingiva into the vestibule at either end of the operation area. These incisions are joined by a horizontal scalloped incision having an 'inverse' or 'reverse bevel' through the gingival margin so that the pocket wall is separated from the rest of the gingival tissue (Fig. 166). This incision is scalloped so that when the flap is replaced the tissue will fit about the necks of the teeth. If the operation area is extensive no releasing incisions are needed.
2. On the lingual aspect a conventional gingivectomy may be carried out (or flap if necessary).
3. Any tissue of the pocket wall still attached to the teeth is curetted away with all granulations.
4. The teeth are carefully scaled, but the root surfaces are not planed excessively.
5. Any bone surgery is carried out.

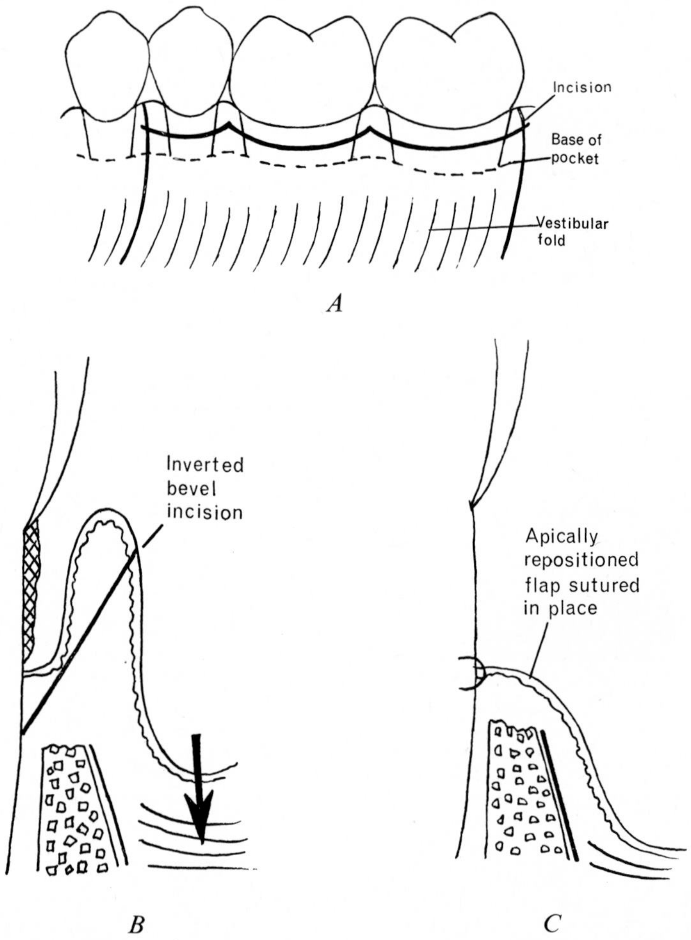

FIG. 166.—The apically repositioned flap technique.
(*A*) Three incisions are made so that a full flap can be raised. (*B*) Gingival tissue is conserved and the pocket wall is separated by using an inverted bevel when making the horizontal incision. After freeing the flap from its attachment to the periosteum it is repositioned deeper in the vestibule. (*C*) After removing all calculus and granulation tissue the flap can be sutured over the wound.

6. Remaining attachments from the periosteum to the base of the flap are incised so that it can be placed more deeply in the vestibule with its edge just covering the alveolar margin (Figs. 166*C* and 167).
7. Modified mattress or sling sutures are placed so that they hold the flap firmly over the bone margin. The suture is inserted from the lingual side into the edge of the flap and then brought back through the same interdental space, carried around the lingual surface of the tooth and through the next interdental space where the flap is caught up again. The suture is then tied on the lingual aspect of the tooth (Fig. 168).

   If instead of a lingual gingivectomy a lingual flap has been raised in order to treat lingual bone defects, the interdental suturing presents little difficulty.
8. A periodontal dressing is placed.
9. The dressing and sutures are removed one week later. Healing is usually uneventful and little tissue shrinkage takes place if the flap has been handled with care.
10. Aftercare is the same as for gingivectomy.

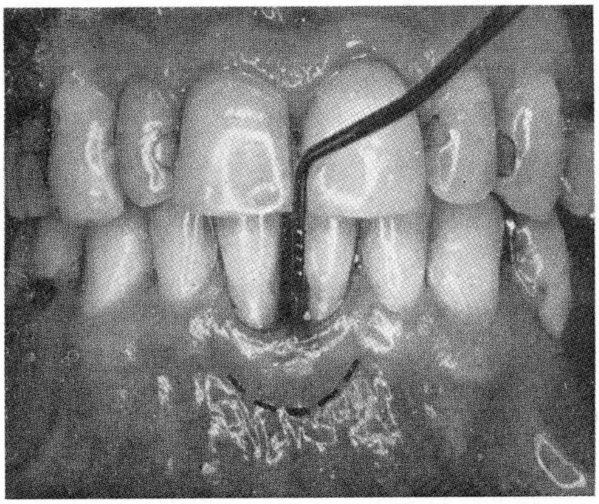

A

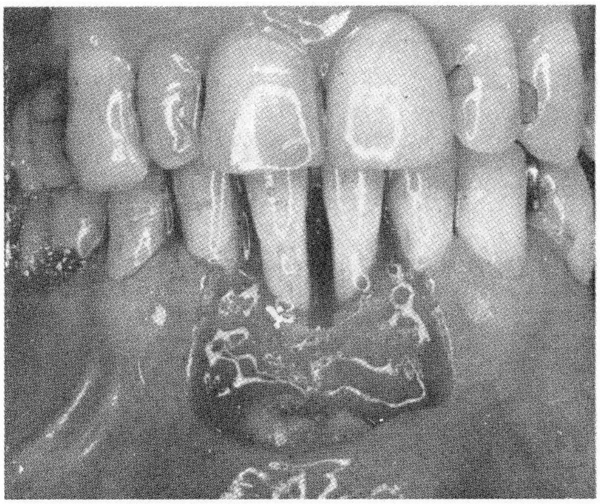

B

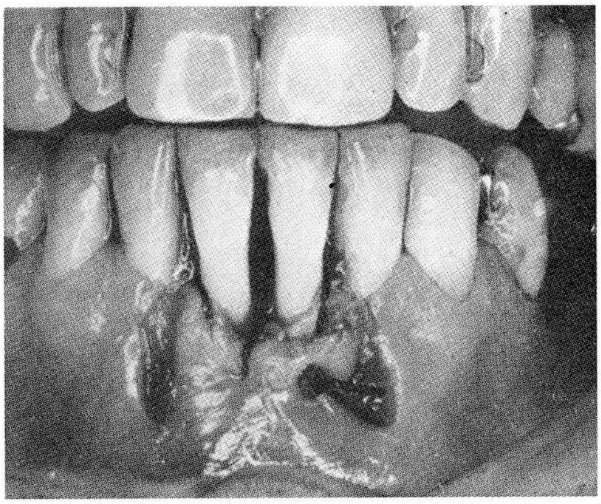

C

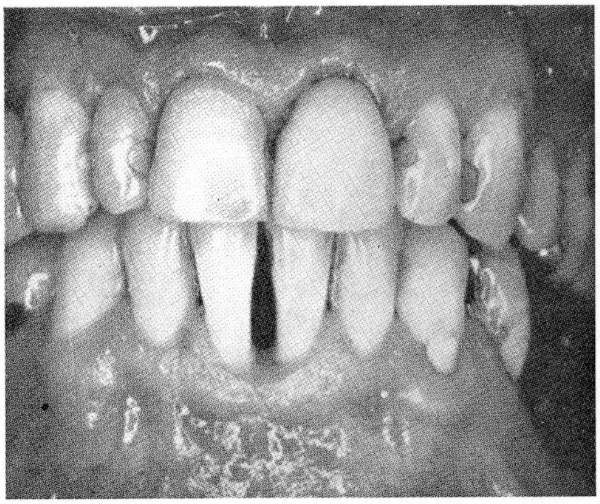

D

FIG. 167.—(*A*) Pocketing extending into alveolar mucosa. (*B*) Flap raised, and calculus and granulation tissue removed. (*C*) Sutures being inserted so that the flap is held over bone margin. (*D*) Six weeks after operation. There is no pocketing, the vestibule is deepened and a zone of attached gingiva has been created.

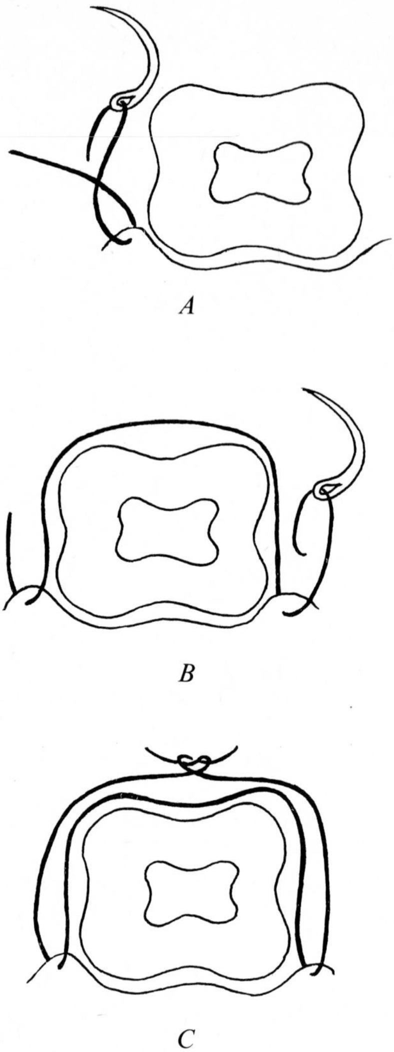

FIG. 168.—The modified mattress suture used to support the apically repositioned flap.

(*A*) The needle is inserted into the edge of the flap from the buccal side. (*B*) The suture is taken around the lingual side of the tooth and the edge of the flap is caught up again, this time from the lingual side. (*C*) The suture is taken back through the interdental space and is tied on the lingual surface of the tooth.

THE APICALLY DISPLACED FLAP

The apically displaced flap and apically repositioned flap techniques are essentially the same. They both aim to produce a zone of attached gingiva and to deepen the vestibule, but in the latter procedure the soft tissue also covers the alveolar process. Where the amount of mucosa is limited, deepening the vestibule and covering the alveolar process become conflicting aims and if deepening the vestibule is the primary aim the alveolar periosteum must remain uncovered to heal by secondary intention. Each area has to be assessed at the time of surgery and the technique modified to the best purpose. Fig. 169 illustrates a case where tissue destruction over the central incisors was much greater than that over the laterals and canines, therefore the alveolar process could be covered in the latter area but not in the former. In those cases where one can predict that there will be insufficient tissue to cover the alveolar process and deepen the vestibule the following technique can be used.

Procedure (Fig. 170)

1. The gingival margin is incised with an inverted bevel. The incision can be straight, there is no need to make a scalloped incision as the flap margin will not be placed around the necks of the teeth.
2. If attached gingiva is left releasing incisions are made over the canines or first premolars (in this case the incision must be short to avoid the metal nerve) and the attached gingiva is lifted with a periosteal elevator. This blunt dissection must be done with care to avoid tearing the flap.
3. Sharp dissection is carried out (No. 15 Bard-Parker blade) to separate the loose alveolar mucosa connective tissue and mentalis muscle from the periosteum to the required depth.
4. In the base of the wound a horizontal incision about $\frac{1}{2}$-inch in length is made through the periosteum to bone. This creates a 'fenestration' which heals with a scar and is meant to prevent contraction of the vestibule past this point.
5. The edge of the flap is then sutured down to the underlying tissue in the depth of the vestibule. Several interrupted sutures with black silk (3–0) are used.

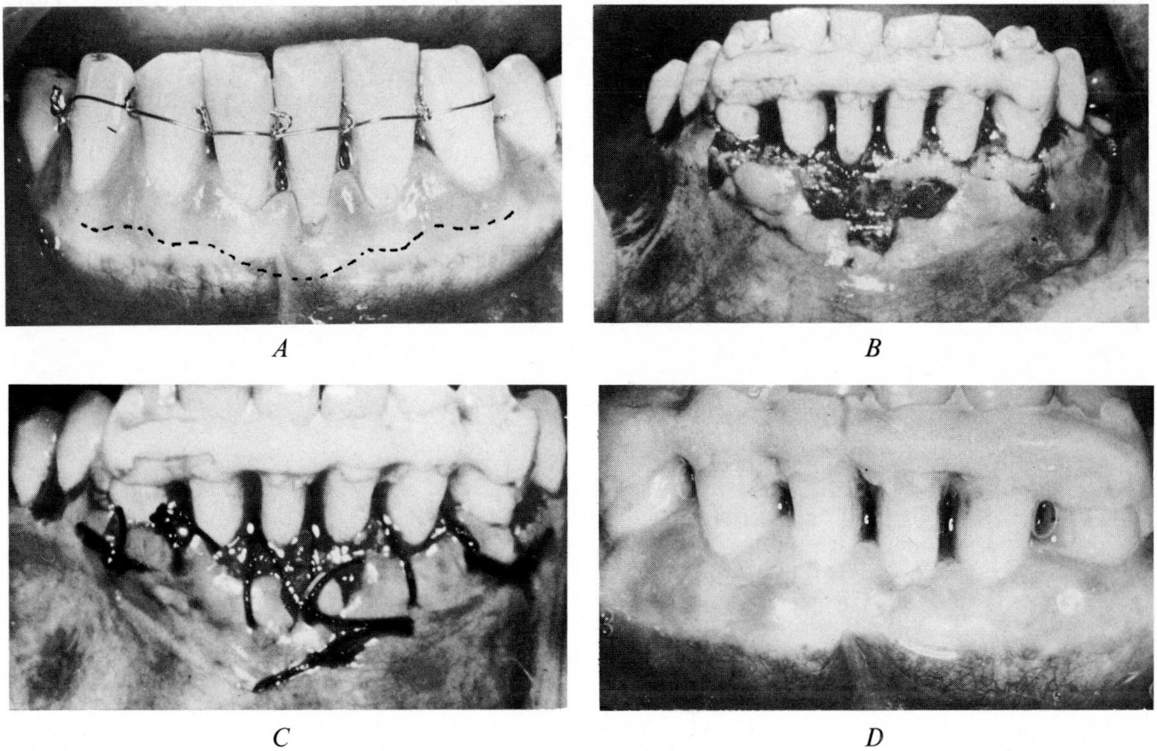

Fig. 169.—Case demonstrating both apically repositioned flap at $\overline{3/3}$ and apically displaced flap at $\overline{21/12}$ where amount of tissue needed to cover alveolar process is inadequate. (*A*) Prior to surgery: deep pocketing apical to muco-gingival line at $\overline{21/12}$. (*B*) Dissection of flap and mentalis muscle. (*C*) Flap sutured: deep suture through mentalis and suspensory sutures holding flap margin: periosteum exposed at $\overline{21/12}$. (*D*) 8-weeks post-operative appearance showing adequate zone of attached gingiva.

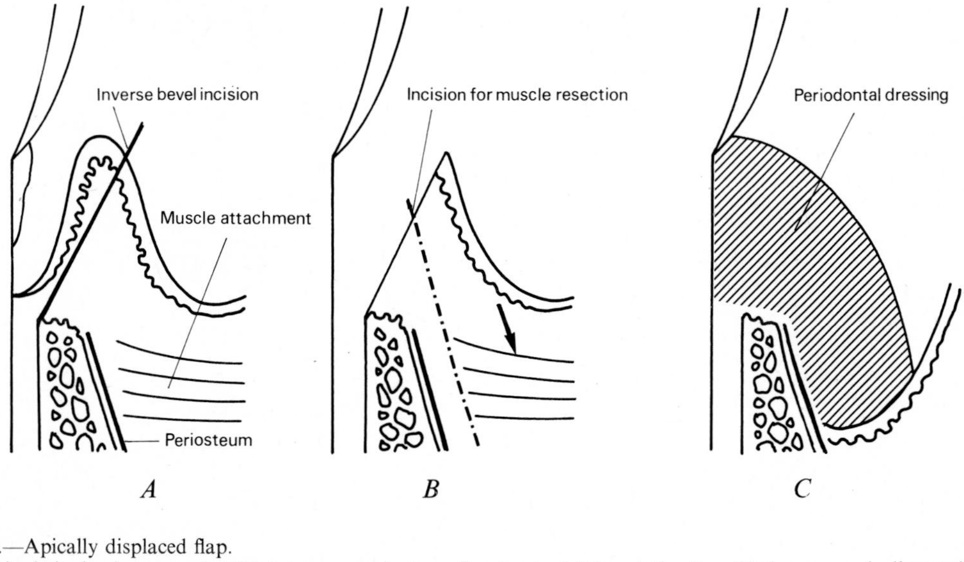

Fig. 170.—Apically displaced flap.

(*A*) Marginal gingiva is removed. (*B*) (a) A mucoperiosteum flap is raised ('denudation') or (b) the mucosa is dissected from the periosteum ('periosteal retention'). Muscle attachments are dissected through so that soft tissue can be moved apically. (*C*) Edge of flap is sutured and dressing placed.

6. A periodontal dressing is placed to cover the wound. Care is taken that the dressing fills the depths of the vestibular wound.
7. The dressing is changed after one week. The original dressing is gently removed. The wound is irrigated with warm water, gently dried and then coated with a topical anaesthetic. A second dressing is placed. As the wound can be very sensitive the dressing must be applied while still soft and care taken before the patient is dismissed that the dressing has not been displaced coronally.
8. Dressings are changed at weekly intervals for two or three weeks by which time the wound should be well epithelialized.

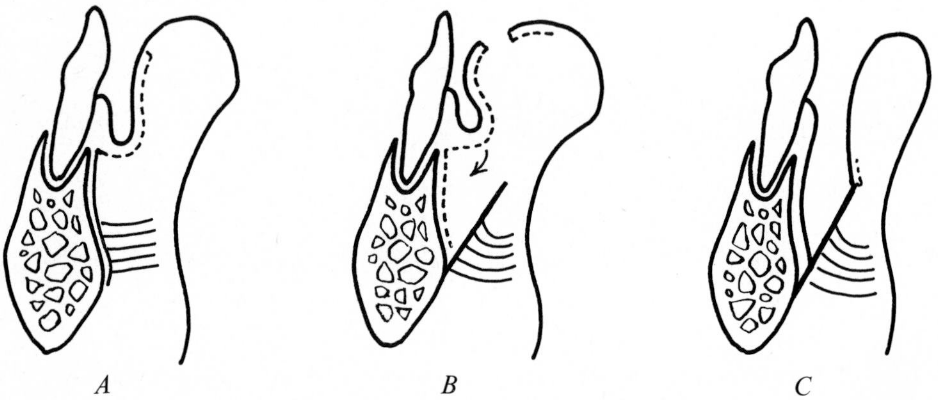

FIG. 171.—The Edlan technique for vestibular deepening.
(*A*) Lip mucosa is dissected as far back as the alveolar process. (*B*) Periosteum is lifted so that lip mucosa can fall back on bone. (*C*) The periosteum is sutured to the edge of the lip wound to create the new labial aspect of the vestibule.

THE EDLAN TECHNIQUE

This technique was devised by Edlan and Mejchar (1963) to help improve denture retention where the lower labial vestibule was shallow. It involves a different approach to the problem of deepening the vestibule. Tissue from the inside of the lip is dissected back as far as the alveolar process. Periosteum is then dissected and the position of the lip mucosa and periosteum exchanged so that the lip mucosa can fall back on to the bone. The periosteum is then sutured to the edge of the lip wound to form the labial aspect of the new vestibule (Fig. 171).

The depth of the vestibule is effectively increased by this technique but while it is a useful procedure in prosthetic surgery its application to the treatment of periodontal disease is limited.

THE LATERALLY REPOSITIONED FLAP

This procedure has been devised for covering isolated areas of exposed root with gingival tissue (Grupe and Warren, 1956). Gross gingival recession about one tooth is a fairly common condition found most frequently on the labial aspect of a lower incisor. In many cases the tooth is placed labially so that initially the buccal plate of bone may have been very thin or even absent. In some cases a labial frenum is inserted into the margin of the gingival defect and may have contributed to its formation (Fig. 172). The defect is generally full of debris and calculus and quickly refills after scaling. Frequently the tooth involved suffers excessive occlusal stress in protrusive excursions, and when this is so the occlusion should be adjusted prior to surgery.

A laterally repositioned or 'sliding flap' procedure is indicated when there is little or no pocketing in the region, and the defect is deep and localized to one tooth. It becomes unnecessary when there is deep pocketing on adjacent teeth, as the general surgical procedure normally involves the defect. When a frenum is present frenectomy may be carried out first and the resulting contour re-appraised.

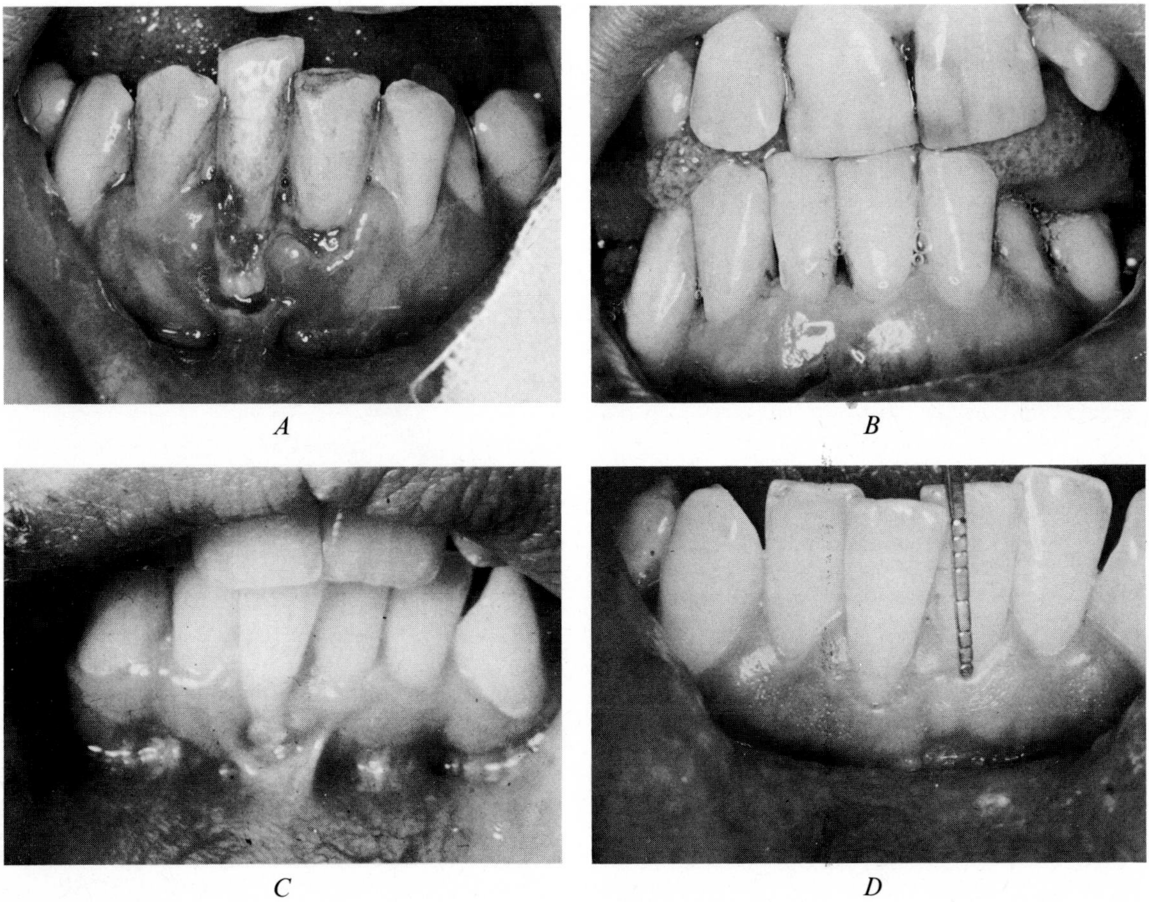

FIG. 172.—(*A*) Isolated gingival recession, gross calculus plus inflammation. (*B*) Three-month's post-scaling and laterally repositioned flap. (*C*) Isolated gingival recession in a 19-year-old youth. The involved lower incisor is placed slightly labially and a labial frenum may interfere with proper cleaning of the area. (*D*) Four years later. Slight recession has occurred but no pocket was discernible.

Procedure

1. All debris and calculus is removed from the gingival defect.
2. The edges of the defect are excised (Fig. 173).
3. The exposed root is thoroughly planed and all tissue tags carefully curetted so that the bone margins of the defect are exposed.
4. At a point two teeth distant from the defect a vertical incision is made from the gingival margin into the vestibule. The vertical incisions are joined by a horizontal incision through the margin (Fig. 173*B*). The mucous membrane flap is very gently freed from the underlying periosteum. If it tears failure is inevitable. The dissection must be carried deep into the vestibule so that the flap is freely movable and can be swung over the defect without any tension at its base (Fig. 173*C*).
5. If the initial incisions are made correctly exact apposition of the flap presents no problem and the flap can be sutured into its new position. Very great care must be taken to ensure that the flap fits tightly around the neck of the affected tooth, and that no 'eye-let' defect is left in the vestibule.
6. A light dressing is applied over the whole area; pressure might cause the flap to necrose. 'Orabase', a soft periodontal dressing like Coe-pak, or a cyanoacrylate dressing may be applied directly over the wound, or on top of a layer of dry-foil which is placed over the closed incision.

The patient is instructed to be careful not to traumatize the wound and not to extend his lip too vigorously. Post-operative pain is rare, and any swelling can be controlled by applying ice-packs. The sutures are removed after five days. Even after this short period healing at the suture line is advanced and the denuded area is covered by granulations. Two weeks after the operation this area is well epithelialized and the incision line has almost faded. At this time it is important not to probe for a gingival crevice in the area of the defect. When the patient is seen a month later gentle probing generally fails to detect a pocket.

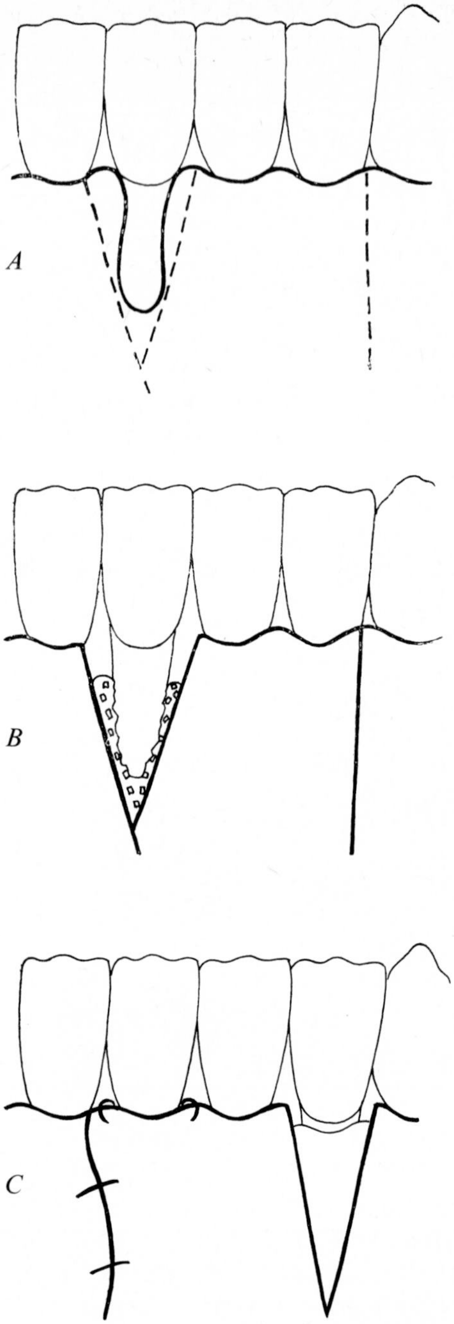

FIG. 173.—The laterally repositioned flap procedure.
(*A*) Three incisions are made; one each on either side of the defect and a third far enough away to maintain a good blood supply to the flap. (*B*) The marginal tissue of the defect is removed and all calculus and granulation tissue removed. (*C*) The flap is swung over and sutured into place.

Comment

It is reasonable to think that the procedure must replace a gingival defect by a deep pocket. In practice, if a suitable case is chosen, *i.e.* a single gross defect in an otherwise fairly healthy area, and the procedure is carried out carefully, a detectable pocket is only occasionally produced (Fig. 172*C*). Although it is not possible to say that a fibrous attachment between flap and tooth has been created, a very close adaptation certainly results in many cases. Given a good standard of oral hygiene a healthy margin can be maintained for several years, and even where some recession of the gingival margin recurs the situation is usually a considerable improvement on the original condition.

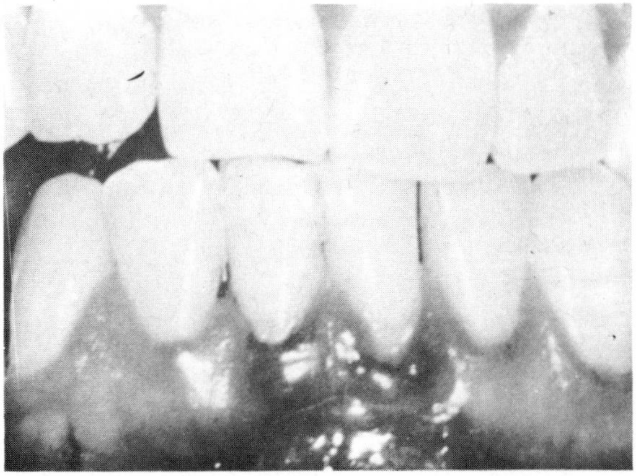

A

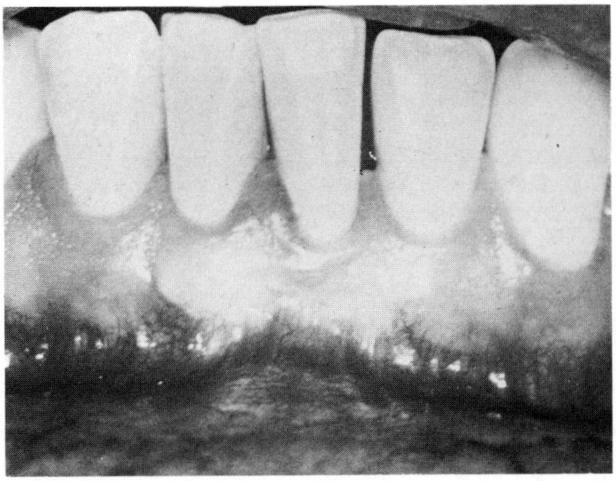

B

FIG. 174.—Free gingival graft. (*A*) Inflammation and pocketing extending through zone of attached gingiva into aveolar mucosa. (*B*) Tissue replaced by free graft from palate to form zone of attached gingiva.

FREE GINGIVAL GRAFT

Limitations of the usual methods of obtaining an acceptable zone of attached gingiva, particularly where a muscle attachment or frenum involves the gingival margin, are shrinkage of the vestibule and reformation of the muscle attachment. These difficulties can be overcome and a predictably wide zone of attached gingiva obtained in localized areas by using a graft of oral mucosa obtained from a suitable donor site (Bjorn, 1963; Nabers, 1966).

Procedure

1. Where pocketing is present it may be removed by simple gingivectomy and curettage. Where pocketing is shallow or absent and the aim is simply to widen the zone of attached gingiva the gingival margin can be left intact.
2. Vertical incisions are made in either side of the area to be deepened. If the gingival margin is to be left intact a horizontal incision is made at the level of the mucogingival junction. If a gingivectomy has been carried out a muco-periosteal flap is raised in the usual way. The alveolar mucosa is dissected back from the underlying periosteum to about twice the width of attached gingiva required, *i.e.* about 10 mm (Fig. 174).
3. Bleeding is controlled by pressure with a swab, and a pocket measuring probe is used to determine the dimensions of the wound. A template of tinfoil can also be cut to size.
4. A donor site is picked. The graft must be made of masticatory mucosa and suitable tissue is found at either (a) the palate, (b) an edentulous area or (c) a neighbouring site with a broad zone of attached gingiva. The graft is outlined on the donor site with a No. 15 Swann-Morton Blade, and a partial thickness graft (2 mm thick) of epithelium and connective tissue is carefully dissected.

   Control of the graft is greatly facilitated by placing sutures through the edges of the graft as it is raised.

   Once the graft is free any tags are trimmed and if it seems too thick the under-surface can be scraped gently to thin the tissue.

5. With as little delay as possible the graft is transferred to the recipient site. It is essential that the graft is firmly adapted to the underlying connective tissue with a minimum thickness of blood clot. The graft is immobilized by suturing it to the edge of the recipient site with very thin silk (5/0: Ethicon 500). In doing this the graft should be fully extended but not stretched. Pressure with a swab on the graft is maintained for 3 minutes to ensure close adaptation of the tissues.
6. The graft and donor site are covered with a periodontal dressing, *e.g.* a cyanoacrylate for one week after which the sutures can be removed from the graft and the wounds left uncovered. Post-operative instructions are the same as for gingivectomy.

Revascularization of the graft begins to take place after 2–3 days but the graft remains morphologically distinct for several months.

The graft shrinks to some extent and, therefore, it is necessary to overestimate the width of attached tissue required, but it does effectively maintain an acceptable width of attached gingiva and vestibular depth (Fig. 175).

Attempts have been made to cover denuded root surface but except for narrow clefts, without success. In this situation the blood supply is inadequate and the graft becomes necrotic re-exposing the root surface. In the treatment of isolated gingival recession the laterally repositioned flap technique remains the method of choice.

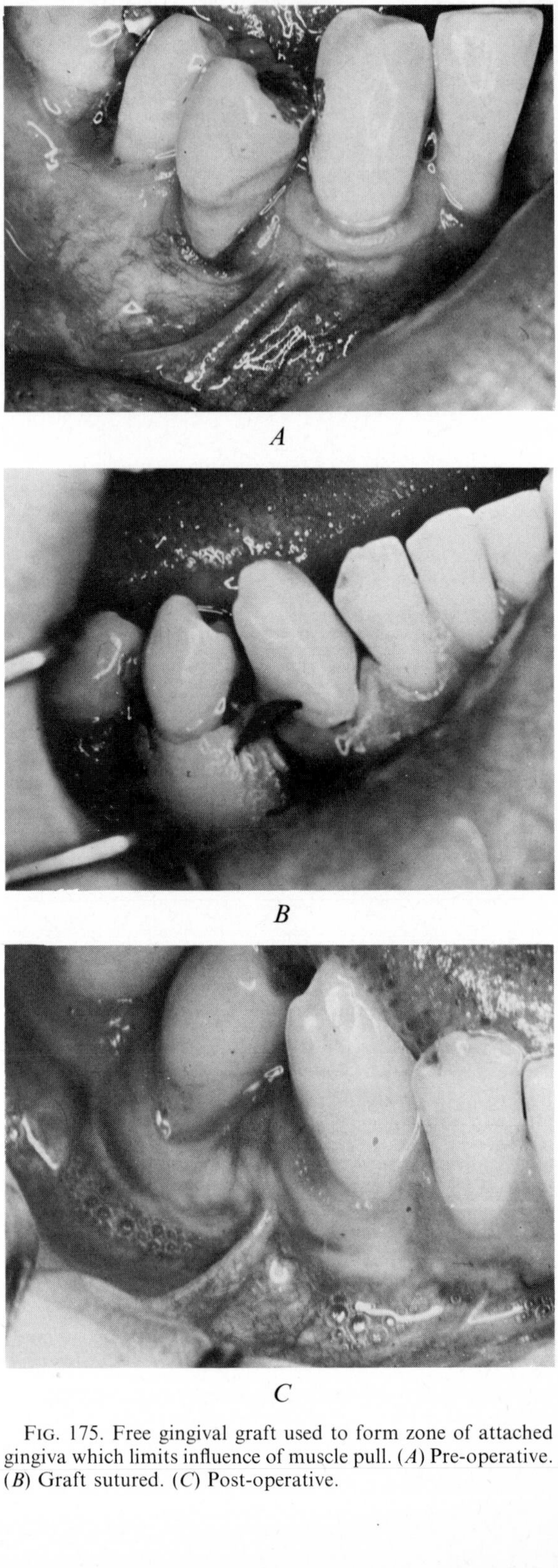

A

B

C

FIG. 175. Free gingival graft used to form zone of attached gingiva which limits influence of muscle pull. (*A*) Pre-operative. (*B*) Graft sutured. (*C*) Post-operative.

REFERENCES

BERGENHOLTZ, A. and HUGOSON, A. (1967). Vestibular sulcus extension surgery in cases with periodontal disease. *J. periodont. Res.*, **2**, 221.
BJORN, H. (1963). Free transplantation of gingiva propria. *Sveriges Tandlak. T.*, **22**, 684.
BOHANNAN, H. M. (1962a). Studies in alteration of vestibular depth. I. Complete denudation. *J. Periodont.*, **33**, 120.
BOHANNAN, H. M. (1962b). Studies in alteration of vestibular depth. II. Periosteal retention. *J. Periodont.*, **33**, 354.
BOHANNAN, H. M. (1963). Studies in alteration of vestibular depth. III. Vestibular incision. *J. Periodont.*, **34**, 209.
BOWERS, G. M. (1963). A study of the width of the attached gingiva. *J. Periodont.*, **34**, 201.
EDLAN, A. and MEJCHAR, B. (1963). Plastic surgery of the vestibulum in periodontal therapy. *Int. dent. J.*, **13**, 593.
FRIEDMAN, N. (1962). Mucogingival surgery. The apically repositioned flap. *J. Periodont.*, **33**, 328.
GOTTSEGEN, R. (1954). Frenum position and vestibule depth in relation to gingival health. *Oral Surg.*, **7**, 1069.
GRUPE, H. E. and WARREN, R. F. (1956). Repair of gingival defects by a sliding flap operation. *J. Periodont.*, **27**, 92.
NABERS, C. L. (1966). Free gingival grafts. *Periodontics*, **4**, 243.

12. The Periodontal Abscess

Abscess formation may follow physical damage to the periodontal tissues, or occur by extension of infection from a periodontal pocket. A deep periodontal defect is a very narrow and irregular sinus which is easily blocked by tissue swelling, blood clot, food debris or calculus. An abscess forms if there is an obstruction to drainage. It is also possible that micro-organisms are carried from the pocket through blood or lymph vessels into deeper tissues and there cause tissue breakdown and suppuration. Frequently excessive occlusal stress appears to be a contributory factor in the aetiology of an abscess (Fig. 180*A*).

A periodontal abscess is also sometimes caused by incomplete surgical removal of a periodontal pocket. Tissue shrinkage after surgery may result in the remaining tissue of the pocket wall closing over the incompletely removed contents of the pocket so that drainage is impeded. This happens most frequently in relation to pockets at the bifurcation or trifurcation of a molar, and is avoided by radical removal of the pocket wall.

The abscess, initially, is either acute or chronic. After discharge of an acute abscess a chronic abscess remains, and if untreated may undergo recurrent acute changes. With each recurrent episode more alveolar bone is destroyed.

CLINICAL FEATURES

The clinical features are best described according to the stages of abscess development.

Stage I
The onset of abscess formation is signalled by a deep throbbing pain. The associated tooth becomes slightly loose and sensitive to touch. The overlying gingiva may be red, swollen and tender. Associated lymph glands sometimes enlarge. There is *no fluctuation* or discharge of pus.

Stage II
The pus may burst into the periodontal pocket in which case the pain diminishes, or it may track through the alveolar bone and form an abscess under the alveolar mucoperiosteum (Fig. 176). This abscess swelling is red, shiny, fluctuant and sensitive to touch, and most frequently appears on the labial aspect over the tooth involved (Fig. 177). Occasionally a palatal swelling arises (Fig. 178). If untreated the abscess bursts or, less commonly, the infection spreads.

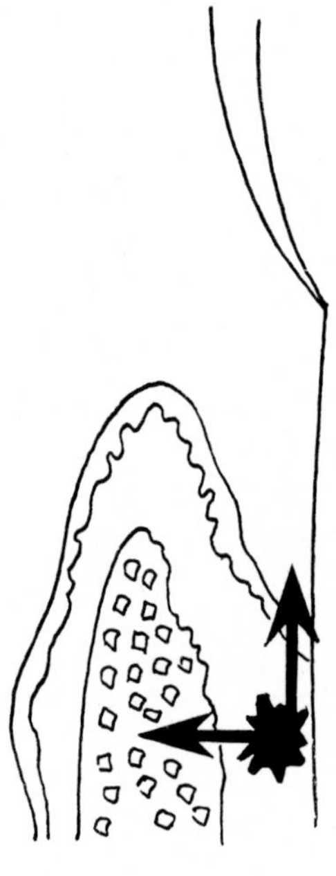

FIG. 176.—The pus may burst into the periodontal pocket, or may track through the alveolar bone.

Stage III
Spread of infection into surrounding tissues and development of a cellulitis may occur if the condition is neglected, or the patient's tissue resistance is low. If the abscess is in the upper jaw the patient will present with a swollen face, swollen lip or even a swollen lower eyelid (depending on the site of origin of the abscess). If there is spread of infection from a lower molar, there may be trismus and difficulty in swallowing apart from facial swelling. Whatever the site, the patient suffers a dull aching pain, is obviously unwell and may have a raised temperature.

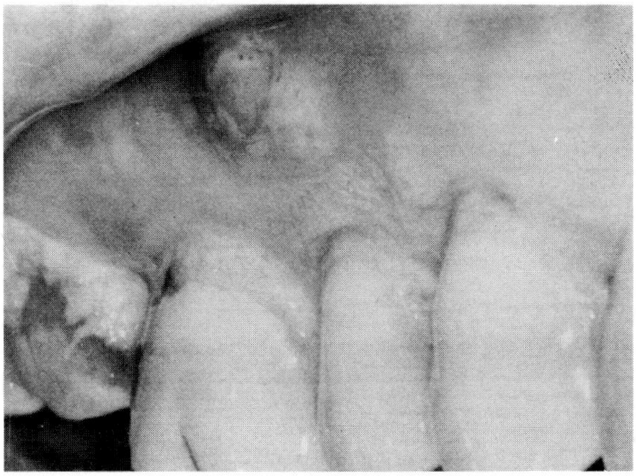

FIG. 177.—Acute periodontal abscess involving an upper first molar.

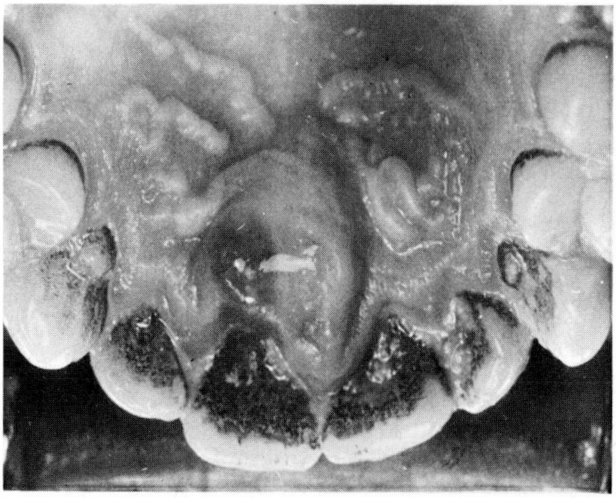

FIG. 178.—Acute periodontal abscess which has tracked through to palatal mucosa.

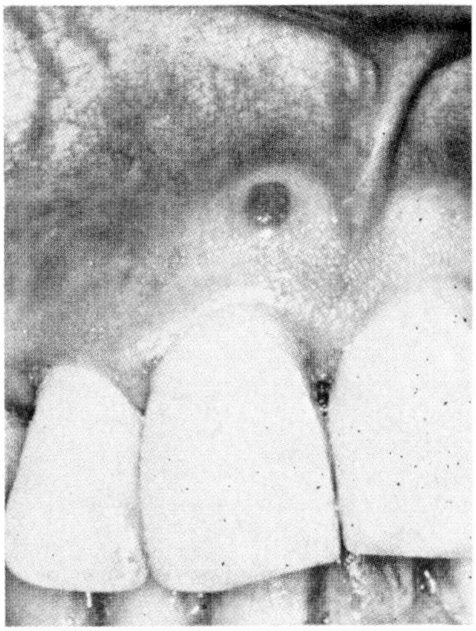

A

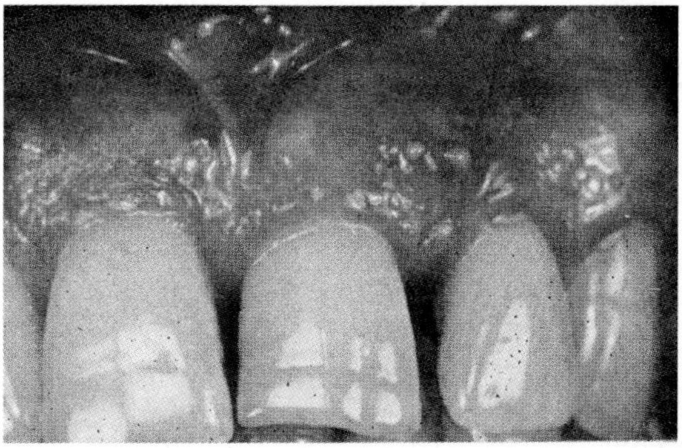

B

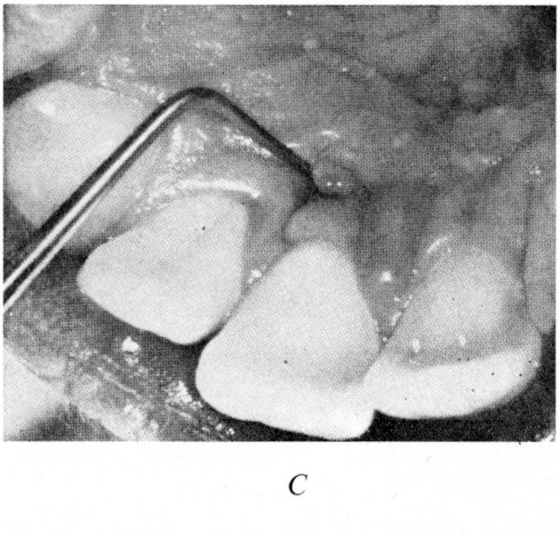

C

FIG. 179.—(*A*) Bead of granulation marking the site of abscess sinus. (*B*) Pus exuding from sinus of abscess between |12. (*C*) Sinus through which the root of the tooth could be probed without discomfort.

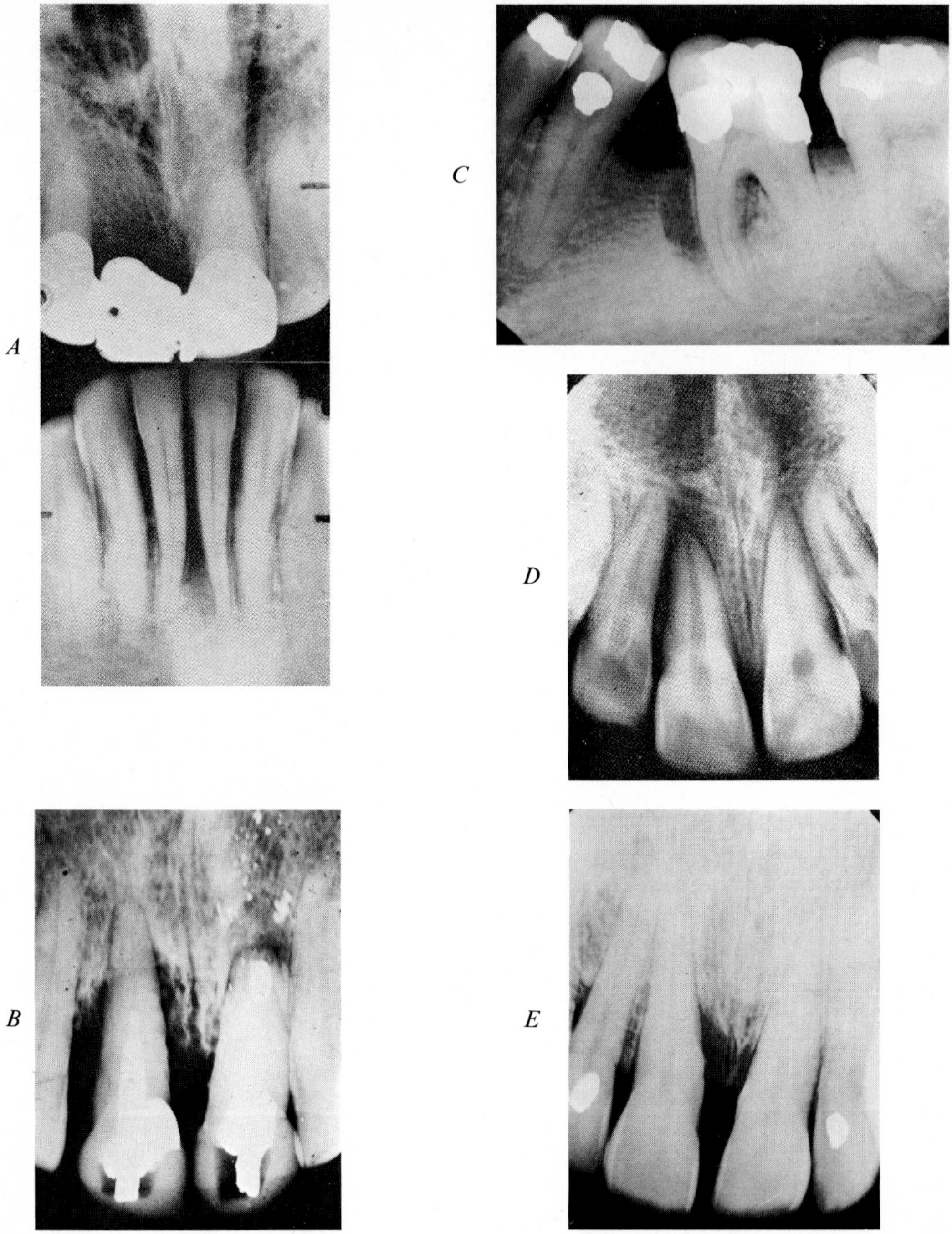

FIG. 180.—The radiographic appearance of a periodontal abscess varies considerably.

(*A*) Diminished radiodensity between lower central incisors marks the site of an abscess. These teeth were traumatized in protrusive excursions by a bridge inserted in the upper jaw one year previously. (*B*) Periodontal abscess on 1| indicated by diminished radiodensity around the root. The crown on this tooth was in traumatic occlusion. (*C*) A periodontal abscess on the buccal aspect of the mesial root of a lower molar. (*D*) The incisor shown in Fig. 179 (*C*). The only sign is widening of periodontal space. (*E*) Typical appearance of abscess which has burst into the periodontal pocket to form an infrabony pocket.

Stage IV
If the abscess bursts and the acute inflammation subsides a chronic abscess with a sinus tract remains. The exit of the sinus is usually marked by a small bead of granulation tissue on the gingival mucosa, from which pus may drain (Fig. 179). Pressure over the area increases the flow of pus. The chronic abscess is frequently asymptomatic except perhaps for some discomfort and mobility of the tooth. Recurrent episodes of acute inflammation are marked by a dull gnawing pain, an increase in tooth mobility and sensitivity, and an inclination on the patient's part to grind on the tooth.

Radiographic Appearance
In the initial stages of abscess formation no bone change is evident on the radiograph. After about one week the abscess is seen as a localized radiolucent area in relation to the side of the root. Its appearance is determined by the site and the amount of bone damage. A recently-formed abscess usually appears as an area of diminished radiodensity, while in long standing cases the abscess may appear as a well-defined area of radiolucency sometimes delinated by a 'lamina dura' (Fig. 180).

Differential Diagnosis
Sometimes it is difficult to distinguish a periodontal (or lateral) abscess from a periapical abscess. This is particularly so in the initial stage of abscess formation before changes have appeared on the radiograph, unless the acute abscess forms at the site of a chronic lesion.

If the tooth is vital the abscess is likely to be periodontal; when the tooth is non-vital it may be either periodontal or periapical. A detailed history and careful examination of the gingival crevice all around the tooth and not merely in the neighbourhood of the abscess swelling, usually makes diagnosis possible; a deep pocket with exudation of pus indicates that the lesion is lateral to the root (Fig. 181). In the later stages of abscess formation, the radiograph provides positive evidence of bone destruction, which is seen to be at the side of the tooth.

Occasionally a periapical abscess spreads up the side of the root, or a periodontal abscess enlarges to involve the periapical region. In either case a definitive diagnosis may not be possible in the initial stages, and in fact is not essential to the establishment of emergency treatment.

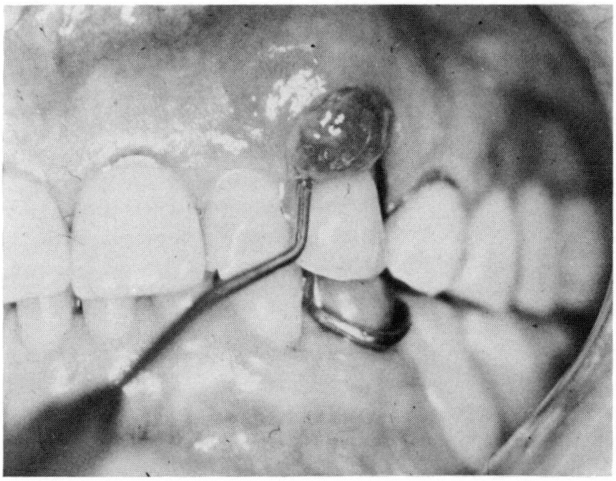

FIG. 181.—A periodontal abscess being probed from the gingival crevice. This case also shows proliferation of granulation tissue from the lesion.

TREATMENT OF THE PERIODONTAL ABSCESS

The development of an acute periodontal abscess is generally regarded as justification for tooth extraction. In fact, where bone destruction is not great, conservative treatment has a high success rate. Treatment is divided into two stages; the acute phase and the chronic phase.

Treatment of the Acute Phase
The aims of this phase of treatment are the relief of pain, the control of spread of infection, and the establishment of drainage. The methods employed depend upon the stage of abscess formation.

Stage I
1. Relieve the occlusion by grinding the *opposing* tooth.
2. Prescribe hot salt water mouthwashes: $\frac{1}{2}$ teaspoonful of salt in a tumblerful of hot water to be used every two hours.
3. Prescribe systemic antibiotic: penicillin V (or tetracycline if the patient has a history of sensitivity to penicillin) – one 250 mg capsule to be taken four times a day for five days.

Stage II

1. Relieve the occlusion by grinding the *opposing* tooth.
2. Prescribe hot salt water mouthwashes as before. Antibiotics are not needed if drainage can be easily established.
3. If the abscess is fluctuant it can be incised under ethyl chloride spray or regional or general anaesthesia, depending on its location and size, the facilities available and the patient's preferences. The incision should be horizontal, parallel with the gingival margin. A vertical incision is likely to result in permanent gingival deformity.

Stage III

1. Immediate intramuscular injection of procaine penicillin (500,000 U) unless penicillin is contraindicated, in which case oral tetracycline is prescribed. Subsequently the antibiotic must be taken by mouth (250 mg capsule) four times a day for five days.
2. Prescribe hot salt water mouthwashes.
3. If the abscess is fluctuant and the patient can open his mouth it may be possible to incise it under ethyl chloride spray. Adjustment of the occlusion can be delayed until the infection is under control.

Once drainage is established and the infection is limited the second stage of treatment may be undertaken.

Treatment of the Chronic Lesion

Treatment depends upon the extent and form of bone destruction. This must be determined as accurately as possible by examination of the pocket and radiographs. There are four possibilities:

(a) The abscess may have drained into the gingival pocket in which case there is an infrabony defect which can be treated as previously described.

(b) The abscess may have broken through the alveolar process so that there is a sinus from the abscess site through the bone with its exit in the attached gingivae or oral mucosa (Fig. 182). Treatment in this case consists of lifting a flap and exposing the defect so that it can be thoroughly curetted; the procedure is similar to the treatment of the infrabony pocket.

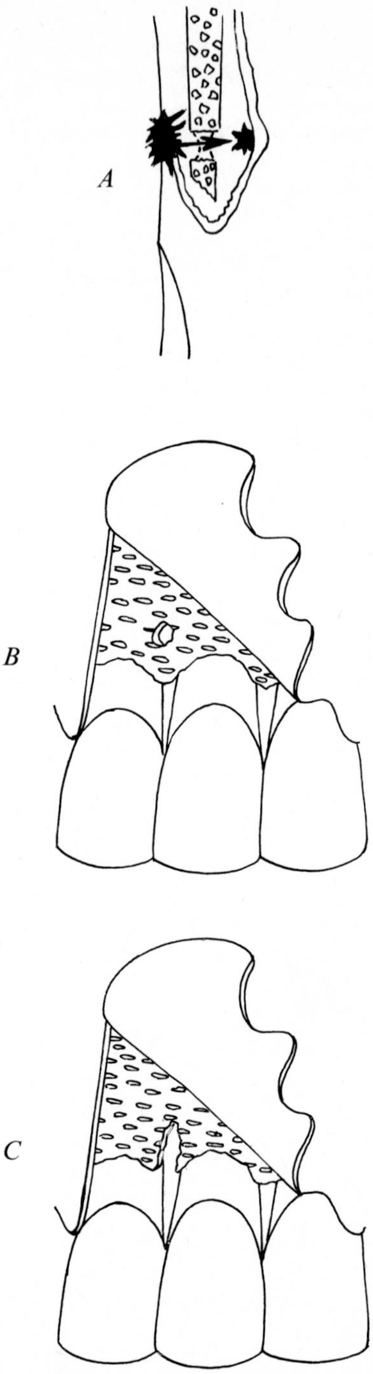

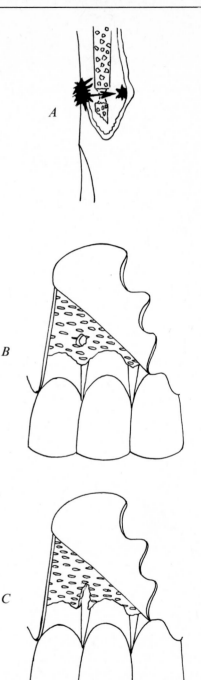

Fig. 182.—(*A*) Perforation of the alveolar process to form a sub-mucoperiosteal abscess. (*B*) Bone destruction may be localized and a marginal bridge of bone remain intact. (*C*) The bone may be destroyed to form a one- or two-walled infrabony defect.

Procedure

1. The occlusion is adjusted to allow mandibular excursions in all directions without stress on the tooth; if necessary the tooth is immobilized with a wire and acrylic splint.
2. After local anaesthesia a flap is lifted so that the defect can be visualized completely (Fig. 183).
3. Root surfaces are cleaned of calculus and granulation tissue (Fig. 184).
4. The bone defect is curetted, great care being taken to ensure that any remaining marginal bone is not further broken down.
5. The lesion is thoroughly irrigated with warm sterile normal saline or boiled water to wash all debris away.
6. The flap is replaced and sutured. If the shape of the gingival margin is poor the flap may be trimmed with scissors before suturing.

The sutures are left in place for one week. Post-operative care is as described for the treatment of the infrabony pocket.

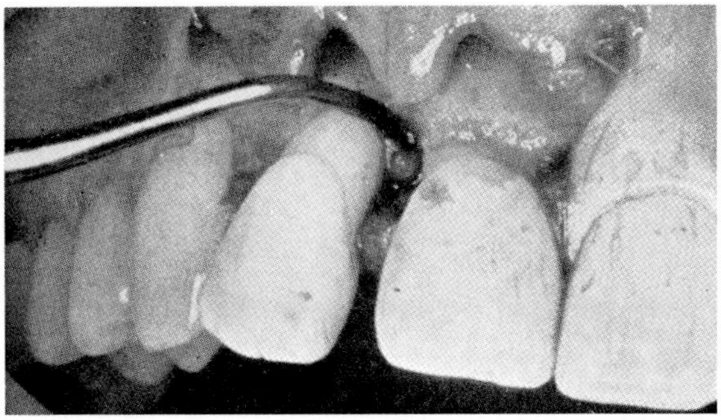

A

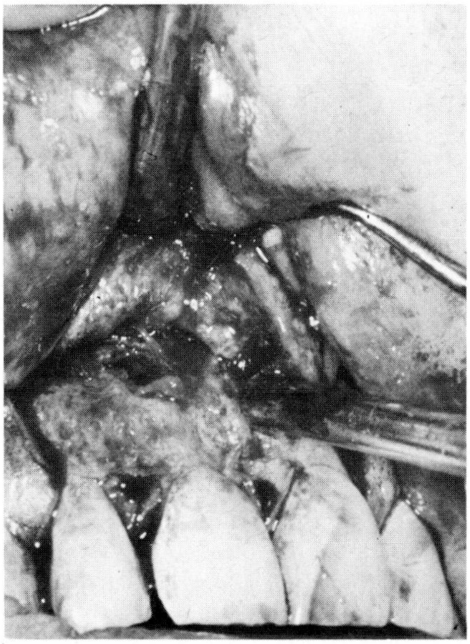

FIG. 183.—The flap is raised to expose both the marginal lesion and any other bone perforation as in Fig. 182 (*B*).

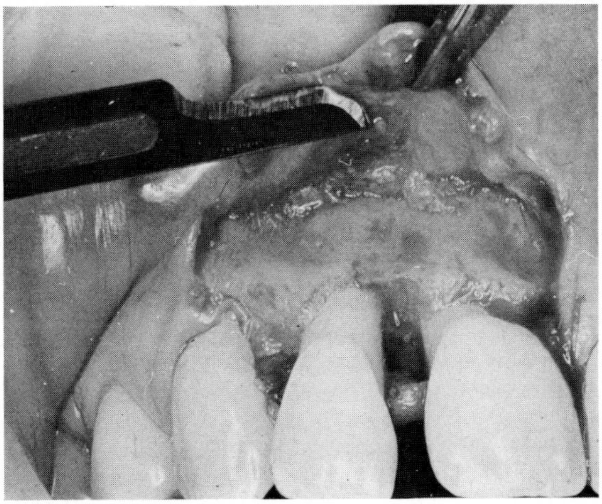

B

FIG. 184.—(*A*) All calculus and granulations are curetted away so that the root surface is clean and the bone defect completely exposed for examination as in (*B*).

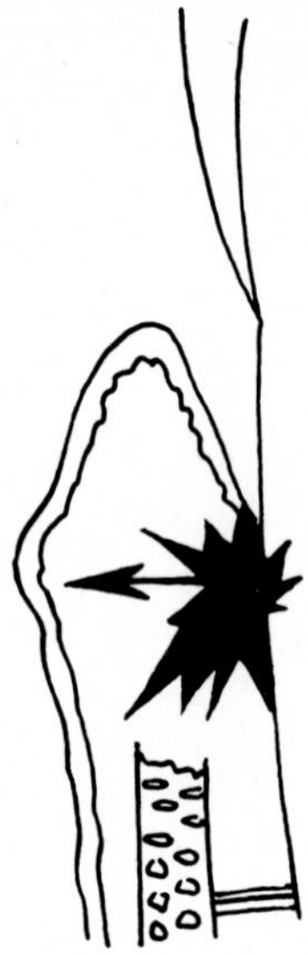

FIG. 185.—A considerable amount of bone may be destroyed so that the abscess is contained within soft tissue. In this situation re-attachment is unlikely to take place after a flap operation.

Procedure

1. The bottom of the pocket is carefully defined and gingivectomy is carried out so that the lesion is completely removed and a gingival shape which allows effective cleansing techniques is attained.
2. The bone defect is explored and curetted.
3. The root surface is planed.
4. If necessary, the shape of the bone margin is altered to allow more effective food shedding and cleansing.
5. A periodontal dressing is placed filling the bone defect. The dressing is replaced at weekly intervals for three weeks.
6. Subsequently special attention has to be paid to devising an oral hygiene technique which will adequately clean the area.

(d) Where the bone damage is extensive and retention of the tooth represents an obvious liability to the health of the neighbouring teeth, it should be extracted. A well designed fixed bridge supported by sound abutment teeth is *always* to be preferred to the retention, even by ingenious means, of a tooth which represents a hazard to the proximal teeth.

(c) Where a considerable amount of alveolar bone has been destroyed the abscess is contained entirely within soft tissue (Fig. 185). This is particularly common on the lingual aspects of molars where the plate of alveolar bone is thin and recession is marked. The form of conservative treatment already described, *i.e.* curettage at flap operation, is almost certainly doomed to failure. As the flap of soft tissue is unsupported by bone, re-attachment and regeneration of bone is highly unlikely and abscess recurrence is almost inevitable. This can be avoided by radical gingivectomy and complete excision of the abscess, but this procedure must result in gross gingival deformity, and extraction is likely to be preferred in the front of the mouth. In the back of the mouth the gingival deformity is not seen, and a multi-rooted tooth is frequently firmly embedded even after considerable bone loss has occurred.

THE COMBINED CHRONIC LATERAL-APICAL ABSCESS

Treatment of a periodontal abscess which has involved the apex, or of a chronic apical abscess which has discharged through the gingival crevice involves both endodontics and periodontal surgery, and results can be rewarding particularly where one root of a multi-rooted tooth is involved (Fig. 186).

Endodontic treatment must be carried out prior to periodontal treatment in order to seal all connections with the involved root and with the apical area.

If the associated bone defect is deep so that it cannot be eliminated by periodontal treatment root resection can be carried out at the time of periodontal surgery (Fig. 187). The bone defect should heal as after a conventional tooth extraction. Care has to be taken that the amputated tooth surface is shaped and polished to allow effective cleaning of the resultant embrasure.

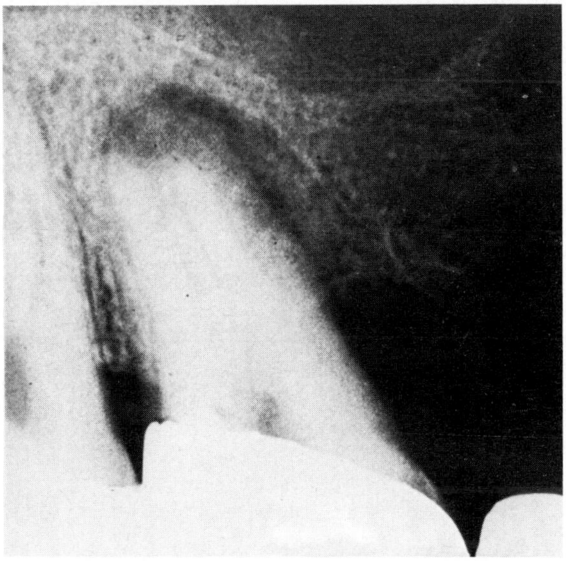

A

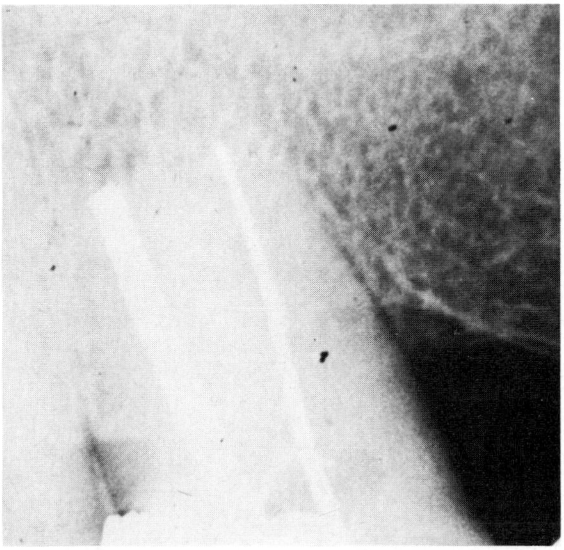

B

FIG. 186.—Radiograph of combined apical-periodontal lesion treated by endodontics and periodontal surgery. (*A*) Pre-treatment. (*B*) 2 years post-operative.

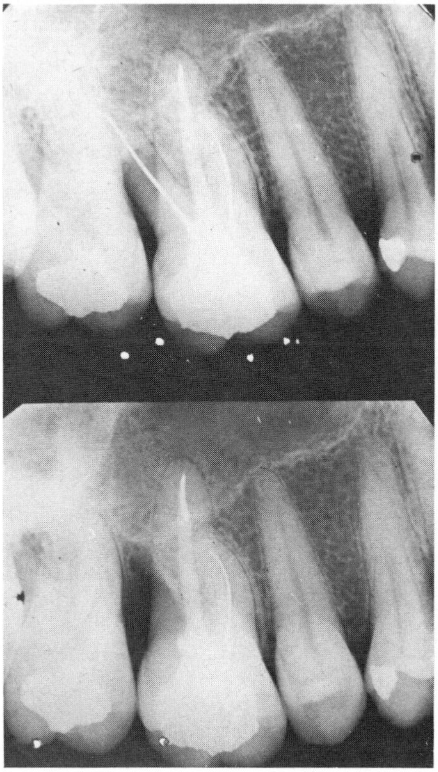

FIG. 187.—Radiographs of combined apical-periodontal lesion treated by endodontics and root resection. (By courtesy of Mr E. Nicholls.)

RECOMMENDED READING

CAHN, L. R. (1961). The pathology and treatment of periapical disease. *Brit. dent. J.*, **111**, 57.
PRICHARD, J. F. (1953). Management of the periodontal abscess. *Oral Surg.*, **6**, 474.
TROTT, J. R. (1959). The acute periodontal abscess. *J. Canad. dent. Ass.*, **25**, 601.

13. Occlusion and the Periodontium

THE NORMAL PERIODONTIUM

The tissues of the periodontium which are apical to the crest of the alveolar housing, the cementum, periodontal ligament and the alveolus itself, have two separate and closely interrelated functions: tooth support and proprioception (Fig. 188).

1. Tooth Support

The first function of the attachment apparatus is the absorption and dissipation of any stress which arises from forces applied to the crown of the tooth. Various theories have been proposed to explain the means by which the supporting tissues actually dissipate masticatory stress. The collagen fibres of the subcrestal part of the ligament make up between 53% and 74% by volume, the blood vessels 1–2% (Götze, 1965) and the remainder is made up of the ground substance and tissue fluid. An analysis of the vascular architecture of the periodontium (Kindlová and Matena, 1962) would seem to indicate a degree of complexity commensurate with some functional significance. One of the earliest theories (Fox, 1833) proposed that the blood vessels act as a hydraulic damping device. The impact of an occlusal force is absorbed and damped down by the extrusion of blood from the ligament, through foramina in the socket wall, or into other vessels in various parts of the ligament. At higher levels of force the alveolus itself distorts, the distortion being dependent upon the areas of tension and compression created in the ligament by the occlusal stress.

There are thus two phases to the movement which a tooth undergoes when an external force is applied, and it would appear that the support mechanism afforded by the periodontal tissues is the same irrespective of the direction of the applied

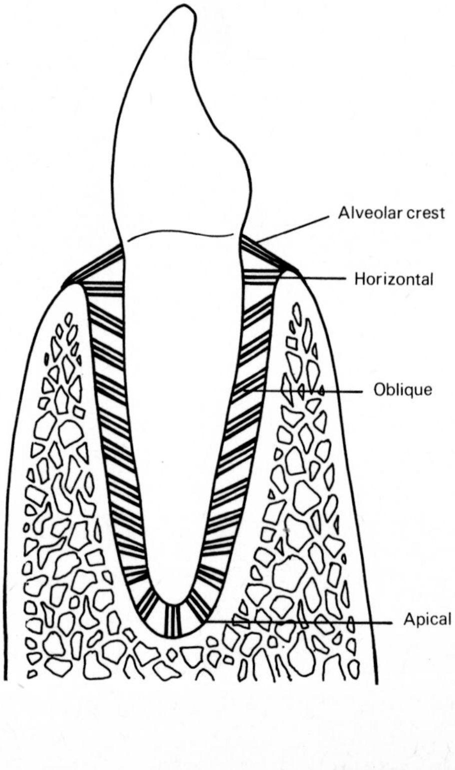

FIG. 188.—The attachment apparatus of the periodontium, consisting of the tissues apical to the crest of the alveolus.

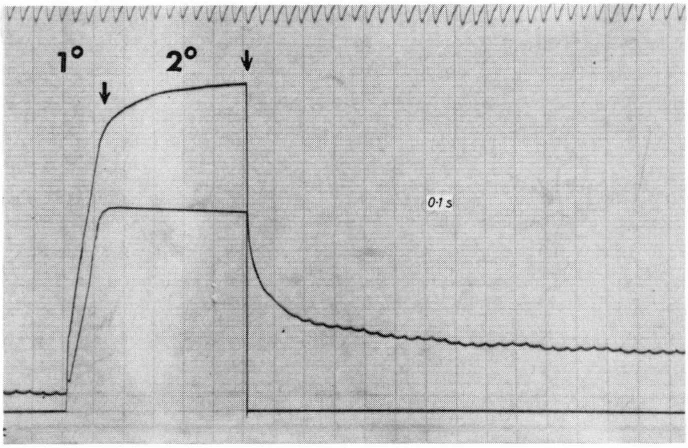

FIG. 189.—Normal tooth mobility curve on application of 250 grams force. Upper trace is tooth displacement and the lower trace is the applied force. The displacement shows the primary and secondary phases of tooth mobility.

force (Fig. 189). There is an almost linear relationship between force and displacement in the initial phase of tooth movement, while in the second phase there is a logarithmic relation with force (Parfitt, 1960). Mühlemann (1967) has interpreted this as a series of events which are:

1. Initial displacement is associated with a redistribution of intra- and extra-vascular fluid contents.
2. Orientation of periodontal ligament fibres to receive tensional or compressive stress.
3. Distortion of the walls of the alveolus and the surrounding bone.
4. Distortion of the dentine of the tooth itself (Fig. 190).

It is evident that the constituent tissues of the periodontal ligament act not only as a tensional system of fibres, as was once thought, but also as a compressive system of support, and both tension and compression appear to be of equal importance (Picton and Davies, 1967). Recent work (Wills, Picton and Davies, 1972) has shown that the supporting structures of the tooth behave in a visco-elastic manner. The behaviour of the complete attachment apparatus can be characterized functionally by at least three visco-elastic Voigt elements (Fig. 191), but it has not been possible to identify specific structural components which correspond to the individual elements. However, the blood vessels, together with the

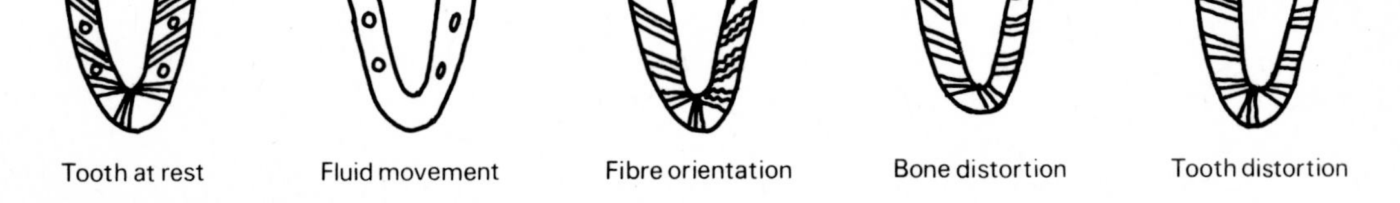

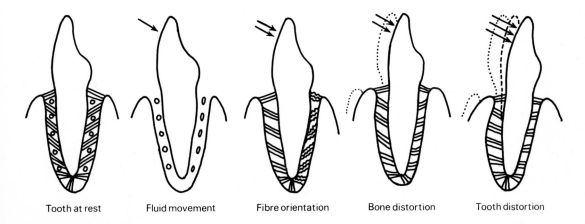

FIG. 190.—Events within the attachment apparatus on increasing levels of applied force.

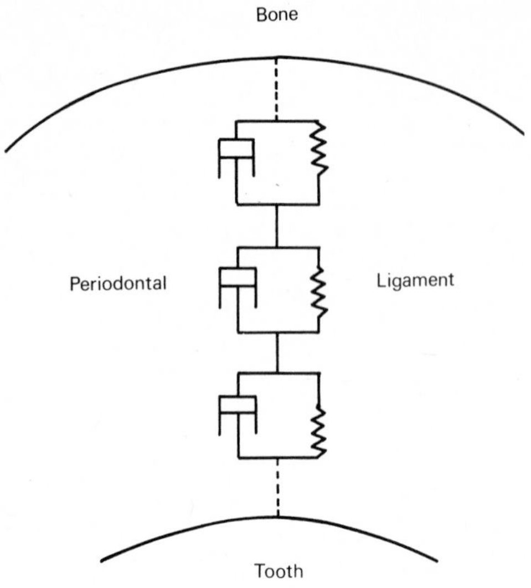

FIG. 191.—The functional characteristics of the attachment apparatus may be simulated by Voigt elements.

tissue fluid and ground substance, subserve the viscous portions of the support system, while bone and fibrous tissue elements account for the elasticity. As would be expected in such a visco-elastic system, the rate of application of the force to the tooth has a marked effect upon the displacement (Körber, 1971). Rapid rates of force application result in a marked reduction in total displacement, and the ligament appears to be more rigid. Forces applied over a longer period of time cause greater displacement as there is 'flow' or 'creep' within the more viscous parts of the ligament, and complete recovery of the equilibrium position on removal of such a force also takes longer. Since the rates of application of forces to teeth varies from the rapidly applied forces of normal mastication to the larger, slowly applied forces of parafunctional activities, such reactions to the rate of force application within the supporting tissues has obvious functional significance.

In the light of this ever-increasing understanding of the physiology of tooth support, it can be seen that every tooth in a healthy periodontium has a physiologic range of normal tooth mobility. If there were not such a 'give' within the system, then the periodontium could not act as a shock-absorbing mechanism. Precise measurement of physiological tooth mobility, while rarely carried out clinically, has shown that there are variations within the normal range. Thus incisor teeth are always more mobile than are premolars and molars (O'Leary, 1969). Tooth mobility is normally greater on awaking and decreases progressively throughout the day, as a tooth is extruded from its socket after a period of sleep, when there is no occlusal contact, and is then gradually depressed into the supporting tissues as function occurs. Similar changes in tooth mobility may be found when comparing mobility values pre- and post-mastication (O'Leary *et al.*, 1967).

The state of the deeper tissues of the periodontium in health is therefore intimately related to function. The variations in physiological tooth mobility are a reflection of changes in the visco-elastic behaviour of the system, which in turn must be attributable to alterations in individual components in the system. Thus, the previous loading history of the teeth might well affect the amount of fluid in the periodontal ligament, be it blood or tissue fluid, and this would cause a reduction in mobility (Picton, 1964). Similar mobility changes would be expected to occur if alterations took place within the collagen fibre system of the ligament.

2. Proprioception

The second function of the periodontal ligament is to form an essential component of the neurophysiological mechanisms which control the activities of the masticatory system, mainly chewing, swallowing and speech. It fulfils this function via the proprioceptive nerve endings which intertwine throughout the various fibres of the ligament proper.

It is essential to realize that the periodontium forms but one part of the whole masticatory or stomatognathic apparatus. This apparatus consists of the mandible and maxilla with their respective teeth embedded in the periodontal tissues, joined by the temporomandibular articulation and the associated musculature and ligaments. Its activities are co-ordinated largely by one neural network – the Trigeminal Nerve. The neuromuscular activities involved in controlling the functions of the masticatory system have been shown to be various forms of reflex activity (Thexton, 1974).

There are two basic kinds of reflexes, the innate or unlearned reflex, and the acquired or conditioned reflex. In the former, without any learning or training period being necessary any given stimulus will automatically produce a certain response. Examples of this in the masticatory system are the nociceptive reflex responses and the act of swallowing. Virtually all other activities in mastication and speech involve conditioned reflexes. As the name implies, such activity has to be learned by experience and the maintenance of such activity requires the presence of a conditioning stimulus. The sensory information for conditioning stimuli is obtained from all parts of the stomatognathic system, through sensory endings in the temporomandibular joint, ligaments and muscles, and also the proprioceptive nerve endings of the periodontal ligament itself (Lewinsky and Stewart, 1936).

The trigeminal nerve is largely a sensory nerve with motor branches serving the muscles of mastication running only in the Mandibular Division. The central connections of these motor and sensory branches are integrated within the various parts of the trigeminal nucleus (Fig. 192). Thus the reflex arcs are completed and the synaptic mechanisms within the nucleus allow of a very rapid response to any stimulus (Kawamura, 1967).

This is well exemplified on biting a small piece of hard foreign material when chewing a bolus of food. The excessive pressure on the tooth and hence on the periodontal ligament causes the initiation of a response in the proprioceptors in the ligament, which in turn, reflexly causes an opening movement of the jaws to reduce the excessive forces.

While it can be seen that the masticatory system is a single functional unit controlled by activity within the trigeminal nucleus, it must also be remembered that the nucleus itself is affected by the activity of the higher centres within the central nervous system. The synaptic inhibition or facilitation which follows some forms of cerebral

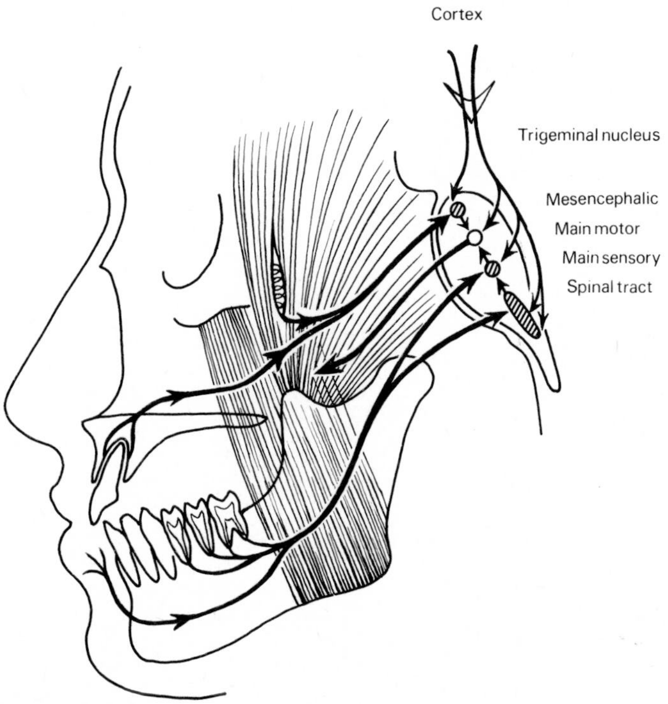

FIG. 192.—A diagrammatic representation of the afferent and efferent connections to the trigeminal nucleus, forming the reflex arcs, which in turn are subject to the activities of the higher centres.

cortical activity can result in altered behaviour during mastication or swallowing (Schärer and Pfyffer, 1970). An alteration of muscle tonus due to the fear of a dental procedure is a familiar example of this form of cortical influence. Within the range of normal function of the masticatory system, however, the important physiological principle of homeostasis is observed and activities of individual components of the system are designed to protect individual parts, as well as the whole unit. As in all neuromuscular behaviour of this kind, there is a degree of tolerance within this system, in the main due to the adaptive capacity of the component structures, so that there is always a range of activity which is 'normal' or 'physiological'.

THE FUNCTION OF THE MASTICATORY SYSTEM

Occlusion is normally taken to mean the static relationship of the two dental arches when the mandible is closed up to the maxilla. Clearly, there are many different relationships of mandible to maxilla which occur during function and the term 'occlusion' must be used to include these various functional activities in a dynamic sense.

The complexity of the masticatory system has resulted in many different research approaches to the analysis of mandibular movements during mastication and other activities, varying from radiographic and photographic methods to sophisticated forms of radiotelemetry. None of the more recent work has superceded that of Posselt (1952) who investigated the total excursive movements of the mandible in the sagittal and horizontal planes and who showed that the limits of movement, 'the border paths' of the mandible, were reproducible (Fig. 193).

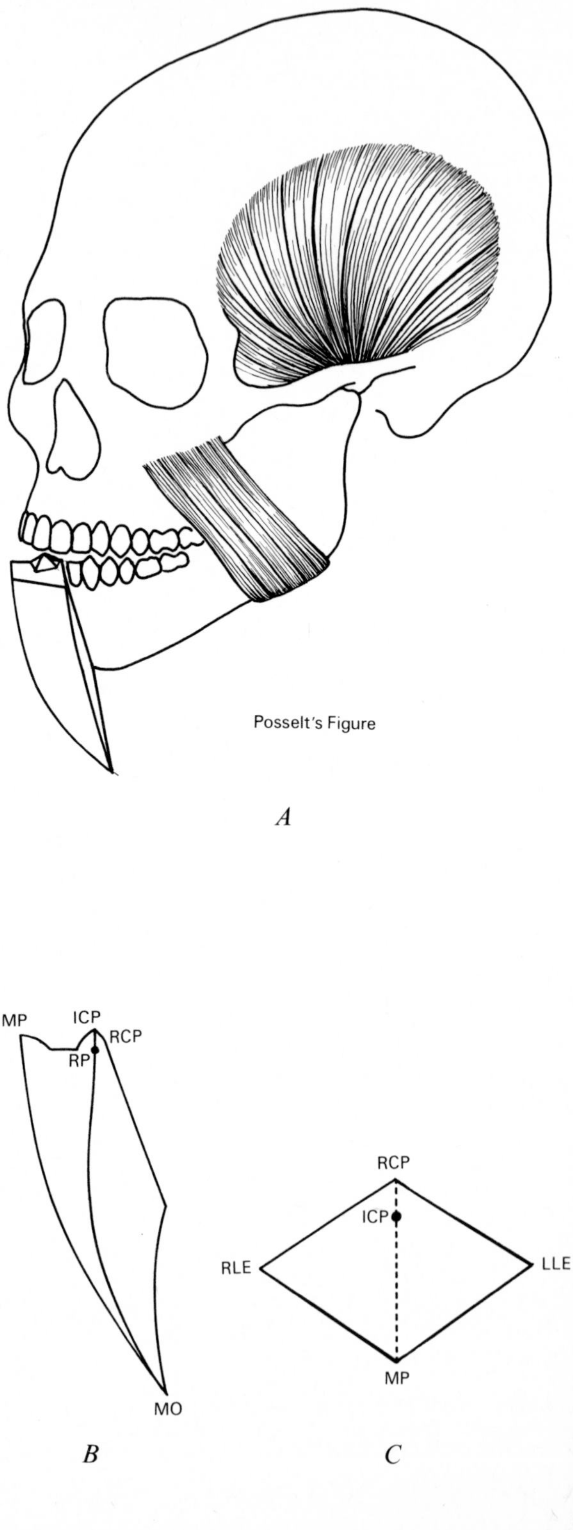

FIG. 193.—(*A*) The masticatory apparatus with the three dimensional Posselt's figure of excursive movements of the mandible. (*B*) Border paths of mandibular movement in the sagittal plane. (*C*) Border paths of the mandible in the horizontal plane. RCP = Retruded Contact Position; ICP = Intercuspal Position; MO = Maximum Opening; MP = Maximum Protrusion; RP = Rest Position; RLE = Right Lateral Excursion; LLE = Left Lateral Excursion.

MANDIBULAR MOVEMENTS

1. The Posterior Border Path

When the mouth is opened there is a range of movement, usually about 2.5 cm, when the condyles are in their most retruded position in the glenoid fossa, and the mandible effectively moves as a hinge about this posteriorly placed intercondylar axis. Such movement is termed the terminal hinge movement and the most superior point on this path, when the teeth make first contact, is the retruded contact position of the mandible (RCP). Opening beyond the terminal hinge movement results in translation within the upper compartment of the temporomandibular joint and a change in axis position for the remainder of the posterior border path, until the point of maximum opening (MO) is reached. The terminal hinge movement can only rarely be performed by the patient without the assistance or guidance of the clinician.

2. The Anterior Border Path

The anterior border path occurs with the condylar heads maintained forward on the articular eminence, so that the intercondylar axis is static and the path traces out a single arc to the position of maximum protrusion (MP) of the mandible. Such movement is virtually never carried out in normal function.

3. The Superior Border Path

The most superior sagittal border path differs from the previous two in that the movements are controlled more by the interdigitation of the two dental arches than by neuromuscular activity, as the two arches are in contact for the whole of this path. In approximately 90% of the dentate population, the position of maximum interdigitation of the two arches occurs at a point anterior to the retruded contact position (Beyron, 1964). The distance between this, the intercuspal position (ICP) and the retruded position is approximately 1 mm. In the remaining 10% of individuals, the intercuspal and retruded contact position are coincident. The protrusive path from maximum intercuspation is then forwards and downwards, until the anterior teeth are in an edge-to-edge position. Continued movement is forward and upwards to the position of maximum protrusion (MP), thus completing the superior sagittal border path.

4. The Horizontal Border Paths

In the horizontal plane, movement from the retruded contact position to extreme right and left lateral excursions of the mandible and then to maximum protrusion will trace out the diamond-shaped figure characteristic of the 'Gothic arch'. The mandible is, in fact, capable of tracing out such a figure of movement at each horizontal level along the vertical border path, with each Gothic arch becoming progressively smaller in area until the point of maximum opening is reached. Putting together the vertical and horizontal border paths will give the outline of a three-dimensional figure, the envelope of mandibular movement, named after Posselt. It is within this figure that all normal functional movements take place and they actually occupy a small proportion of the total volume of Posselt's figure. On a typical vertical functional path, there is a position just inferior to the intercuspal position, where the force of gravity upon the mandible is counterbalanced by the tonus in the elevator muscles of mastication. Such a position is the postural or rest position of the mandible (RP).

The Functional Significance of the Border Paths

The various positions adopted by the mandible in relation to the maxilla are largely governed by neuromuscular activity. The intercuspal position is the end-point of most of the activity of the masticatory system (Pameijer, Glickman and Roeber, 1968). Clearly this is not a fixed position, in that it depends upon the occlusal surfaces of the teeth and the morphology of the dental arches themselves. During eruption of the teeth the position of maximum intercuspation must change, as is also the case after dental treatment such as orthodontics, oral surgery or restorative dentistry. The intercuspal position is then a learned position, the proprioceptors in the periodontium once again enabling conditioning of reflex muscle activity, so that co-ordination of the elevator muscles results in reaching the final position of maximum interdigitation with no interferences occurring between the cusps of opposing arches.

Neither is the rest position fixed. By definition this is a position dictated by reflex neuromuscular activity and as a postural position, it will alter slightly with a change in posture or gravitational pull. On the other hand, the end of the terminal hinge path of closure, the retruded contact position, is a fixed position in that it is dependent not on neuromuscular activity at all, but is limited by anatomic structures, the bones, ligaments and the temporomandibular articulation. As such it is a completely reproducible point.

There has been some difference of opinion as to whether the retruded position is ever adopted during normal masticatory function. Earlier workers reported that, in adults, as the act of deglutition commenced, in order to brace the mandible for a tooth-together swallow, the masticatory muscles tended to draw the mandible distally to a more retruded position. Even the more modern radiotelemetric techniques have failed to completely resolve the issue. One school has reported that tooth contacts in the retruded position are made regularly in swallowing (Jankelson, Hoffman and Hendron, 1953), while other workers have shown this position to be used very infrequently during mastication or swallowing (Graf and Zander, 1963; Glickman *et al.*, 1969). The weight of evidence indicates that the retruded position, or positions intermediate between retruded contact and the intercuspal, occur only during swallowing and possibly in certain parafunctional activity. Stallard (1969) has defined parafunctional activities as any conscious or subconscious act performed by an individual which overrides the protective neurologic mechanisms of the masticatory system.

FUNCTION AND THE PERIODONTIUM

It has already been stated that function and the state of the periodontium in health are intimately related. As teeth erupt it is possible to observe the collagen fibres of the ligament assume the characteristic arrangement of the principal bundles of the adult periodontium. This functional arrangement is in turn greatly influenced by the occlusal forces to which the tooth is subjected. It has, for instance, been shown that in teeth subjected predominantly to vertical stress, the oblique fibres become most distinct, and align themselves almost parallel to the root surface (Kronfeld, 1931). Tooth mobility studies have already proved that occlusal forces, be they axial or horizontal in direction, result in areas of tension and compression occurring at different points in the ligament, and, depending on the duration of these forces, characteristic changes in the components of the ligament may take place. Physiologic horizontal forces have been said to promote the development of the crestal fibres of the periodontium and, as such, are conducive to the health of these tissues. The general arrangement of the principal fibres would, however, seem to indicate that the periodontal ligament is designed to absorb axial forces best with optimal distribution of the stress throughout the ligament (Beyron, 1954).

Adaptation to Altered Function

Since there is an interdependence of form and function within the various parts of the periodontal ligament, it is obvious that a continuous low level of remodelling takes place throughout the life of the teeth. Such remodelling is part of the adaptive capacity of the periodontium, and accounts for such phenomena as mesial drift, wherein bodily movement or tilting of teeth occurs in an anterior direction as wear of the contact points takes place with age (Picton, 1969).

There is a range of adaptation within which the periodontium may still maintain itself in health despite the alteration in function, be it increase or decrease in occlusal stress (Ramfjord and Kohler, 1959).

1. Hypofunction

In hypofunction, certain dystrophic changes occur in the connective tissue of the ligament. The principal fibres become less pronounced, the periodontal space narrows and the collagen fibres that are present are aligned parallel to the root surface rather than obliquely. The layer of cementum is thicker and the alveolar bone presents all the features of lack of functional stimulation with sparse trabeculation and large narrow spaces. The ligament space is narrow.

2. Hyperfunction

As function increases, re-orientation of the fibres occurs, and hyperfunction actually causes an increase in the number of Sharpey's fibres as well as of definition of the fibre bundles. The number of blood vessels within the ligament decreases and the bone trabeculation is better defined with an increase in the thickness of the lamina dura. The periodontal ligament becomes wider and there have been reports that the increase in width varies from area to area of the ligament according to the direction of increased functional demands. This widening of the periodontal ligament space appears to result from an initial resorption of the socket before repair in adjacent areas of the alveolus lays down a more well-defined lamina dura.

In this way, the periodontium is able to tolerate a degree of change in function and while the morphology of components changes, no real breakdown of tissue occurs. These changes are an adaptation, and the degree of adaptation possible must show great individual variation (Weinmann, 1955).

FORCES WHICH EXCEED THE TISSUE TOLERANCE

In certain circumstances, larger forces may be applied to teeth which may be of short or long duration, and which the periodontium is not able to absorb. No longer does adaptation occur and such excessive forces cause damage to the deeper tissues of the periodontium.

A common situation where a very heavy force is applied for a short period of time occurs when a high dental restoration is placed in a tooth with a previously healthy periodontium. An acute apical periodontitis results. The inflammatory changes make the tooth tender to occlusal pressure and increase the overall mobility. Excessive forces applied intermittently over a long period of time give rise to a chronic lesion, because the tolerance of the tissue has been exceeded. The characteristics of this chronic lesion are: (see Orban, 1928; Bhaskar and Orban, 1955; Reitan, 1969)

1. Compression of periodontal ligament fibres.
2. Thrombosis of blood vessels, leading to necrosis of areas of the periodontal ligament.
3. Loss of definition of the collagen fibre bundles, resulting in hyalinization of the ligament.
4. Possible resorption of cementum.
5. Osteoclastic activity, with resorption of the alveolar bone of the socket walls. Both frontal and rear bone resorption have been noted in different parts of the socket.

Such a pathologic lesion in the periodontium is described by the term 'Occlusal Trauma'. This may occur to varying degrees in different areas of the ligament of any one tooth, depending on the severity and direction of the applied forces (Carranza and Cabrini, 1967; Grant and Bernick, 1972).

OCCLUSAL TRAUMA – DEFINITION

In the literature on the subject of 'Occlusion' several semantic difficulties have arisen in defining the term 'Occlusal Trauma'. Some writers have used the term to describe a pathologic lesion, others have used it to describe the forces causing the lesion, leading one to the conclusion that 'occlusal trauma causes occlusal trauma'. To eliminate this problem as suggested by Mühle-

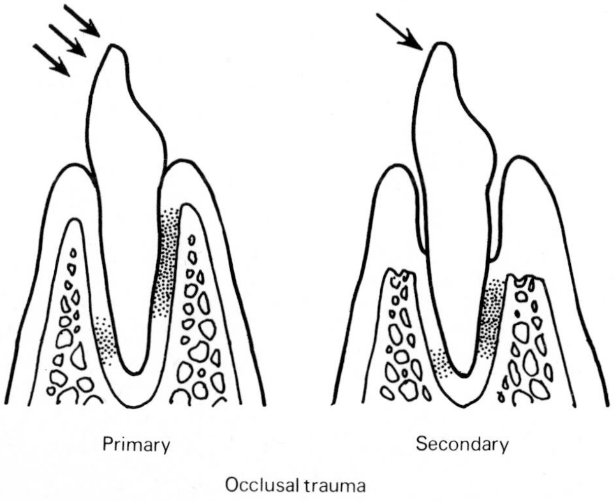

FIG. 194.—The lesions of occlusal trauma.

mann, the term 'occlusal trauma' should be confined to *the lesion* of the supporting structures, the characteristics of which have already been discussed. The lesion arises because of occlusal stress which exceeds the physiologic limit of adaptation of that particular periodontal membrane. The characteristics of the visco-elastic elements are altered, resulting in changes in the mobility of the tooth. Allusion has already been made to the fact that such increased mobility may be due to either a qualitative or quantitative change in the membrane (see Chapter 8). The term 'occlusal trauma' may be divided into two categories, the lesion being the same, but the aetiology being different (Fig. 194).

1. Primary occlusal trauma

This is the lesion produced by excessive forces acting upon a tooth with a normal amount of bone support. There may or may not be inflammatory disease in the marginal tissues of the periodontium, but essentially there has been no loss of alveolar bone.

2. Secondary occlusal trauma

In the presence of pre-existing periodontal disease, a situation is eventually reached when destruction of the supporting tissues causes reversal of the effective crown-to-root ratio. In this situation normal forces dissipated over this greatly reduced amount of supporting tissue may become excessive and cause continued damage.

Clearly the lesion of primary occlusal trauma is completely reversible because elimination of the excessive forces will allow healing of the lesion and a return to normal tooth mobility. This cannot be true of secondary occlusal trauma, as there has been an irreversible loss of alveolar support. These differences can be summarized as in the table (after Abrams and Coslet, 1973):

	Primary	*Secondary*
Aetiology	Excessive forces	Normal forces
State of periodontium	Normal amount of periodontal support	Reduced support due to periodontal disease
Healing	Potential for reversibility	Essentially irreversible

It must be emphasized again that excessive force has no bearing upon the aetiology of the gingival lesion, and the pre-existing periodontal disease in secondary occlusal trauma has been a consequence initially of plaque irritation, not of occlusal stress *per se*. The exception to this is the direct trauma from the occlusal table onto the gingival soft tissues, for example in deep overbite cases (Fig. 195). This is quite a different entity from the lesions produced via excessive forces acting upon the teeth.

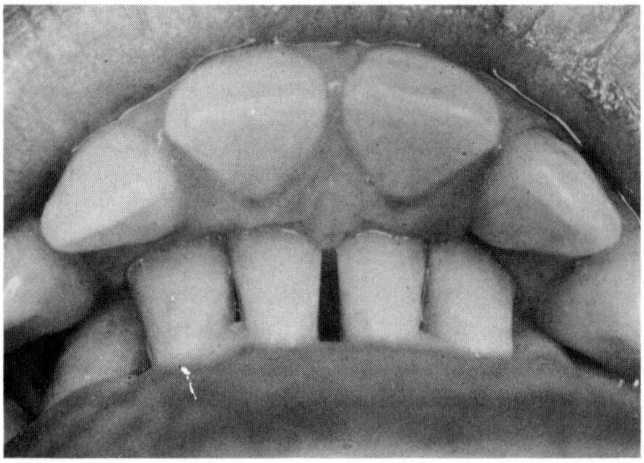

Fig. 195.—Direct trauma to the palatal gingivae 3|3 in a severe Class II Division I Malocclusion.

The effect of trauma from occlusion as a destructive or co-destructive aetiologic factor in patients with chronic periodontal disease has been fully discussed in Chapter 8. Even the most careful evaluation of previous research fails to completely resolve whether and how occlusal trauma affects the progression of a periodontitis. It is, however, pertinent to note that occlusal function and the state of component tissues of the periodontal ligament are related, and that such altered components may change, or impair, the tissue resistance to pre-existing inflammation.

AETIOLOGY OF TRAUMATOGENIC FORCES

The origin of the excessive forces which produce the lesion of occlusal trauma must be considered before any occlusal treatment can be performed to treat the lesion.

Clearly a knowledge of the functional anatomy of the masticatory system indicates that the neuromuscular mechanisms involved protect the component parts from injury. During mastication, the forces generated between the dental arches depends to a large extent on the texture and consistency of the food. Yurkstas and Curby (1953) reported peak forces from 0.4 to 1.8 kilograms per tooth, while Anderson (1956) found average peak pressures only up to about 0.6 kilogram on the lower first molar in adults. For most of the chewing cycle the teeth are in fact separated by the bolus of food and only contact each other at the end of the cycle and during swallowing. The loading rates involved can only result in a functional stimulation to the periodontal tissues, and the total time in a period of twenty-four hours when there is direct occlusal force application to the periodontium is less than twenty minutes (Graf, 1969). Since it is unlikely that normal function could generate traumatic forces, the damaging forces are produced outside the normal functional range, during the parafunctional activities.

There are many types of parafunction associated with the masticatory system, with many different causes, but a useful classification is that of Abrams and Coslet (1973):

1. Parafunction with a direct tooth-to-tooth contact.
2. Parafunction with a soft tissue-to-tooth contact.
3. Tooth-to-foreign body habit patterns.

Examples of the second category are patients with lip or cheek biting habits and also those with some form of anterior tongue thrust (Fig. 196). There are a number of foreign bodies used in some parafunctional activities, including pencil chewing, hairgrip opening, finger sucking, nail biting and pipe smoking (Fig. 197). In such situations the total force of the masticatory muscles may be distributed over very few periodontal ligaments, hence resulting in traumatogenic forces.

Tooth-to-tooth habits probably form the commonest sort of parafunction of the masticatory system. Ramfjord and Ash (1971), while noting that prevalence figures for bruxism vary between 20 and 80 per cent, depending on the method of clinical assessment, state that with careful examination methods, a 'very high percentage' of patients with periodontal disease have bruxism. Other forms of parafunction within this tooth-to-tooth category include the day-time clenching and grinding habits, which may involve the whole dental arch or individual groups of teeth. Forces generated in tooth-to-tooth parafunction are not only much greater than those of mastication, but they are also of long duration.

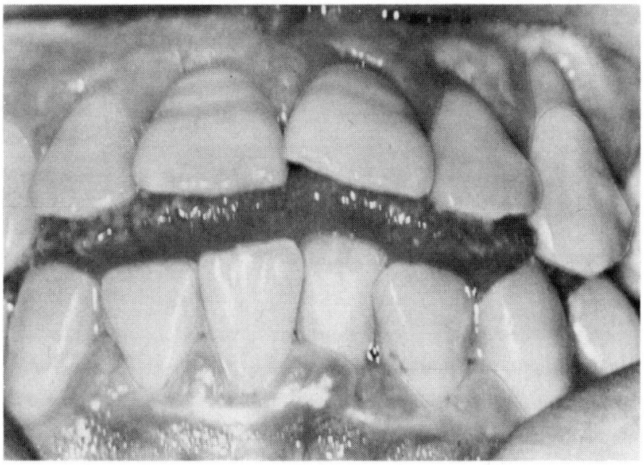

FIG. 196.—A tongue thrusting habit with flaring of the upper incisor segment.

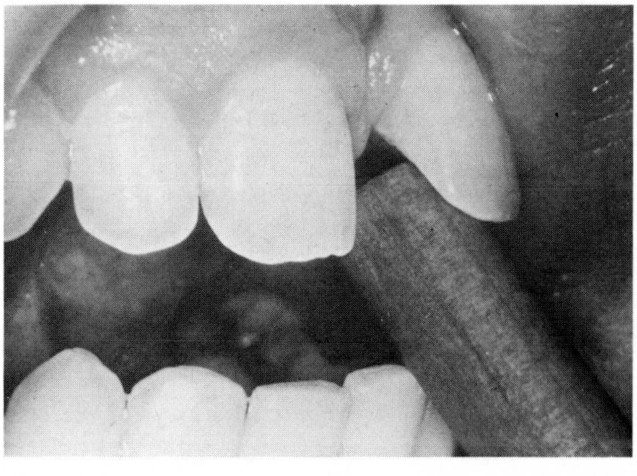

FIG. 197.—A pencil chewing habit resulting in increased mobility of |1 and consequent migration.

Posselt (1966), basing his observations on the results of three separate research reports, noted that during bruxing and clenching activities, individuals could achieve biting forces of over 20 kilograms and that in some instances intermaxillary contacts extended for up to 2.5 seconds. Such increased magnitude, frequency and duration of occlusal stress must result in a pronounced 'creep' or 'flow' within the visco-elastic periodontium, increased distortion of the alveolus and prolonged recovery times for the teeth to reach their equilibrium intra-socket positions. The threshold for the proprioceptive sensory endings in the supporting tissues is lowered by this excessive force and the protective reflexes are no longer effective in preventing further damage. Asynchronous electromyographic activity is found in the muscles of mastication (Jarabak, 1956) which perpetuates the unfavourable forces, so that they continue to act as a potentially traumatogenic insult to the periodontium.

Such forces from bruxing, clenching and grinding habits remain only potentially damaging, as in some young individuals, the periodontium responds by adapting to the hyperfunctional demands. It must, however, be conceded that the lesion of primary occlusal trauma is commonly the outcome of such parafunctional activities.

BRUXISM AND RELATED ACTIVITIES – THEIR AETIOLOGY

The relationship between psychic or emotional stress and tooth clenching and grinding is familiar to all and it would appear that there are two aetiologic factors in such forms of parafunction (Ramfjord, 1961):

1. The presence of an occlusal interference

Those interferences which are most capable of initiating a bruxing/clenching activity are, primarily, centric prematurities distal to the intercuspal position, *i.e.* between retruded contact and maximum intercuspation. Non-working or so-called 'balancing' contacts and, to a much lesser extent, working side interferences have also been incriminated.

2. The presence of psychic tension

The trigeminal nucleus does not exist in isolation, and must be subject to cortical influences. The muscles of mastication themselves react to psychic stress by an increase in tonus, resulting from altered fusimotor activity.

This nervous tension then leaves the neuromuscular threshold of the system in a hypersensitive state and there seems to be a subconscious attempt to seek out the occlusal interference and to grind it in, through the parafunctional activity. It has been shown that when the occlusal interference is eliminated the bruxism may be alleviated.

Such destructive habits are quite contrary to the normal protective reflexes, where an avoidance reaction would usually occur in the presence of an occlusal interference (Fig. 198). However, these avoidance phenomena in themselves may initiate asynchronous electromyographic activity which might become a detrimental influence on components of the masticatory system.

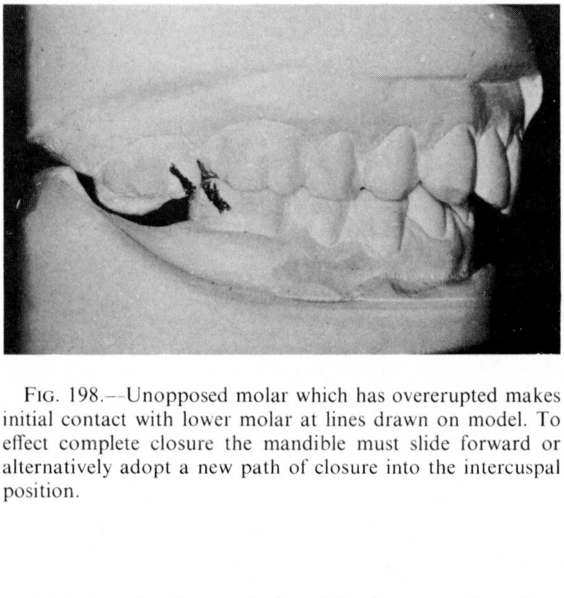

FIG. 198.—Unopposed molar which has overerupted makes initial contact with lower molar at lines drawn on model. To effect complete closure the mandible must slide forward or alternatively adopt a new path of closure into the intercuspal position.

Clearly, the interrelationship between bruxism and psychic tension will mean that bruxism will be more evident at times of emotional stress. Indeed it has been suggested (Posselt, 1962) that there is a spectrum of activity which results in bruxism or clenching. Thus, there can be severe psychic tension with a minor occlusal interference or a pronounced occlusal interference with mild psychic stress, with varying combinations of the aetiologic factors reacting together at different times in the patient's life.

Although, in this text, the effect of parafunctional activities upon the periodontium is the prime consideration, it must be realized that the periodontal ligament is but one part of the whole masticatory system. Excessive forces generated within the system may not only cause damage to the ligament, but to the teeth themselves, the muscles and the temporomandibular joint.

Excessive and abnormal wear patterns are a common sign of parafunction. Such wear facets are often referred to as pernicious wear as it is not commensurate with normal attrition. Teeth themselves are more mobile (O'Leary, 1969) (Fig. 199), or they may migrate; pulpal changes including complete necrosis have been reported (Ingle, 1960), and even fracture of the crown or root has occurred (Ramfjord and Ash, 1971).

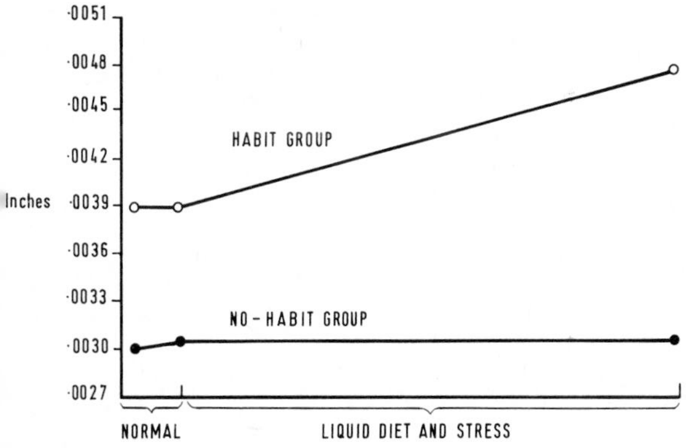

FIG. 199.—Mobility patterns for two groups of subjects exposed to a standard liquid diet and to a stress situation, the group with evidence of parafunction exhibiting a pronounced increase in mobility when compared with that without any occlusal habits. (After O'Leary.)

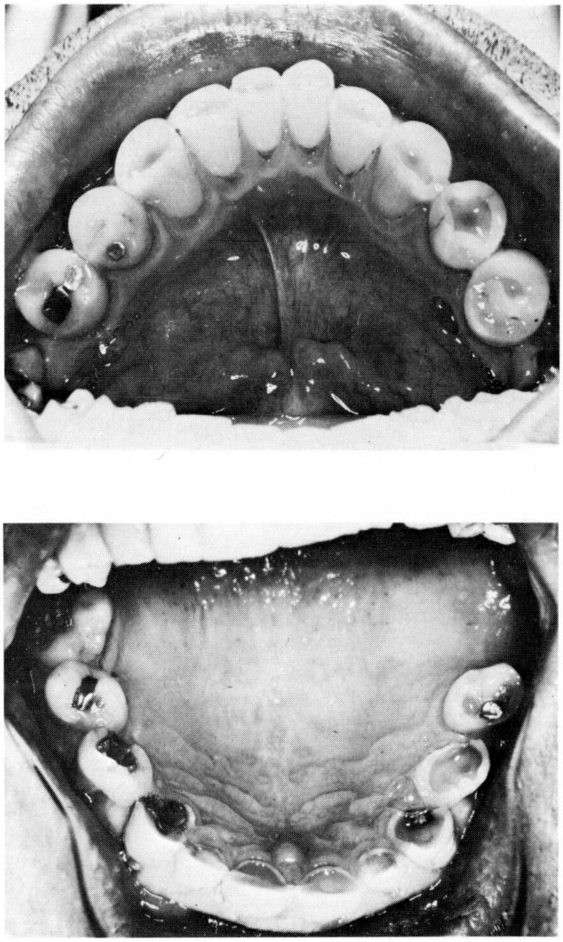

FIG. 200.—Advanced attrition caused by bruxism.

PARAFUNCTION – DIAGNOSIS

As patients are often not aware of their occlusal habit, establishing a diagnosis of bruxism or another type of parafunction depends upon a careful history and a thorough clinical examination including an analysis of occlusal function (see Chapter 14). Sometimes the pattern of wear or migration will give a very obvious clue (Fig. 200), at other times it is necessary to collate several different signs, which may be summarized as (after Graf, 1969):

1. Increased mobility patterns.
2. Migration of individual teeth or segments of the dental arch.
3. Presence of abnormal, pernicious wear facets. They generally have sharp edges and antagonistic pairs of facets can be matched, sometimes only in extremes of mandibular excursions.
4. The presence of occlusal interferences, especially in the retruded contact to intercuspal range.
5. Hypertonicity of the muscles of mastication, which may be tender to palpation.

6. Dullness of the teeth to percussion and tenderness to pressure, especially on awaking.
7. Temporomandibular joint pain.
8. The history, yielding evidence of an occlusal habit, for example, the audible sounds of nocturnal bruxism in the past.

Since bruxism and other forms of parafunction are of such importance in the aetiology of primary occlusal trauma all the above clinical features should be noted and their cumulative effects analysed. Ideally, since these conditions have two basic causes, both should be eliminated in therapy, but the treatment of psychic tension rarely falls within the purview of a dentist, so the elimination of occlusal disharmonies is the most important contribution of the dentist in eliminating these damaging forces.

OTHER FACTORS DIRECTLY OR INDIRECTLY CAUSING EXCESSIVE OCCLUSAL STRESS

A number of the causes of occlusal disharmonies seem to relate to dental treatment. Dental restorations, from a simple Class II amalgam to the most complex bridge, all have the potential to act as occlusal interferences. The fact that few of the prematurities so caused give rise to permanent periodontal damage gives some indication of the adaptive capacity of the masticatory system. However, persistent forces will cause damage.

A. **Removable Prostheses**

The tissue-borne acrylic denture covering the gingival margins has been rightly condemned as an initiator of gingival inflammation, but partial dentures with clasps and rests can be equally damaging if every care is not taken with the design of the denture. Excessive lateral stresses on abutment teeth may result in tissue breakdown and migration of the teeth (Fig. 201). A particular problem is the abutment tooth in a free-end saddle partial denture. Poorly designed clasps, especially without any occlusal rests, can result in large lateral and distal forces on the abutment tooth as the denture sinks into the soft tissues (Fig. 202). The all too familiar pattern of gradual periodontal destruction about the abutment tooth, its extraction, followed by additions to the

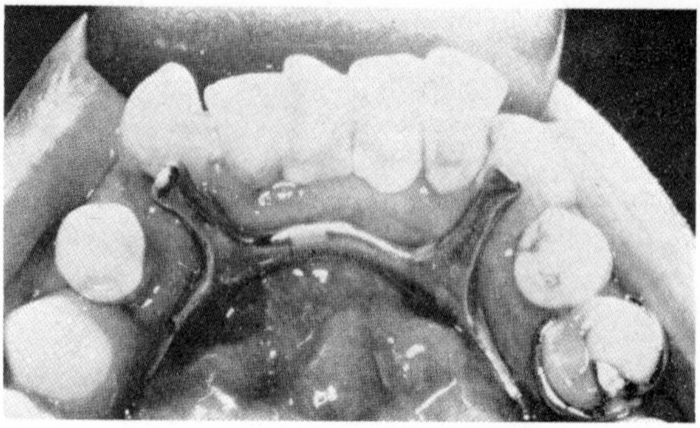

A

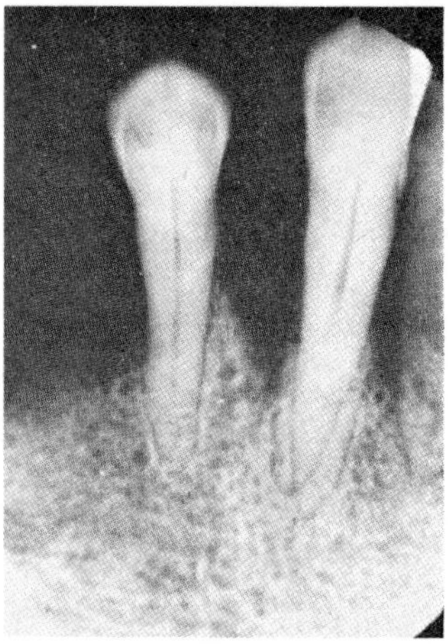

B

Fig. 201.—(*A*) Lower denture in which a rest has created excessive stress on a canine tooth. (*B*) Radiograph of the canine shows considerable bone loss about this tooth which migrated labially.

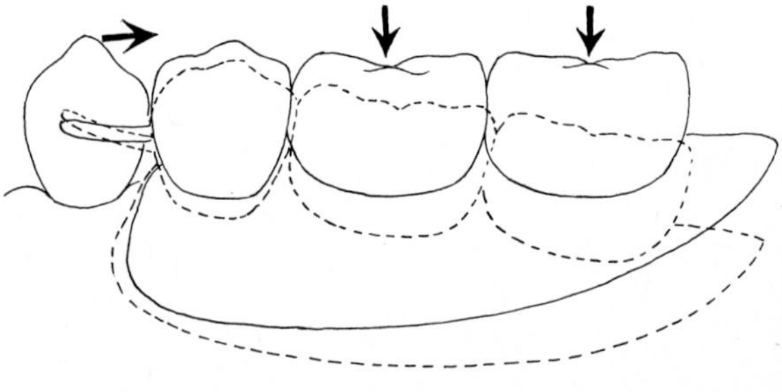

Fig. 202.—The forces exerted on an abutment tooth for a lower free-end denture without occlusal rests.

partial denture, is the outcome of this kind of dentistry. When designing removable prostheses, the periodontal implications should lead to the use of occlusal rests, so that forces are directed axially over several sound abutment teeth.

B. Fixed Restorations

Improper occlusal contouring may result in an occlusal interference. The result of this interference may be one of several clinical possibilities:

(i) Adaptation, with change in the mandibular path of closure to avoid the interference, or, possible wear of the offending part of the occlusal anatomy.

(ii) Excessive force on the tooth, with the interference resulting in primary occlusal trauma (Fig. 203). In this regard, all excursive movements of the mandible must be considered when carving the occlusal table, not simply maximum intercuspation (Fig. 204). This is especially true with gold

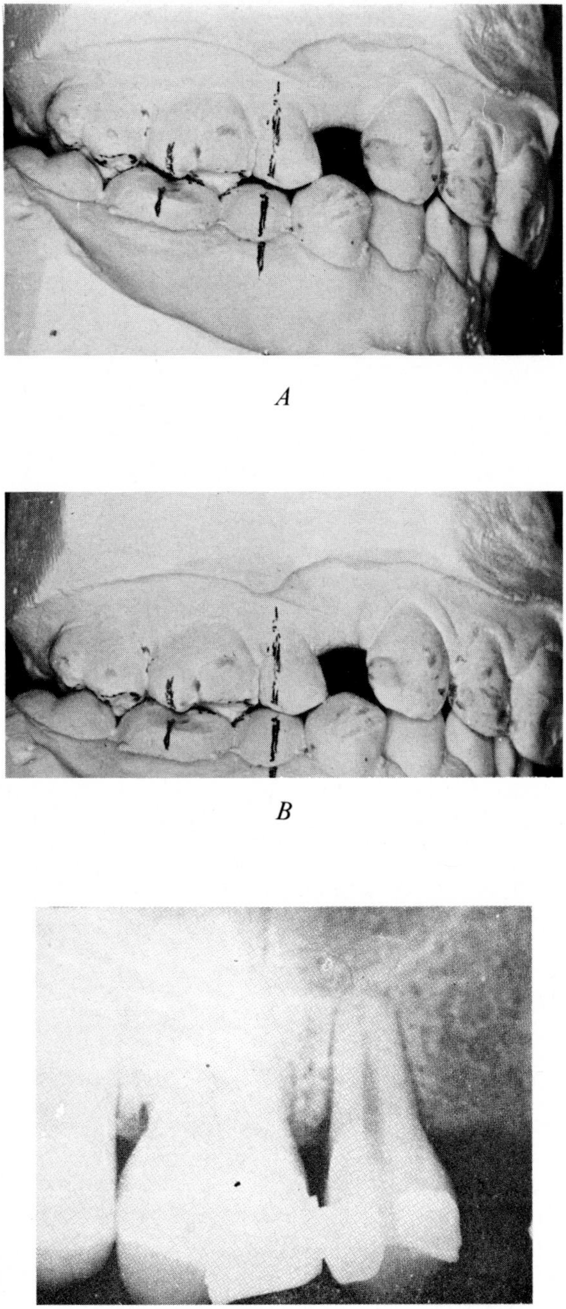

A

B

C

FIG. 203.—(*A*) Models in the retruded contact position, with a premature contact on the mesial slope of the palatal cusp of the upper second premolar. (*B*) Contacts after a forward slide into the intercuspal position. (*C*) Radiograph showing widened periodontal space around the premolar involved.

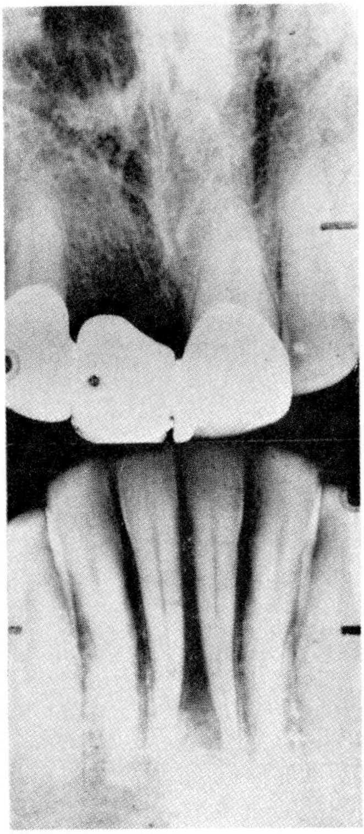

FIG. 204.—Bone loss associated with an acute periodontal abscess between $\overline{1|1}$, which were the sole teeth in contact with an upper bridge in protrusive movements. There was no hyperfunction in the intercuspal position.

restorations, and it is patently impossible to register all the potential occlusal contacts for a restoration on a simple hinge articulator.

(iii) The convenience path of closure of the mandible may cause excessive forces on other segments of the dental arch. This is most likely to occur in the anterior segments with a forward posturing of the mandible. The anterior teeth may then migrate under the influence of these forces, or they may show signs of primary occlusal trauma, or both may be found simultaneously.

(iv) The initiation of parafunctional activities, dependent to a large extent upon the patient's emotional stress.

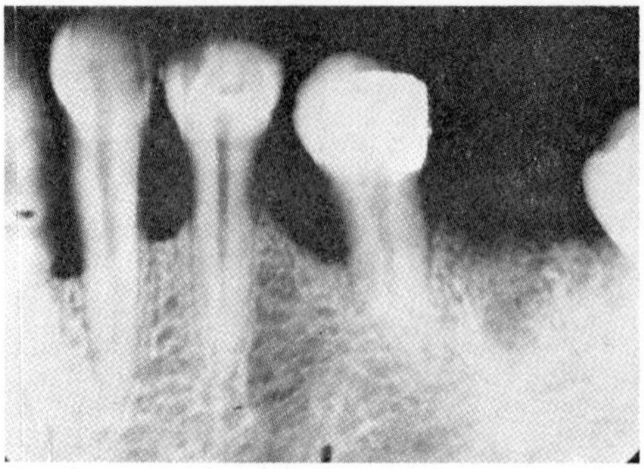

FIG. 205.—Wide clinical crown and tapering root of lower first premolar, together with short root of second premolar would make these undesirable abutment teeth.

Care should be taken in selecting abutment teeth for fixed prostheses which must be capable of withstanding the increased occlusal stress. Single cantilever bridges need particularly careful assessment in this regard. Crown and root morphology must play a part in judging the suitability of abutment teeth, as teeth with large crowns and short, tapered roots (Fig. 205) always have a predeliction for occlusal traumatic lesions.

Lack of replacement of lost teeth also results in changes within the dental arches conducive to the formation of occlusal disharmonies. The over-eruption, drifting and tilting which may ensue (Fig. 206) may give rise to many periodontal problems which are discussed elsewhere (Chapter 4). In fact, a common presenting sign of such a collapse of the posterior occlusion is the migration of the incisor teeth consequent upon the excessive forces placed on the incisor segment (Fig. 207). Although it may be unrealistic to expect every lost tooth to be replaced, it is incumbent upon the dentist to observe and follow the results of an extraction with no prosthetic replacement very carefully. There can be no excuse for supervized neglect, with potentiation of periodontal breakdown with the passage of time.

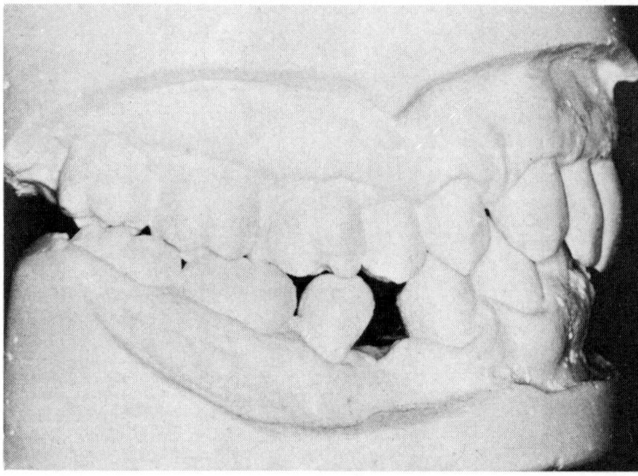

FIG. 206.—Typical case in which arch collapse has occurred after extractions.

Over-eruption of teeth with no antagonists can often lead to abnormal paths of closure due to centric prematurities. The wear facets that are found on such teeth can only occur in movements from a retruded contact to intercuspal position (Fig. 208). Such interferences are a common cause of temporomandibular joint dysfunction.

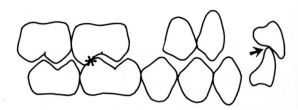

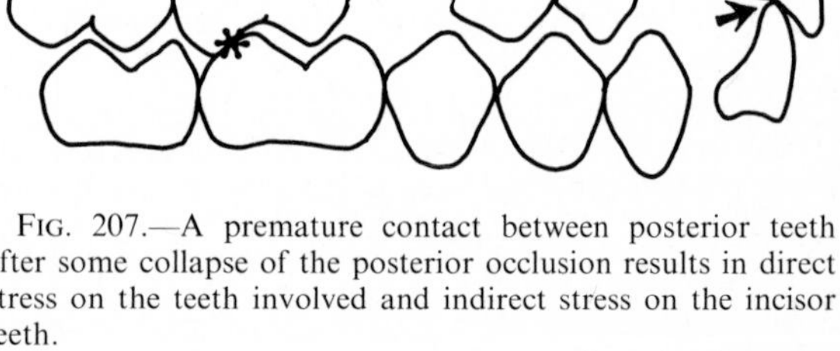

FIG. 207.—A premature contact between posterior teeth after some collapse of the posterior occlusion results in direct stress on the teeth involved and indirect stress on the incisor teeth.

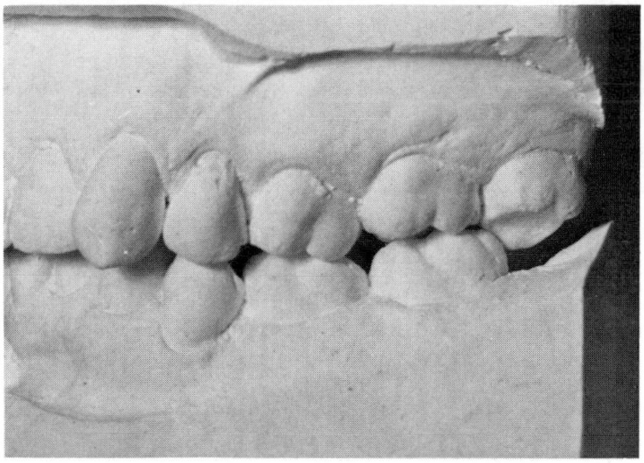

A

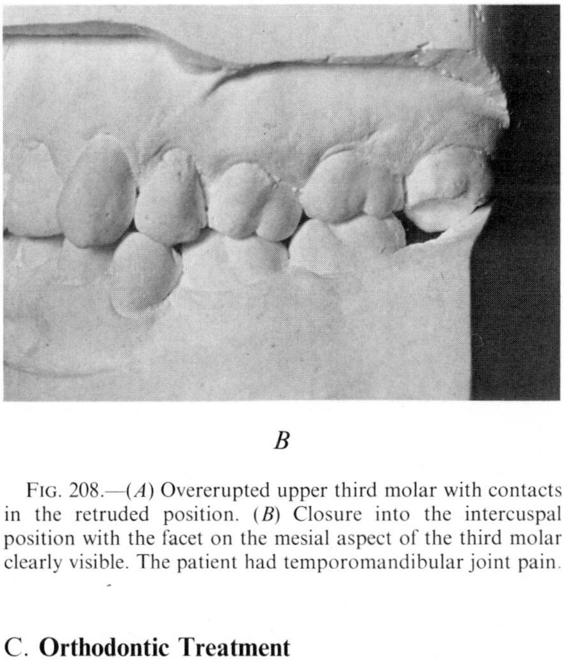

B

Fig. 208.—(*A*) Overerupted upper third molar with contacts in the retruded position. (*B*) Closure into the intercuspal position with the facet on the mesial aspect of the third molar clearly visible. The patient had temporomandibular joint pain.

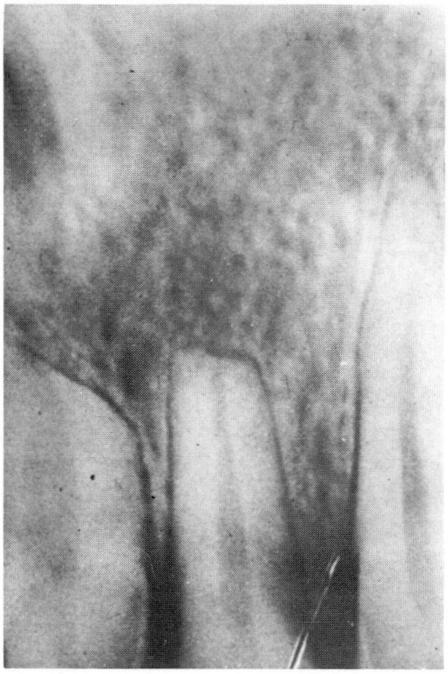

Fig. 209.—Intermittent forces, caused by a retainer worn at night, have resulted in increased mobility patterns and resorption of the roots.

C. **Orthodontic Treatment**

To maintain stability of an orthodontic result, it is important to ensure that the dental arches after therapy are in complete harmony with the neuromuscular activities of the masticatory system (Moyers, 1949). Simply producing an acceptable aesthetic result is not sufficient, and retaining a result incompatible with physiologic neuromuscular mechanisms with an appliance can be positively damaging to the supporting structures (Fig. 209). Careful occlusal analysis followed by any necessary treatment should always complete a course of orthodontic therapy.

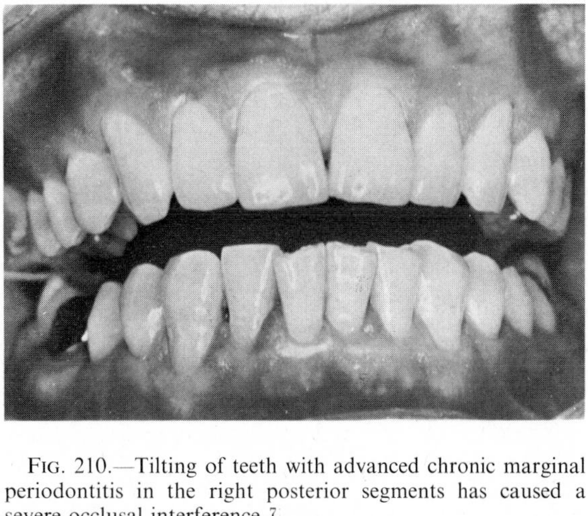

Fig. 210.—Tilting of teeth with advanced chronic marginal periodontitis in the right posterior segments has caused a severe occlusal interference $\frac{7|}{7|}$.

D. Oral Surgery

The occlusion may well be deranged following surgical reduction of a fracture. Any gross disharmonies should be eliminated to enable the patient to bring his teeth into a harmonious, functional relationship.

E. Periodontal Disease

In advanced chronic marginal periodontitis, the tilting and migration of teeth which have lost a considerable amount of their supporting tissue may themselves give rise to occlusal interferences (Fig. 210) and the treatment of such conditions involves a consideration of secondary occlusal trauma, which is described elsewhere (Chapter 14).

REFERENCES

ABRAMS, L. and COSLET, J. G. (1973). Occlusal adjustment by selective grinding. *In* Goldman, H. M. and Cohen, D. W., Periodontal Therapy, 5th ed. C. V. Mosby Company, St. Louis.

ANDERSON, D. J. (1956). Measurement of stress in mastication II. *J. dent. Res.*, **35**, 671.

BEYRON, H. L. (1954). Occlusal changes in the adult dentition. *J. Amer. dent. Ass.*, **48**, 674.

BEYRON, H. L. (1964). Occlusal relations and mastication in Australian aborigines. *Acta odont. scand.*, **22**, 597.

BHASKAR, S. N. and ORBAN, B. J. (1955). Experimental occlusal trauma. *J. Periodont.*, **26**, 270.

CARRANZA, F. A., Jr. and CABRINI, R. L. (1967). Histometric studies of periodontal tissues. *Periodontics*, **5**, 308.

FOX, J. (1833). Natural History and Diseases of Human Teeth, 3rd ed. E. Cox, London.

GLICKMAN, I., PAMEIJER, J. H. N., ROEBER, F. W. and BRION, M. A. M. (1969). Functional occlusion as revealed by miniaturized radio transmitters. *Dent. Clin. N. Amer.*, **13**, No. 3, 667.

GÖTZE, W. (1965). Uber Atemsveranderungen des Paradontiums. *Dtsch. zahnärztl. Z.*, **15**, 465

GRAF, H. and ZANDER, H. A. (1963). Tooth contact patterns in mastication. *J. prosth. Dent.*, **13**, 1055.

GRAF, H. (1969). Bruxism. *Dent. Clin. N. Amer.*, **13**, No. 3, 659.

GRANT, D. A. and BERNICK, S. (1972). The periodontium of aging humans. *J. Periodont.*, **43**, 660.

INGLE, J. L. (1960). Alveolar osteoporosis and pulpal death associated with compulsive bruxism. *Oral Surg.*, **13**, 1371.

JANKELSON, B., HOFFMAN, G. M. and HENDRON, J. A. (1953). The physiology of the stomatognathic system. *J. Amer. dent. Ass.*, **46**, 375.

JARABAK, J. R. (1956). An electromyographic analysis of muscular and temporomandibular joint disturbances due to imbalances in occlusion. *Angle Orthodont.*, **26**, 170.

KAWAMURA, Y. (1967). Neurophysiologic background of occlusion. *Periodontics*, **5**, 175.

KINDLOVÁ, M. and MATENA, V. (1962). Blood vessels of the rat molar. *J. dent. Res.*, **41**, 650.

KÖRBER, K. H. (1971). Electronic registration of tooth movement. *Int. dent. J.*, **21**, 466.

KRONFELD, R. (1931). Histologic study of the influence of function on the human periodontal membrane. *J. Amer. dent. Ass.*, **18**, 1242.

LEWINSKY, W. and STEWART, D. (1936). The innervation of the periodontal membrane. *J. Anat.*, **71**, 98.

MOYERS, R. E. (1949). Temporomandibular muscle contraction patterns in Angle Class II, Div. I. malocclusions: An electromyographic analysis. *Amer. J. Orthodont.*, **35**, 837.

MÜHLEMANN, H. R. (1967). Tooth mobility: A review of clinical aspects and research findings. *J. Periodont.*, **38**, 686.

O'LEARY, T. J. (1969). Tooth mobility. *Dent. Clin. N. Amer.*, **13**, 567.

O'LEARY, T. J., RUDD, K., NABERS, C., and STINUPF, A. (1967). The effect of mastication and deglutition on tooth mobility. *Periodontics*, **5**, 26.

ORBAN, B. (1928). Tissue changes in traumatic occlusion. *J. Amer. dent. Ass.*, **15**, 2090.

PAMEIJAR, J. H. N., GLICKMAN, I. and ROEBER, F. (1968). Intra-oral occlusal telemetry II. Registration of tooth contacts in chewing and swallowing by intra-oral electric telemetry. *J. prosth. dent.*, **19**, 151.

PARFITT, G. J. (1960). Measurement of the physiological mobility of individual teeth in an axial direction. *J. dent. Res.*, **39**, 608.

PICTON, D. C. A. (1964). Some implications of normal tooth mobility during mastication. *Arch. oral Biol.*, **9**, 565.

PICTON, D. C. A. (1969). The effect of external forces on the periodontium. *In* Melcher, A. H. and Bowen, W. H., Biology of the Periodontium. Academic Press, London.

PICTON, D. C. A. and DAVIES, W. I. R. (1967). Dimensional changes in the periodontal membrane of monkeys (Macacca Irus) due to horizontal thrusts applied to the teeth. *Arch. oral Biol.*, **12**, 1635.
POSSELT, U. (1952). Studies in the mobility of the human mandible. *Acta odont. scand.*, **10**, Suppl. 10, 19.
POSSELT, U. (1962). Physiology of Occlusion and Rehabilitation. Blackwell, Oxford.
POSSELT, U. (1966). Occlusion related to periodontics. Section V. World Workshop in Periodontics. University of Michigan Press, Ann Arbor.
RAMFJORD, S. P. (1961). Bruxism, a clinical and electromyographic study. *J. Amer. dent. Ass.*, **62**, 21.
RAMFJORD, S. P. and KOHLER, C. A. (1959). Periodontal reaction to functional occlusal stress. *J. Periodont.*, **30**, 95.
RAMFJORD, S. P. and ASH, M. M., Jr. (1971). Occlusion. W. B. Saunders Company, Philadelphia.
REITAN, K. (1969). Biomechanical principles and reactions. *In* Graber, T. M., Current Orthodontic Concepts and Techniques, Vol. 1. W. B. Saunders Company, Philadelphia.
SCHÄRER, P. and PFYFFER, G. (1970). Comparison of habitual and cerebrally stimulated jaw movements in the rabbit. *Helv. odont. Acta*, **14**, 6.
STALLARD, R. E. (1969). Occlusion and periodontal disease. *Dent. Clin. N. Amer.*, **13**, No. 3, 599.
THEXTON, A. J. (1974). Some aspects of neurophysiology of dental interest. I. Theories of oral function. *J. Dent.*, **2**, 49.
WEINMANN, J. P. (1955). The adaptation of the periodontium to physiologic and pathologic changes. *Oral Surg.*, **8**, 977.
WILLS, D. J., PICTON, D. C. A. and DAVIES, W. I. R. (1972). An investigation of the viscoelastic properties of the periodontium in monkeys. *J. periodont. Res.*, **7**, 42.
YURKSTAS, A. and CURBY, W. A. (1953). Force analysis of prosthetic appliances during function. *J. prosth. Dent.*, **3**, 82.

14. The Diagnosis and Treatment of Primary Occlusal Trauma

Clinical treatment of any kind can only be justified in occlusal therapy if it can be demonstrated that the occlusal forces are causing or contributing to a pathological lesion. There is no evidence to support clinical intervention during periodontal treatment simply because an occlusion does not conform to a pre-conceived 'ideal' or 'normal' occlusion. Indeed there is strong justification from the periodontal standpoint for adopting the suggestions of Amsterdam (1973) that: A physiologic occlusion is one in which the occlusal forces generated can be demonstrated to be causing no damage to the teeth, their supporting structures or any other component of the stomatognathic system. A pathologic occlusion is one in which there is evidence of disease which can specifically be attributed to occlusal activity.

There is thus no biological basis for prophylactic occlusal adjustment, which presupposes that the clinician can predict which type of occlusion will definitely result in damage. Considering the almost ubiquitous incidence of occlusal premature contacts and the range of tissue tolerance to the prematurities, it is obviously impossible to assess the pathogenic potential of the interference with any accuracy.

The decision as to whether an occlusion is pathologic is based upon a thorough and systematic clinical examination, after obtaining relevant facts from the patient's history.

THE DIAGNOSIS OF PRIMARY OCCLUSAL TRAUMA

The signs and symptoms of this lesion in the deeper tissues of the periodontium constitute almost a syndrome, some of the clinical features of which have already been discussed in the previous chapter, (see the section on parafunction). To establish a diagnosis it is necessary to find several of these signs and symptoms together, and not to depend upon any one clinical feature.

1. The cardinal clinical manifestation of primary occlusal trauma is increased tooth mobility. Although there are mechanical and electronic instruments for accurate measurement of tooth mobility (Mühlemann 1967), none have achieved routine clinical usage. The assessment is usually entirely subjective, teeth being assigned a mobility score on a zero to three scale as in Miller's classification (see Chapter 8). To achieve some consistency in scoring, the tooth movement is best tested using the blunt handles of two instruments (Fig. 211). Since the mobility pattern may be a reflection of qualitative or quantitative change, the increased mobility must be related to other clinical or radiographic evidence of pocket depths and amounts of bone lost.

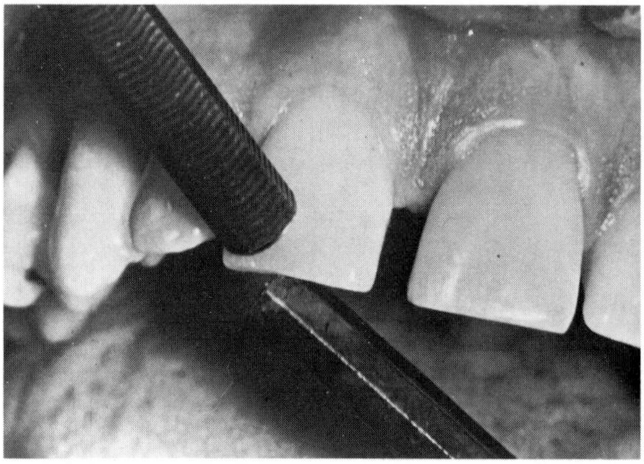

FIG. 211.—Testing the clinical mobility of an upper central incisor.

A distinctly damaging kind of tooth movement is fremitus, which is defined as detectable movement of a tooth on tooth to tooth contact of the two dental arches. It can be detected by lightly palpating the buccal aspects of the teeth with the tip of the finger, as the mandible performs various functional movements. The degree of fremitus can be graded from slight, when the tooth movement can only just be detected, to moderate and severe, when such movement is visible.

2. The presence of excessive occlusal wear, which cannot be attributed to any abnormalities of the patient's diet and which is not commensurate with the patient's age.
3. The tilting and migration of individual teeth or of complete segments. This should be related to some functional position of the mandible, or to such a clinical feature as posterior bite collapse (Fig. 212). The rate of drift and the consequent opening of diastemas between the teeth is of significance.

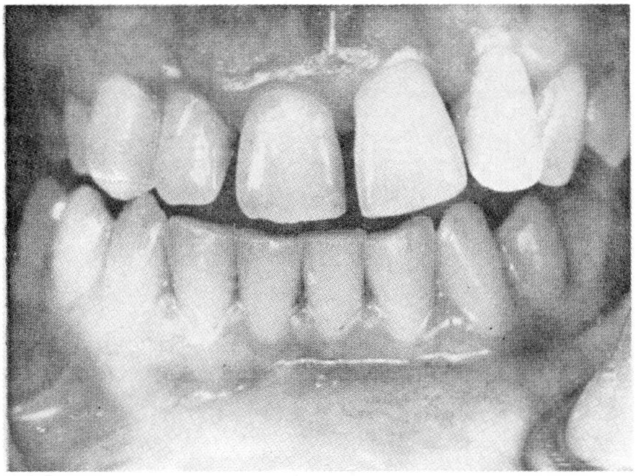

FIG. 212.—The migration of upper anterior teeth in a middle-aged woman with posterior bite collapse.

4. The percussion note of the teeth on tapping with a blunt instrument changes from a resonant note with a healthy supporting structure to a dull note if there is primary occlusal trauma in the attachment apparatus.
5. Careful palpation of the muscles of mastication to ascertain whether there is any hypertrophy or sign of hypertonicity, with possible spasm of one group of muscles.
6. Palpation of the temporomandibular joint and observation of any deviation of the mandible in various paths of closure. Are there any signs of temporomandibular joint pain-dysfunction syndrome?
7. Radiographic investigation, which offers a major contribution in confirming a diagnosis of primary occlusal trauma, provided the radiographic technique is carefully executed, preferably with a long-cone, paralleling device. The various features which are diagnostic of occlusal trauma are:
   (a) Widening of the periodontal ligament space (Fig. 213).
   (b) Loss of definition of the lamina dura (Fig. 214).
   (c) Funnel-like resorption at the crest of the alveolus, or crescentic resorption at the bone margins (Fig. 215).
   (d) In cases of severe occlusal trauma, cemental tears, root fracture, root resorption and pulpal changes might be seen.
8. All these clinical findings are in turn related to various points in the patient's history, and the relationships of the signs to the symptoms in a case of occlusal trauma become apparent. The patient's complaints will indicate the various occlusal problems:

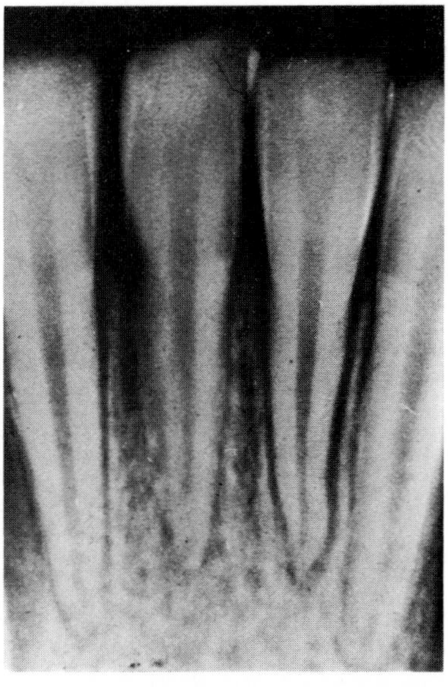

FIG. 213.—Increase in width of the periodontal ligament space in the lower incisor segment is the result of hyperfunction.

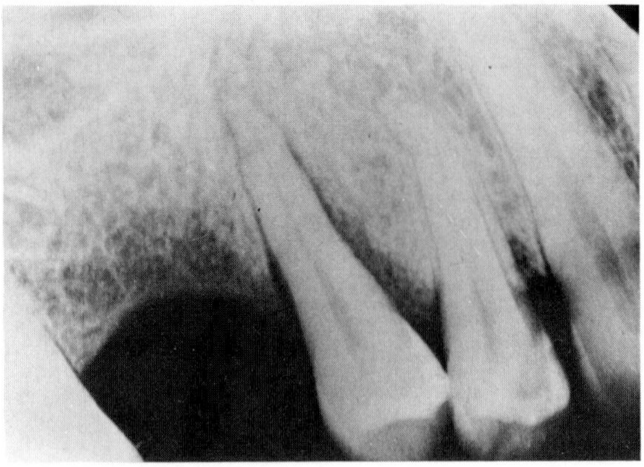

FIG. 214.—Loss of lamina dura mesial to upper second premolar which is highly mobile and is subjected to excessive forces in parafunctional activity.

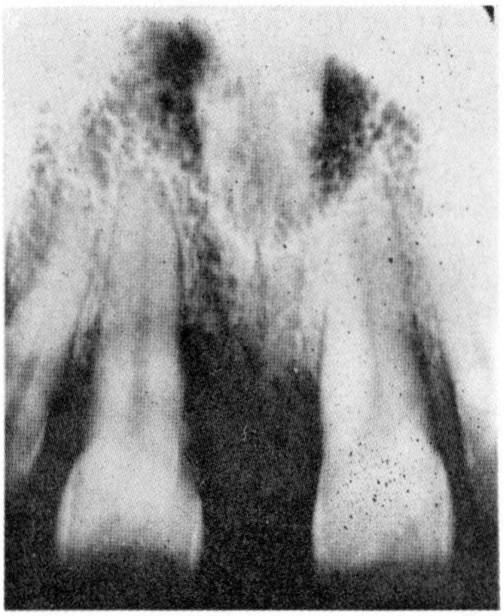

FIG. 215.—Crescentic bone loss about upper central incisors which are subject to abnormal occlusal stress.

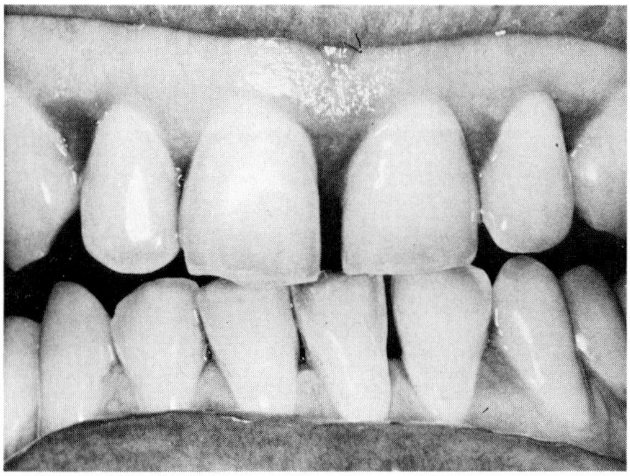

Fig. 216.—Recent opening of median diastema in a 26-year-old woman with signs of occlusal trauma.

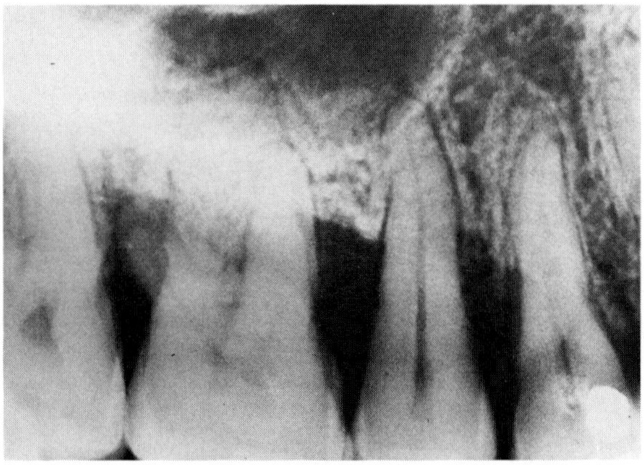

FIG. 217.—Opening of contact area between two upper premolars with considerable loss of support has given rise to food impaction in this area.

(a) Functional difficulties in eating and speech – due to mobile teeth and abnormal paths of closure of the mandible.
(b) Changes in appearance – due to migration and drifting of involved teeth or the excessive wear (Fig. 216).
(c) Tooth sensitivity – either due to wear or to pulpal changes with the traumatic forces.
(d) Food impaction – consequent upon the opening of contact areas with drifting and tilting of teeth (Fig. 217).
(e) Temporomandibular joint symptoms, from clicking noises, to limitation of movement – due to the occlusal disharmonies.
(f) A whole plethora of clinical changes has at one time or another been attributed to the effects of occlusal stress. They range from severe gingival recession and

migraine to obscure facial and neck pain. To a large extent these reports are based upon clinical impressions, which, while valid for that individual case, remain to be substantiated as general propositions.

9. A detailed habit history is taken, in an attempt to delineate and categorize any parafunctional activities. The habit might be quickly revealed, by the wear pattern for instance, but there often has to be repeated questioning on the habit history at several separate appointments. Care must be taken not to use leading questions in this regard.
10. A systematic analysis of the occlusion. This can be performed in the mouth or by using articulated models. The opinions of clinicians differ over this, but it is important to realize that if an articulator is to be used in analysis, it must be at least semi-adjustable, and the techniques for bite registrations and the mounting of the models must be meticulously carried out, or 'interferences' can be created by the very procedures of analysis. Simple study models can be invaluable in this part of the examination as they do enable one to obtain an extra perspective in observing the interdigitation of the teeth (Fig. 218).

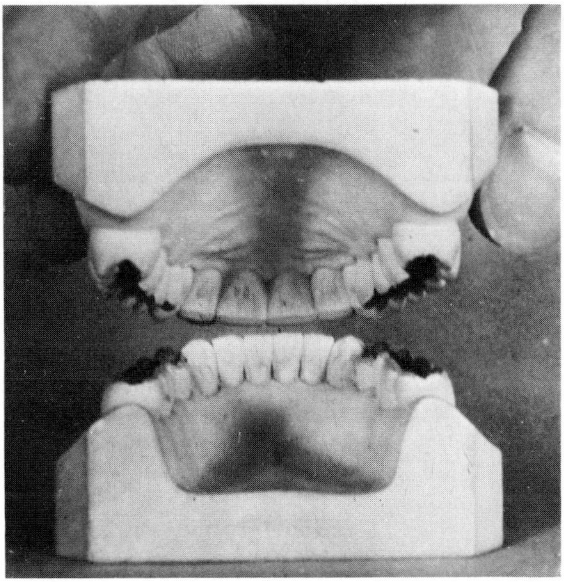

FIG. 218.—Study models enable observation of the interdigitation of the two arches to be made from the lingual aspect.

OCCLUSAL ANALYSIS

The static inter- and intra-arch relationships are first examined, with particular reference to the following features:

A. **Intra-arch examination**
- (i) The integrity of both arches.
- (ii) The alignment of teeth.
- (iii) Drifting and migration of teeth.
- (iv) Over-eruption and plunger cusps.
- (v) Tilting and alterations in the level of the occlusal tables.
- (vi) Wear patterns and open contacts.

B. **Inter-arch examination**
- (i) Angle's orthodontic classification.
- (ii) Amount of overbite and overjet.
- (iii) Form of the planes of occlusion.
- (iv) Gross malpositioning such as cross-bite relationship.
- (v) In maximum intercuspation, the cusp to fossa relationships.

The occlusal examination is then continued with a study of the functional relationships of the two arches. The point from which such a functional analysis should start has been the subject of some debate. It is obvious from the discussion in the previous chapter that the intercuspal position is the end-point of most functional movements of the mandible. As a reference point in analysis, however, it does have a major disadvantage. In so far as it is a neuromuscular position, it is not fixed, and dependent as it is on occlusal morphology, the position will be altered by the very methods used in occlusal adjustment.

The one fixed, reproducible point for occlusal analysis is the end of the terminal-hinge arc of closure, the retruded contact position. To include this in the study of a patient's functional relationships in no way implies that RCP has to be used more extensively during normal function by that patient. Nor should it be taken to mean that all patients receiving occlusal therapy for periodontal reasons should have IC and RCP coincident. The major reason for its use is the reliability with which this point can be achieved by different clinicians at different times. There are two other reasons which justify its inclusion. One is that the more retruded positions are used by some patients with certain swallowing patterns, and the other is the evidence implicating centric prematurities in the IC to RCP range, as initiators of damaging parafunctional activities.

Clinical Procedures in Occlusal Analysis

The analysis of the occlusion starts from the retruded contact position and in order to reach this point, it is essential to have the patient seated in a comfortable, relaxed position. Placing one hand on the chin, with the thumb resting at the incisal edge of the lower anterior segment, the patient is instructed to relax the lower jaw and to allow it to become quite loose in the operator's hand (Fig. 219). When the masticatory muscles do relax the mandible can be moved smoothly about its hinge axis. The thumb, which up to this time has prevented tooth-to-tooth contact is now moved away and the arches allowed to come together. At no time is direct distal pressure put upon the mandible.

The occlusal contacts may be marked with articulating paper, when two different colours are useful; with thin, soft occlusal indicator wax and grease marking pencil, or the cusp contacts can be demarcated with a length of dental floss (Figs 220–222).

From this first contact, a number of inter-arch relationships are noted, together with some observations on the patient's swallowing pattern:

(i) Teeth making contact in RCP.
(ii) Direction and amount of mandibular movement from RCP to IC.
(iii) Tooth contacts on the working and non-working sides during lateral excursions.
(iv) Tooth contacts during protrusion.
(v) An estimation of the free-way space.

Examination of these fractures will reveal the presence of occlusal disharmonies, which must then be related to the signs of occlusal trauma: the lesion is in turn related to the function or parafunction of the masticatory system.

Having established a diagnosis of occlusal trauma, various forms of occlusal therapy are now open to the clinician:

1. Occlusal adjustment by selective grinding.
2. Restorative dentistry to restore or replace the occlusal table.
3. Orthodontic treatment to re-align teeth to better cusp-to-fossa relationships.

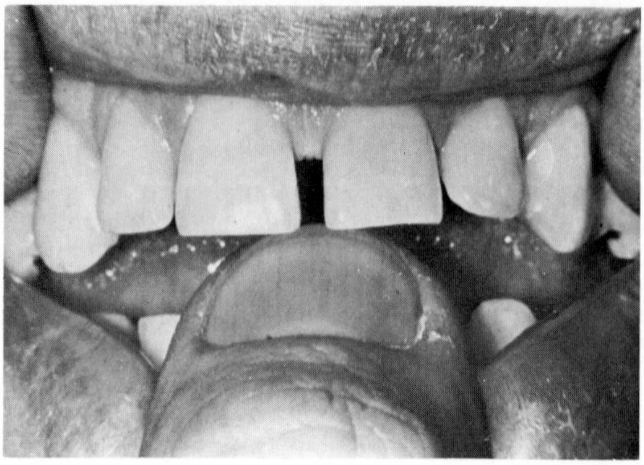

A

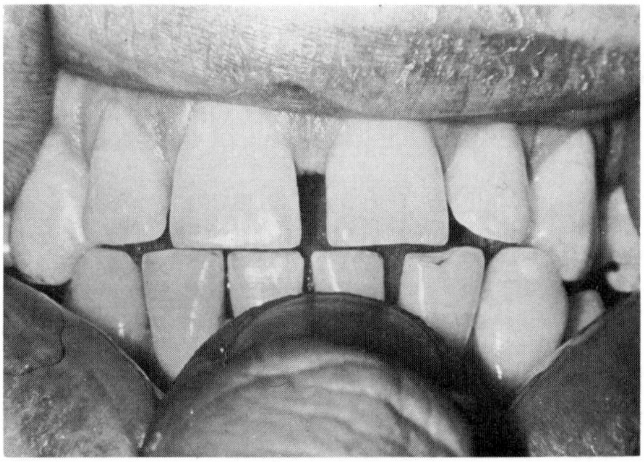

B

FIG. 219.—(*A*) Thumb in position to prevent tooth contact when seeking the terminal hinge path of closure. (*B*) Thumb removed to examine tooth contacts in the retruded position.

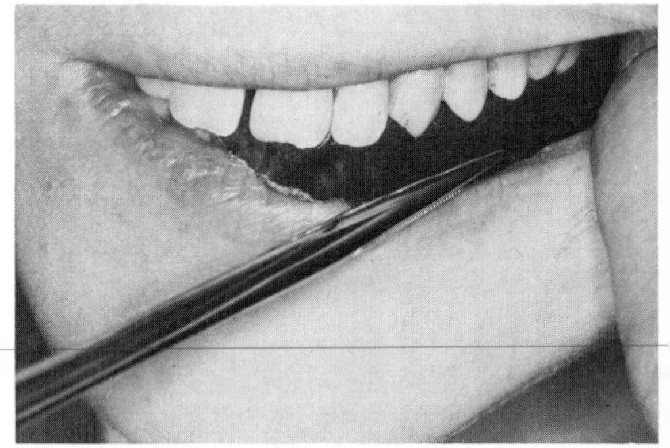

FIG. 220.—Marking occlusal contacts with articulating paper.

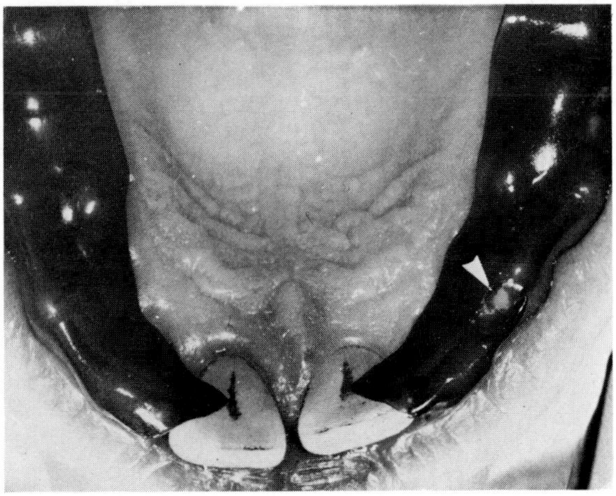

A

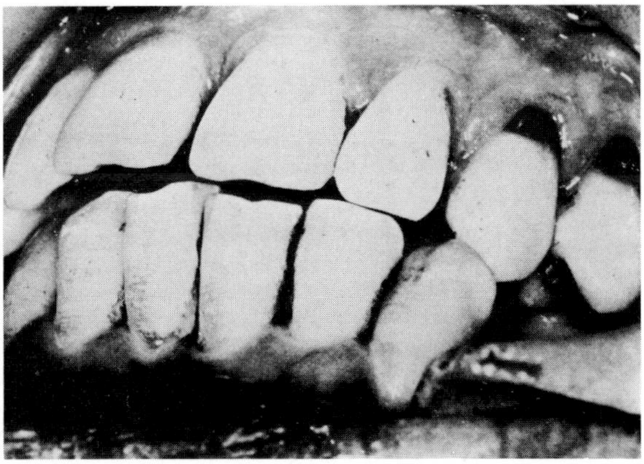

B

FIG. 221.—(*A*) Occlusal indicator wax in place showing perforation (arrowed) indicating premature contact between canines in (*B*).

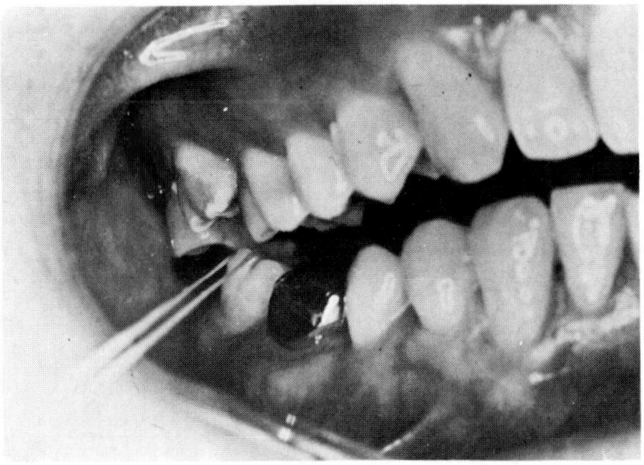

FIG. 222.—Dental floss encircling premature contact.

It is sometimes found necessary to stabilize the final occlusion by a splinting appliance, either fixed or removable. The choice of therapy depends entirely upon the clinical features of the case, and each form of treatment has its own limitations. Occlusal adjustment by grinding away tooth substance is an entirely subtractive procedure, and, as there is only a finite amount of tooth to be ground away with impunity, it is almost self-limiting. Occlusal discrepancies causing deflections of the mandible of 3 mm and over are not really suitable for a subtractive form of occlusal treatment alone.

OCCLUSAL ADJUSTMENT – OBJECTIVES

The basic objectives can be stated reasonably succinctly, but there would appear to be many ways of achieving these objectives during adjustment.

The objectives of occlusal adjustment, in part after Beyron (1969) are:

1. To distribute occlusal forces, as far as possible, in the long axis of the tooth, because this is the direction of force application which is best absorbed and dissipated in the periodontal ligament. It must be equally evident that lateral torque upon the tooth should be minimized.
2. Forces should be distributed over as many teeth as possible in maximum intercuspation.
3. Bilateral contact between posterior teeth in the retruded contact position. If IC and RCP are not coincident, they should lie on a sagittal line, and the distance between them should ideally be less than 1 mm.
4. Chewing may be performed with equal ease on right and left sides. This is facilitated by simultaneous gliding contact between teeth on the working side – group function. This group function is equally applicable to protrusive movements.
5. All this must be achieved at an acceptable occlusal vertical dimension.

6. There should be an improvement in the patient's presenting symptoms, *e.g.* problems in aesthetics, mastication and speech are the most common.

This is by no means the only concept of occlusal adjustment. There are others which for instance strive to achieve bilateral balance, an objective arising out of the prosthetic need to keep denture bases stable (Schuyler, 1935). Biologically there is no justification for translating such a concept to the natural dentition. Similarly the canine-protected occlusion (D'Amico, 1961), while it is perfectly acceptable as part of a physiological occlusion, should not be inflicted upon all patients with occlusal trauma, as the 'ideal' occlusion.

OCCLUSAL ADJUSTMENT – TECHNIQUES

Having arrived at the decision that an occlusion requires some therapeutic intervention, including occlusal adjustment, there must be some kind of logical sequence by which to achieve the objectives of adjustment. Unfortunately, the range of presenting occlusal features is almost infinite, and the rules for adjustment which have been suggested in the past inevitably contain an element of a mechanistic approach to deviations from an ideal kind of interdigitation. Rather than perpetuate this mechanistic series of laws and formulae for occlusal grinding, a sequence of steps to be used therapeutically is suggested purely as a very loose framework which will enable each case to be considered on its own merits and will closely relate the therapy to an understanding of functional oral anatomy as described in Chapter 13.

Although each step is considered as a separate item of treatment, not a single part of the occlusal anatomy should be removed before completing the whole occlusal analysis. The treatment is subtractive, and the effect of each spot grinding on all functional mandibular positions should be studied, not simply the effect upon a single path of closure. Before any indiscriminate grinding is performed, the function of the various families of cusps which exist in the dentition must be considered (Fig. 223).

The interdigitation of cusps and fossae which will be described concerns an Angle's Class I occlusion, but it is possible to extrapolate the functional occlusal anatomy from this, which can then be applied to any given clinical situation (Kraus, Jordan and Abrams, 1969).

As teeth reach the point of maximum interdigitation, in the posterior segments, only two groups of cusps have a potential for contact – the palatal cusps of the maxillary teeth and the buccal cusps of the mandibular teeth. At maximum interdigitation, the tip of the palatal cusp of the upper tooth meets the central fossa of the lower, and the tip of the buccal cusp of the lower meets the central fossa of the upper (Fig. 224). Between these cusps and fossae are the inclines of the Supporting Cusps, so called because their main function is the support of the vertical dimension. Unless there is good reason to do so, removal of cusp height of supporting cusps should not be carried out as it will close the vertical dimension, or take teeth out of occlusion. Neither of these results is part of the objectives of adjustment.

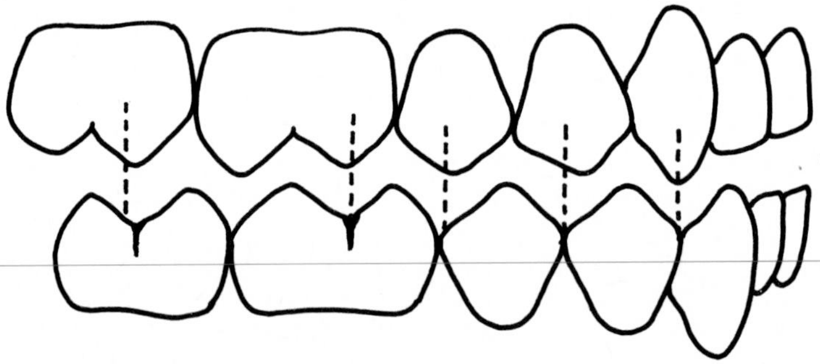

FIG. 223.—Lateral view of the two arches reaching maximum interdigitation, with upper buccal cusps related to marginal ridge and buccal groove areas.

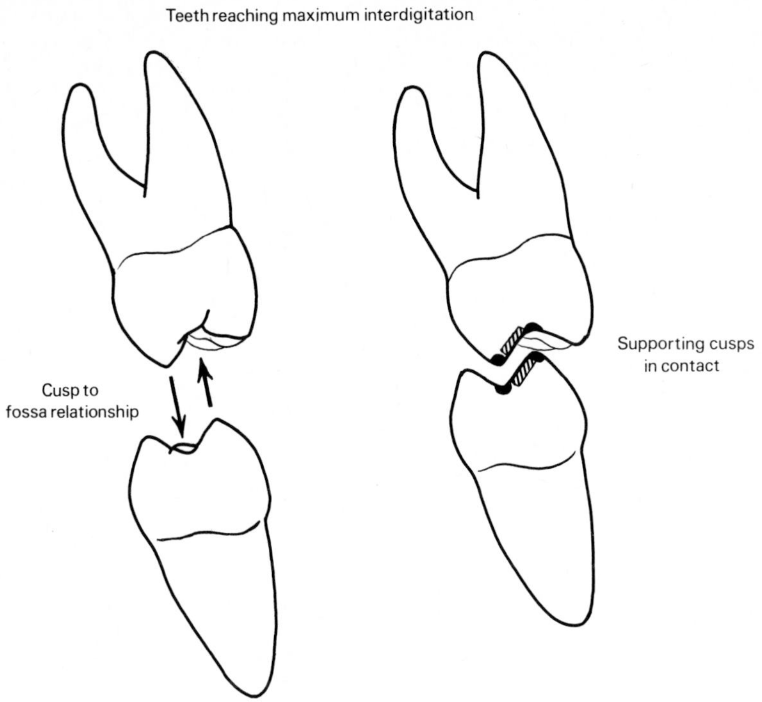

FIG. 224.—The supporting cusps and their inclines.

The other cusps have a potential for contact only in lateral excursion, when the buccal aspect of the tip of the lower buccal cusp glides down the inner incline of the upper buccal cusp (Fig. 225). Clearly, the other family of cusps can influence the lateral excursions of the mandible and as such are called Guiding Cusps, which make up the remainder of the occlusal table.

A separation of function of cuspal families has, of course, given rise to such rules as the BULL rule for occlusal grinding, designed to preserve the cusps supporting the vertical dimension.

In lateral excursions, therefore, there is a small area on the outer aspect of the supporting cusp which contacts the inner incline of the guiding cusp. A similar area of contact can be extended around onto the anterior segments of the arch, when, in protrusive, the outer aspect of the incisive edge of the lower incisors glides down the palatal aspect of the upper incisors. The incisal guidance can in many respects be regarded as a 'guiding cusp' (Fig. 226). Just as the guiding cusps on the working side influence mandibular position in lateral excursion, so does the incisal guidance influence posterior tooth contact in protrusive.

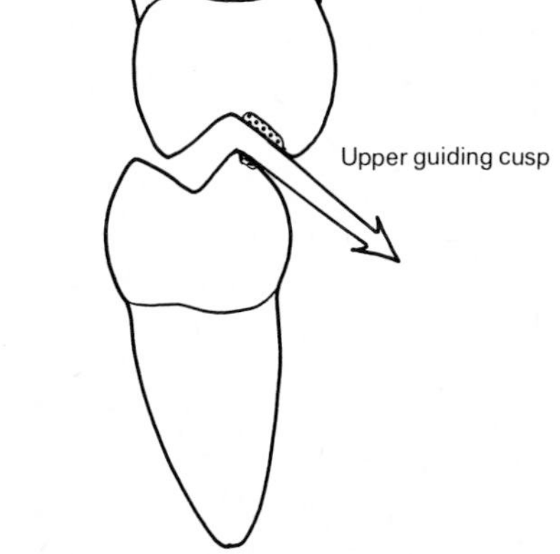

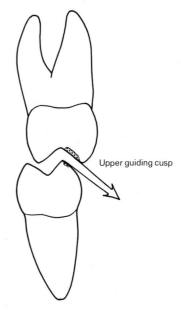

FIG. 225.—The outer aspect of the lower supporting cusp contacting the incline of the upper guiding cusp.

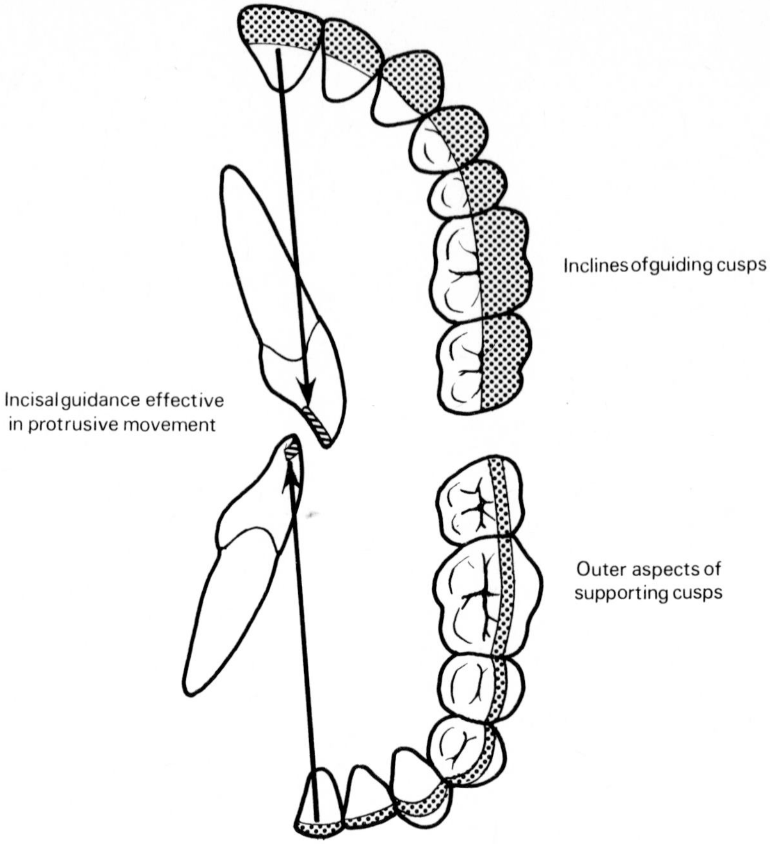

FIG. 226.—The 'guiding cusp' function of the palatal aspects of the upper anterior teeth, in continuity with the guiding cusp inclines of the posterior segments.

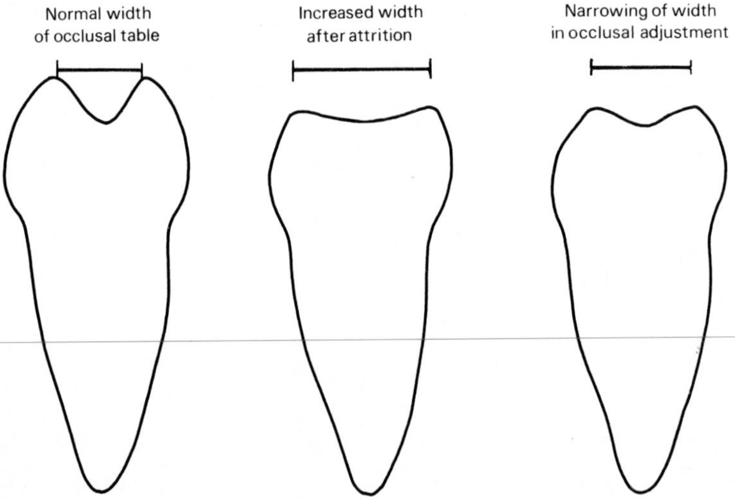

FIG. 227.—Narrowing of bucco-lingual diameters.

With these cuspal functions very much in mind, a sequence of grinding may then be embarked upon, using a handpiece and diamond points.

1. Elimination of gross occlusal disharmonies. Although these are very obvious discrepancies, they should not simply be removed without any reference to their possible implications when attempting to retain tooth structure for future, more definitive occlusal adjustment. Into this category falls the reduction of plunger cusps, the reduction in length of extruded teeth, the narrowing of bucco-lingual diameters, correction of discrepancies in marginal ridge heights and elimination of severe fremitus patterns (Fig. 227).

2. Correcting for prematurities in the retruded contact position. By and large, the objective of simultaneous contact between a number of posterior teeth on both sides in RCP may be accomplished by grinding of involved cuspal inclines, rather than cusp tips. In that manner supporting cusp tips can be brought into alignment with the central fossae of the opposing teeth. The usual finding is that either a mesial incline of an upper tooth or the distal incline of a lower tooth needs grinding. The decision as to whether to grind cusp or fossa of the teeth in premature contact may be resolved by reference to tooth contacts in excursive movements of the mandible (Schuyler, 1935). When there is a prematurity in RCP which results in no disharmonies in lateral excursions, the fossa may be deepened (Fig. 228). Conversely, when two teeth make premature contact in both RCP and lateral excursions, the inclines of the cusps should be reduced (Fig. 229).

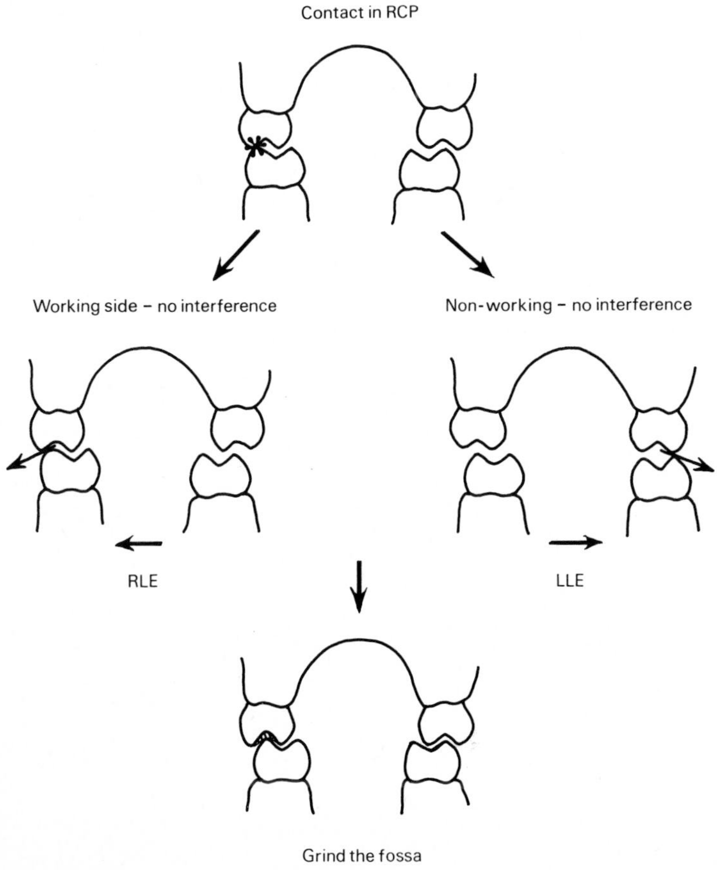

FIG. 228.—Correction of premature contact in the retruded position, with no prematurities in lateral excursion. RCP = Retruded Contact Position; RLE = Right Lateral Excursion; LLE = Left Lateral Excursion.

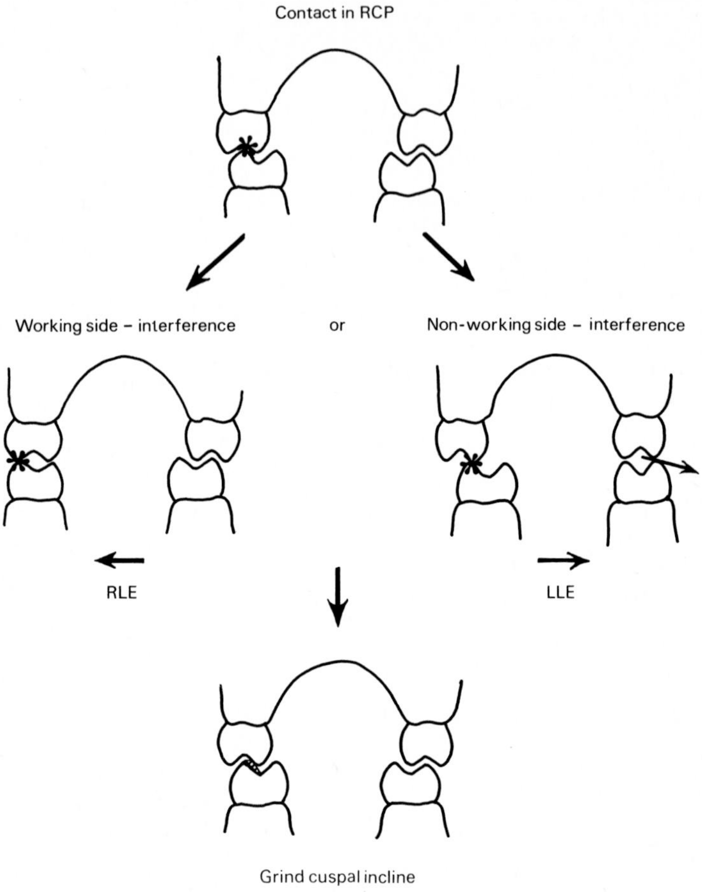

FIG. 229.—Correction of premature contact in the retruded position which also causes prematurities in lateral excursions.

Should the first contact occur in the anterior segment in RCP, the same principles can be applied, with careful reference to protrusive movements of the mandible before a decision is reached as to whether to grind the upper or lower incisors.

It may well be found that the positions of maximum intercuspation and retruded contact will become co-incident during this adjustment if the original discrepancy between the two points is small. Should the difference be large, a great deal of tooth substance would have to be removed to achieve co-incidence. It has already been stated that such co-incidence has not been proved to be a prerequisite for periodontal health, and a bilaterally symmetrical, sagittal slip can be entirely acceptable. However, in the intercuspal position there should be a maximum number of stable occlusal contacts distributing force in the long axes of the teeth. From this position of maximum intercuspation, the mandible now performs the various excursive movements.

3. Correction of protrusive disharmonies. In the protrusive movement, the anterior segments of the dental arches are the effective working areas and the posterior segments are the non-working. Thus the contact between the incisors and canines should be a smooth glide to the edge-to-edge position, with as many incisors as possible in contact at that point. At the same time, the posterior teeth should be out of contact. To achieve this, the adjustment should usually be confined to the lingual aspects of the upper teeth,

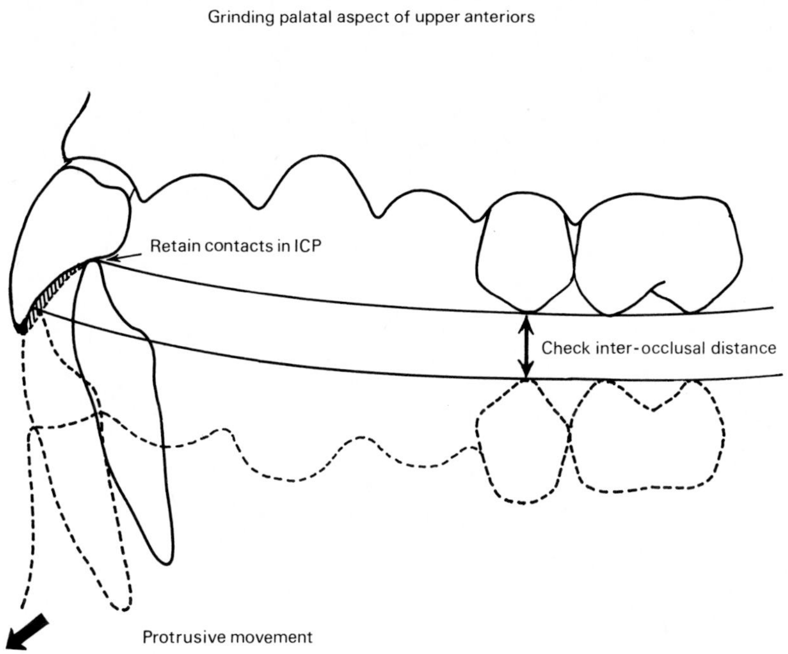

FIG. 230.—Correction of prematurities in protrusive movements, maintaining centric holds and related to posterior inter-occlusal distance.

taking care to retain the intercuspal contacts, and also to relate this grinding to the amount of posterior interocclusal space (Fig. 230).

4. Correction of disharmonies in lateral excursions. The objectives during these mandibular movements are group function on the working side and disarticulation on the non-working side. The concept of 'balance', as has been stated, derives from the world of prosthetics and has no place in the therapy of the natural dentition. Such 'balancing' contacts have, on the contrary, been shown to have a possible aetiologic role in temporomandibular joint dysfunction. Teeth with non-working contacts also exhibit a greater incidence of deep periodontal defects (Yuodelis and Mann, 1965).

To eliminate working side interferences, the BULL rule can normally be applied, so that the small area on the outer aspects of the tips of the lower supporting cusps glides down the guiding cusps of the upper posterior teeth. Cross-tooth balance is not needed, and, once again, the amount of tooth substance to be removed must be related to the interocclusal distance on the non-working side (Fig. 231).

Non-working contacts pose something of a problem, in that they occur on the supporting cusps, usually tracing out an area of contact on the buccal inclines of upper supporting cusps, against the lingual inclines of the lower supporting cusps. Their elimination demands very precise adjustment of cuspal inclines, making every effort to retain the very cusp tip, to maintain the occlusal vertical dimension. Sometimes the cusp has to be grooved to allow passage of the offending cusp tip of the antagonist on the non-working side. In certain circumstances the cusp-tip has to be sacrificed and the area is kept under surveillance to ensure that tipping and tilting of the tooth without a supporting cusp tip does not cause a further interference (Fig. 232).

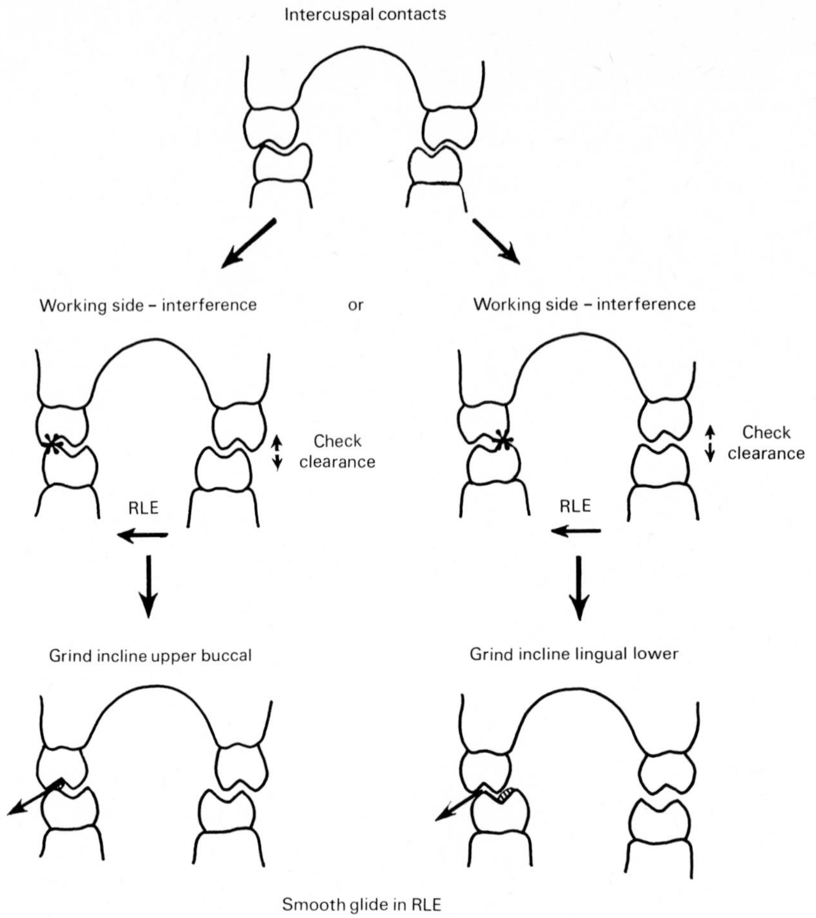

FIG. 231.—Removal of working side interference according to the BULL rule.

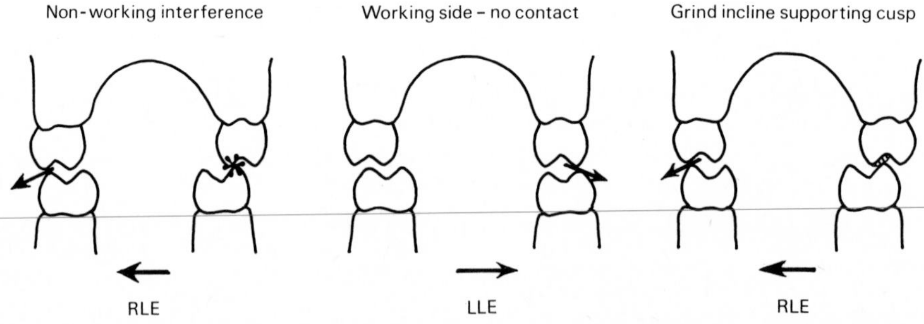

FIG. 232.—Correction of incline of upper supporting cusp to eliminate non-working interference.

At the conclusion of the occlusal adjustment, the areas which have been ground are polished with a rubber wheel. The stability of the occlusion which has been attained, is checked in all functional positions of the mandible, the patient's presenting occlusal symptoms should have been eliminated and, above all, the patient at the end of the adjustment should have a negative occlusal sense, *i.e.* he must be unaware of his occlusion in normal function.

THE ROLE OF ORTHODONTICS IN OCCLUSAL THERAPY

Migration of individual teeth and of complete segments of the dental arches may occur in advanced periodontal breakdown. Parafunctional activities such as tongue-thrust or pencil-chewing may cause tooth migration; the granulation tissue in deep periodontal pockets has been said to cause teeth to migrate as it proliferates; posterior bite collapse commonly results in migration of anterior teeth (Fig. 233). As bone loss occurs in chronic periodontitis, the mobility of teeth increases, resulting in an imbalance of forces upon these teeth, which begin to move out of their equilibrium positions. The teeth, in moving out of alignment, can initiate traumatogenic forces through parafunction, while the forces on the malaligned teeth themselves deviate more and more from the long axes of the teeth. In this way a progressive situation ensues with the tooth malalignment being caused by, and contributing to, the furtherance of the periodontal breakdown. In these circumstances minor tooth movement becomes an integral part of the occlusal therapy. Before such treatment is instituted, however, the cause of the tooth migration *must* be clearly defined, and consideration given to the need for retention of the teeth in their new positions after tooth movement (Ramfjord and Ash, 1971).

Reitan has included the following in the objectives of orthodontic therapy during periodontal treatment:

1. To upright teeth as far as possible, and so to obtain optimal force distribution in the supporting tissues.
2. To minimize the horizontal force components on the teeth.
3. Correction of discrepancies in the occlusal plane.
4. Correction of cusp-to-fossa relationships.
5. Occlusal equilibration, which must be included in the orthodontic therapy, followed by careful retention of the corrected tooth position.

To these must be added the obvious requirements that there be correction of the patient's presenting symptoms, such as problems in aesthetics, mastication or phonetics. Orthodontic treatment is also often necessary prior to the construction of complex restorations such as periodontal splints. Minor tooth movement may produce a favourable response in bony defects, and assist in changing their morphology or even result in filling in of infrabony pockets.

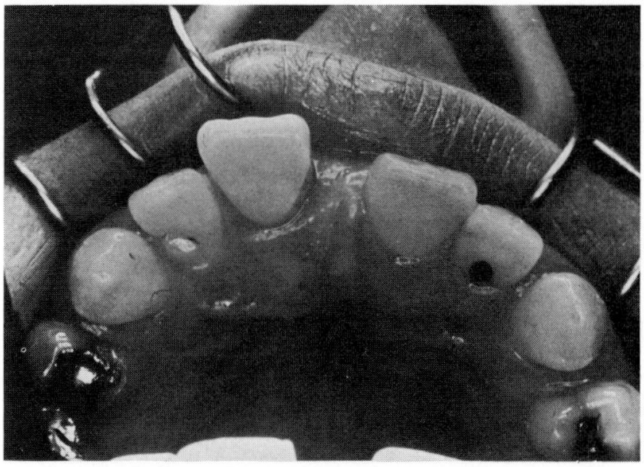

FIG. 233.—Migration of upper central incisor in patient with a lip biting habit.

TECHNIQUES IN MINOR TOOTH MOVEMENT

Both fixed and removable appliances may be used, but in adult orthodontics it will be found that removable appliances are more readily acceptable to the patients. All the basic principles of orthodontic appliance design are applicable to the problems of minor tooth movement in periodontal therapy and great care must be taken to include sufficient anchorage when dealing with teeth which have lost substantial amounts of their supporting tissues. Similarly, the pressures exerted by the active portion of the appliance should be very light and be judiciously applied.

Periodontally involved teeth can often move back into alignment remarkably quickly, and the orthodontic phase of treatment is usually not prolonged. There must, of course, be space into which the teeth can be moved and this may sometimes have to be created by slight stripping of the contact areas.

One of the most useful appliances in minor tooth movement is the Hawley appliance, which, although it can be used in both the mandible and the maxilla (Fig. 234), is most often constructed for the upper arch (Fig. 235). Such an appliance consists of an acrylic palatal plate, some form of posterior anchorage, such as clasps or cribs, and a labial arch. This labial arch can be activated to retract upper incisors (Fig. 236), or the Hawley can be used for the application of elastics, to the same effect. Springs may also be attached to move individual teeth both bucco-lingually (Fig. 237) and mesiodistally (Fig. 238).

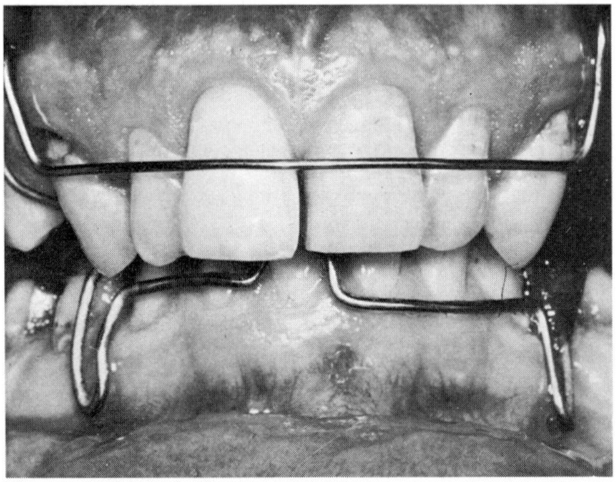

FIG. 234.—Upper and lower Hawley appliances *in situ* for minor tooth movement of the labial segments.

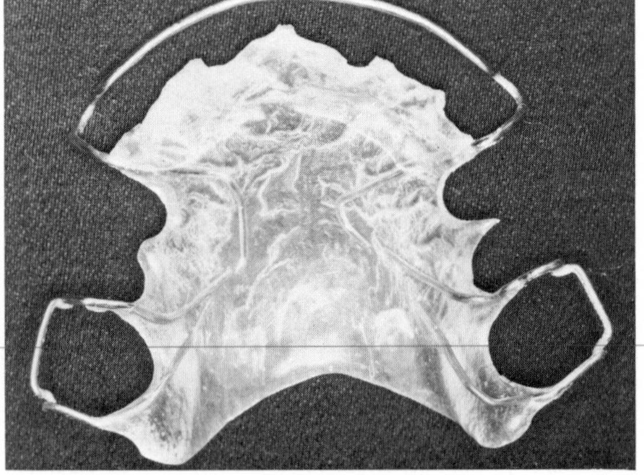

FIG. 235.—An upper Hawley appliance.

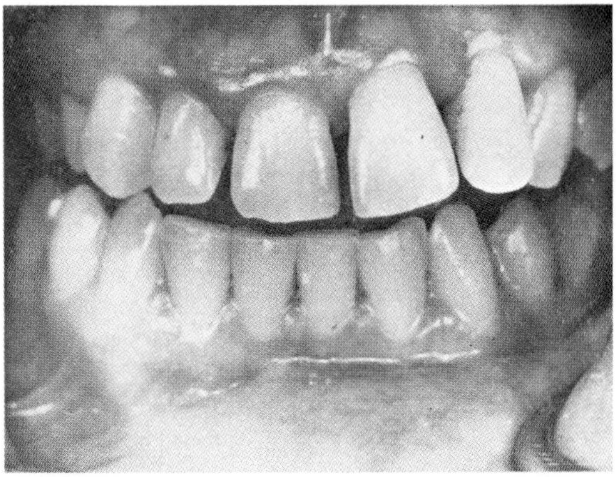

A

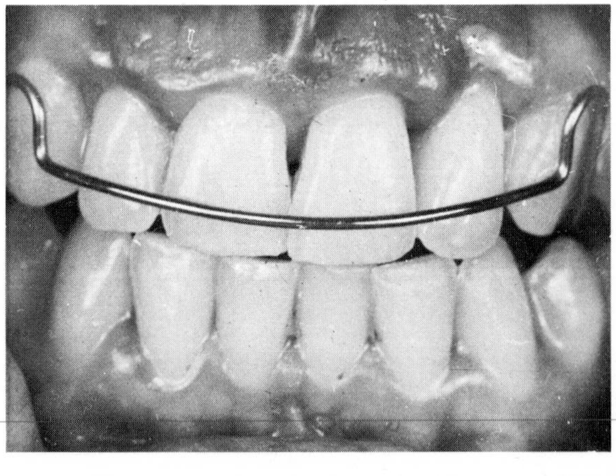

B

FIG. 236.—(*A*) Migrated upper incisors before treatment. (*B*) After retraction with a Hawley appliance.

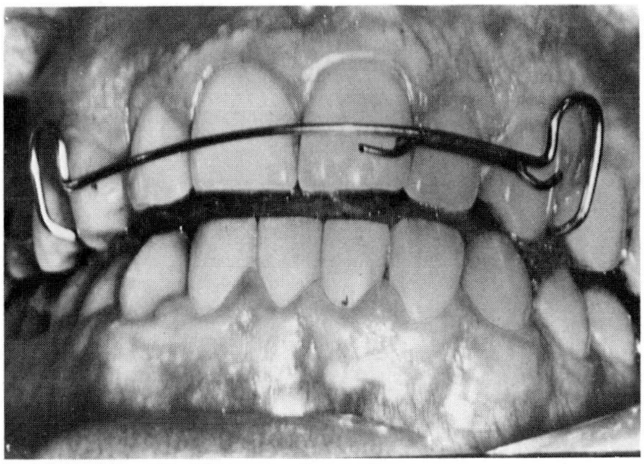

FIG. 237.—Lingual movement of individual anteriors with an upper Hawley appliance and finger springs.

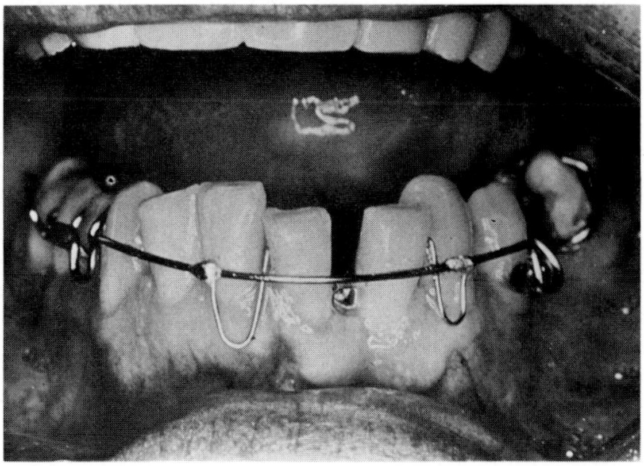

FIG. 238.—Mesial movement of two migrated lower central incisors.

Modification of the basic Hawley to include an anterior palatal bite plane, just posterior to the upper incisor teeth, will allow this appliance to be used to alter the plane of occlusion. The posterior disarticulation caused by the bite plane may result in some slight eruption in the premolar/molar segments, altering the curve of Spee while at the same time, this lack of posterior contact will allow of alterations in the cusp-to-fossa relationships during treatment. When using a palatal bite plane it must be carefully adjusted to produce minimal posterior disarticulation, so that there is no drastic encroachment on the free-way space.

These removable appliances need frequent checks and adjustments until the desired tooth alignment has been produced. The longer the patient is able to wear the appliance initially, the quicker will the result be achieved, and the same appliance, with suitable modifications, can act as a temporary retention plate after the minor tooth movement is complete.

Fixed appliances also have their place in minor tooth movement, but are restricted to their simplest forms. The grassline ligature can, for instance, be used to re-align incisors, while bands and elastics are used to correct cross-bite relationships, when necessary (Figs 239, 240).

Throughout the orthodontic phase of treatment special care should be taken to maintain a very high standard of plaque control, as the appliances can be plaque-retentive. Too rapid movement of periodontally involved teeth may result in a lateral periodontal abscess, which is usually amenable to local therapy. However, such an event can be avoided by careful assessment of the forces involved in the minor tooth movement.

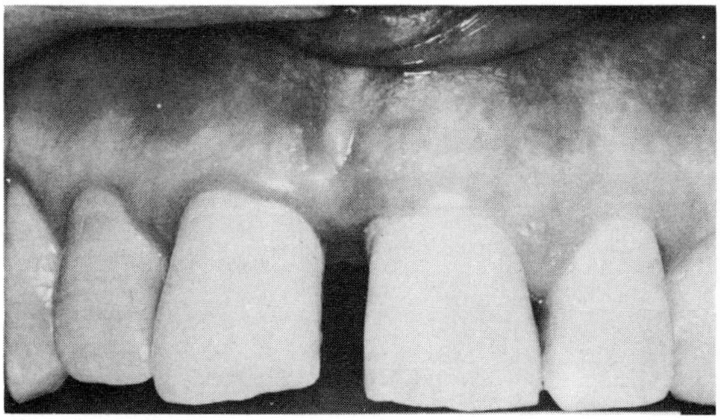

A

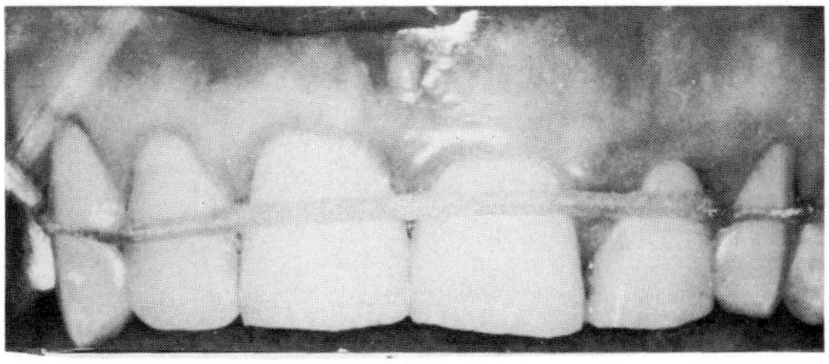

B

FIG. 239.—(*A*) Teeth prior to minor tooth movement (36-year-old woman). (*B*) Teeth after 5 weeks treatment with grassline ligatures.

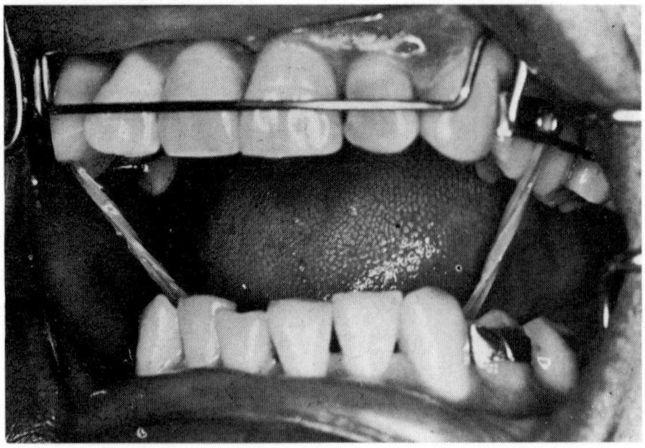

FIG. 240.—Correction of premolar crossbites with fixed bands, crossbite elastics and a Hawley appliance for disarticulation.

SPECIAL PROBLEMS IN TREATING BRUXING AND CLENCHING HABITS

The local dental measures employed in treating a bruxing or clenching habit usually involve the procedures of occlusal adjustment that have already been outlined, but the complex nature of the aetiology in many of these cases may well necessitate additional means of treatment. The psychotherapy needed to diminish the psychic tension does not form part of the dental treatment, but may obviously greatly assist in eliminating these damaging parafunctional activities (Ramfjord and Ash, 1971). The use of tranquillizing drugs has sometimes been recommended, but their use should be strictly confined to bruxists who show signs of muscle spasm or temporomandibular joint symptoms. In this regard, low doses of Diazepam are effective, but the prolonged use of such medications in occlusal therapy cannot be justified.

When confronted with a patient in severe muscle spasm with resultant trismus, alleviation of the acute symptoms may be achieved by inserting a Hawley appliance with a palatal bite plane. The lack of posterior occlusal contact effectively eliminates any premature contacts, thus breaking the reflex activity causing the muscle spasm. This appliance will also enable sufficient relaxation of the muscles of mastication to occur to allow occlusal analysis and adjustment to be commenced. Various modifications of the Hawley have been devised for occlusal therapy, including the Sved plate, which uses acrylic to stabilize the anterior segment, rather than a labial arch (Fig. 241).

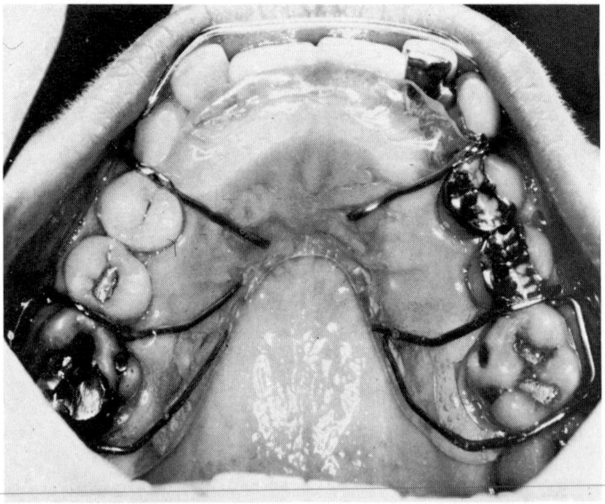

A

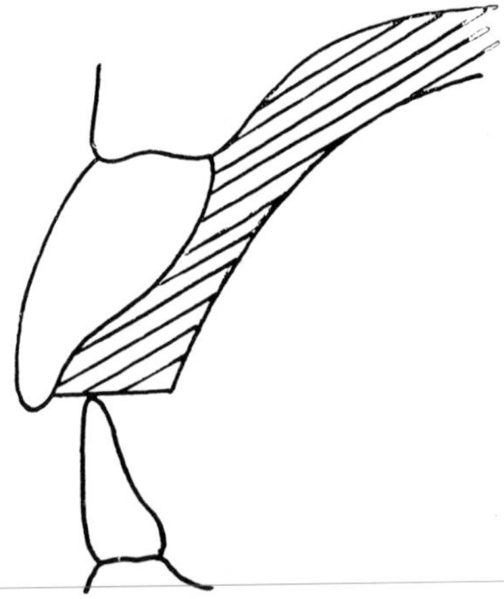

B

FIG. 241.—(*A*) A Hawley appliance *in situ*, with an anterior bite platform. (*B*) Used during the treatment of severe bruxism in a 31-year-old woman.

The prolonged use of such bite-plates cannot be recommended, as jiggling movements of the teeth will result in occlusal traumatic lesions. In cases of intractable bruxing and clenching activity which does not respond to normal treatment, an occlusal guard may be constructed. This usually covers all the occlusal table of the maxillary teeth with clear acrylic and should be so adjusted that there is complete freedom of movement in all excursions of the mandible (Fig. 242). Excessive involvement of the free-way space must be avoided, especially if the bite-guard is replaced by a metal onlay on the posterior teeth. Such appliances, which are designed to open the bite have resulted in severe periodontal problems (Fig. 243). The acrylic occlusal guard may, however, be used over long periods of time, when the bracing action of the splint stabilizes the teeth, and the occlusal coverage prevents occlusal wear while at the same time diminishing the tendency for bruxism.

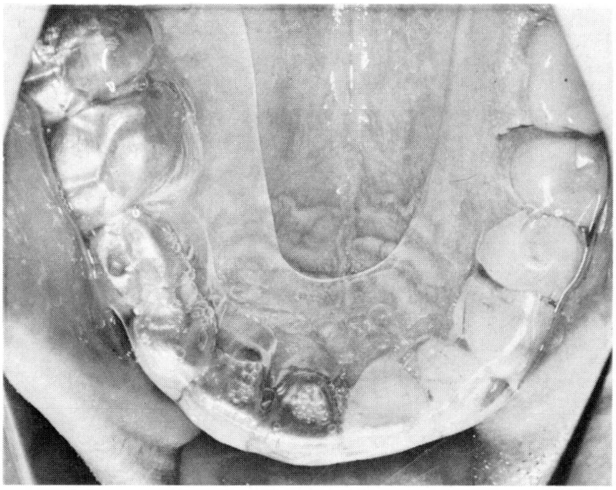

A

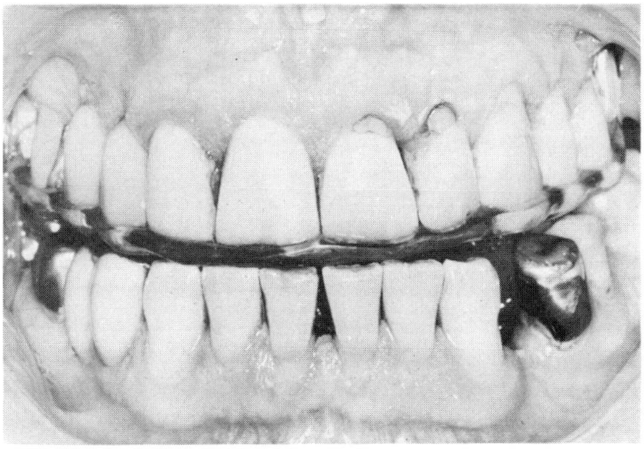

B

Fig. 242.—(*A*) Occlusal bite-guard with palatal and occlusal coverage. (*B*) Bite-guard in position, with complete freedom of movement during excursions of the mandible.

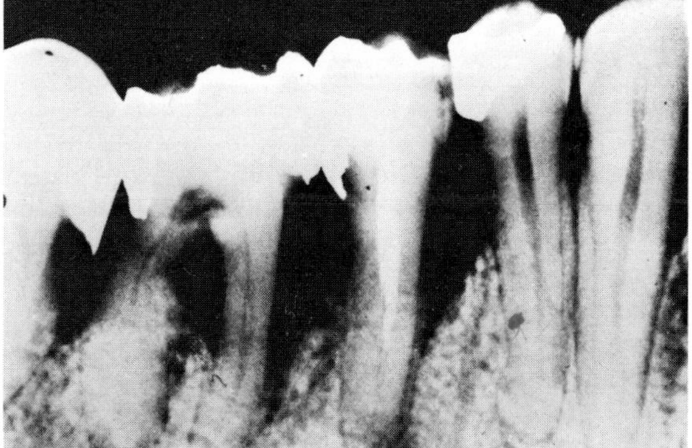

Fig. 243.—Bone destruction associated with a metal bite-guard encroaching on the free-way space, worn for several years.

THE PLACE OF OCCLUSAL THERAPY IN PERIODONTAL TREATMENT

While alteration of the occlusal patterns is carried out for many reasons, including the treatment of temporomandibular joint disorders, the preparation of the mouth for restorative dentistry, and the elimination of parafunctional activities, the techniques outlined in this Chapter have been basically concerned with the treatment of the lesion called occlusal trauma. The various types of occlusal therapy have in no way been concerned with the treatment of inflammatory changes in the gingivae, but only with a pathological process of the attachment apparatus.

When occlusal adjustment is deemed to be an essential part of the treatment plan, it is usually divided into two parts:

1. The preliminary or gross occlusal adjustment. This forms part of those stages of therapy concerned with the elimination of all the aetiologic factors. Any minor tooth movement would also be carried out at this time, after the plaque control has reached the required standard. In this manner, excessively mobile teeth can be stabilized and the normal function of the masticatory system is restored.
2. The definitive or fine occlusal adjustment.

This occurs after any pocket elimination found necessary has been carried out, and it results in an occlusion which has no clinical signs of primary occlusal trauma, is in harmony with the neuromuscular activities of the masticatory system and can demonstrably be maintaining itself in health.

It must be apparent that the dynamic nature of the occlusion will necessitate continued clinical assessment with the passage of time, and, if any sign of further primary occlusal trauma occurs in the future, steps must be taken to treat the new occlusal disharmonies, the underlying objective ultimately being to increase the longevity of the dentition.

REFERENCES

AMSTERDAM, M. (1973). Periodontal prosthesis. *In* Goldman, H. M. and Cohen, D. W., Periodontal Therapy, 5th ed. C. V. Mosby Company, St. Louis.

BEYRON, H. (1969). Optimal occlusion. *Dent. Clin. N. Amer.*, **13**, No. 3, 537.

D'AMICO, A. (1961). Functional occlusion of the natural teeth of man. *J. prosth. Dent.*, **11**, 899.

KRAUS, B. S., JORDAN, R. E. and ABRAMS, L. (1969). Dental Anatomy and Occlusion. Williams & Wilkins, Baltimore.

MÜHLEMANN, H. R. (1967). Tooth mobility: A review of clinical aspects and research findings. *J. Periodont.*, **38**, 686.

RAMFJORD, S. P. and ASH, M. M. Jr. (1971). Diagnosis and treatment of bruxism and minor orthodontic therapy. *In* Occlusion. W. B. Saunders Company, Philadelphia.

SCHUYLER, C. H. (1935). Fundamentals in the correction of occlusal disharmony, natural and artificial. *J. Amer. dent. Ass.*, **22**, 1193.

YUODELIS, R. A. and MANN, W. V. (1965). The prevalence and possible role of non-working contacts in periodontal disease. *Periodontics*, **3**, 219.

15. Splinting

When the periodontal tissues are no longer capable of withstanding the stresses of normal function teeth become mobile. In many cases local treatment of the periodontal lesions and occlusal adjustment is all that is required to strengthen the periodontal tissues and rehabilitate the teeth. In other cases, *i.e.* where there is secondary occlusal stress, teeth must be joined together in some fashion so that the resultant unit of several teeth is capable of withstanding forces too great for the individual teeth.

The value of splinting loose teeth has been questioned on the grounds that when the splint is removed the teeth are found to remain mobile. However the aim of splinting is not simply to make loose teeth firm: it is (1) to protect the tooth-supporting tissues during a healing period after an accident or after surgery, (2) to bring into function teeth which cannot be used to eat efficiently or in comfort without artificial support. If splinting is carried out incorrectly it may make firm teeth loose. Thus if a loose upper central incisor is splinted to a firm central incisor it is most likely that in twelve months both teeth will be loose.

Splints may be temporary or permanent. Many types of splint, both fixed and removable, have been devised. Every splint should meet certain requirements:

1. It should hold the teeth rigidly.
2. It should not subject the teeth to torsional stresses and thereby act as an orthodontic appliance.
3. It should not impose excessive stresses on any supporting tooth.
4. It should not cause pulp damage although elective pulpotomy may be resorted to during tooth preparation for a splint.
5. It must be sufficiently strong to withstand the stresses of mastication.
6. It must not interfere with function.
7. It should be designed so that it can be kept clean.
8. It should be aesthetically acceptable.

In splint construction two rules should be applied:

1. As many teeth as possible should be incorporated in a splint.
2. The splint should extend around the arch, *i.e.* it should include the canine tooth or the teeth on both sides of the canine. In this way the diverse angulation of the roots of the teeth incorporated in the splint forms a rigid buttress against forces from several directions (Fig. 244).

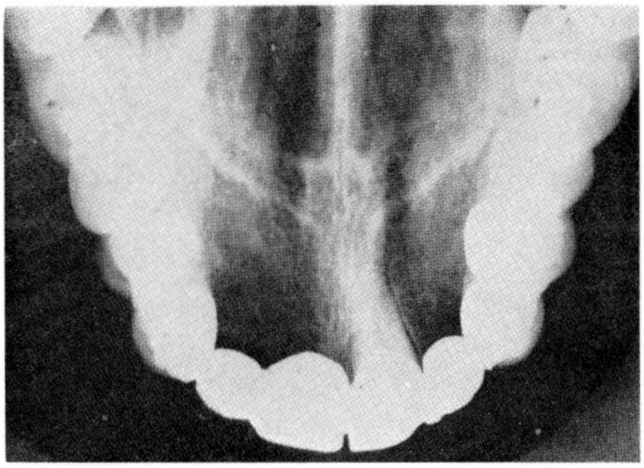

FIG. 244.—A fixed splint which goes around the arch and extends from 5| to |4, stabilizes the teeth incorporated, and replaces 21|2.

THE TEMPORARY SPLINT
(see Friedman, 1953)

Indications

Where tooth immobilization is required so that wound repair can take place as in:

1. Acute periodontitis as a result of a blow on a tooth.
2. Where an infrabony defect is to be treated by curettage to attempt to obtain some bone filling-in and reattachment.
3. As preparation for the insertion of a permanent splint.
4. During the surgical phase of treatment when mobility increases.

The Wire and Acrylic Splint (or Extracoronal Ligation)

Perhaps the most satisfactory of all temporary splints is the fixed wire and acrylic splint. It fulfils all the above criteria and has the added advantages of being simple to make and easy to remove. Five or six teeth are generally incorporated in order to immobilize one or two teeth. A length of stainless steel wire (0.25 mm soft) is looped around all the teeth to be included in the splint and its ends are loosely twisted. It is positioned just apical to the contact points (Fig. 245). Interdental wires (0.2 mm soft) are cut to about 2 inches in length, bent into a hairpin shape with one leg longer than the other and inserted between the teeth from the lingual side (Fig. 245*B*). The ends are gripped in a fine haemostat, maintained under tension and twisted until tight about the loop wire. When all the interdental wires have been placed the loop wire is finally tightened making sure that this is

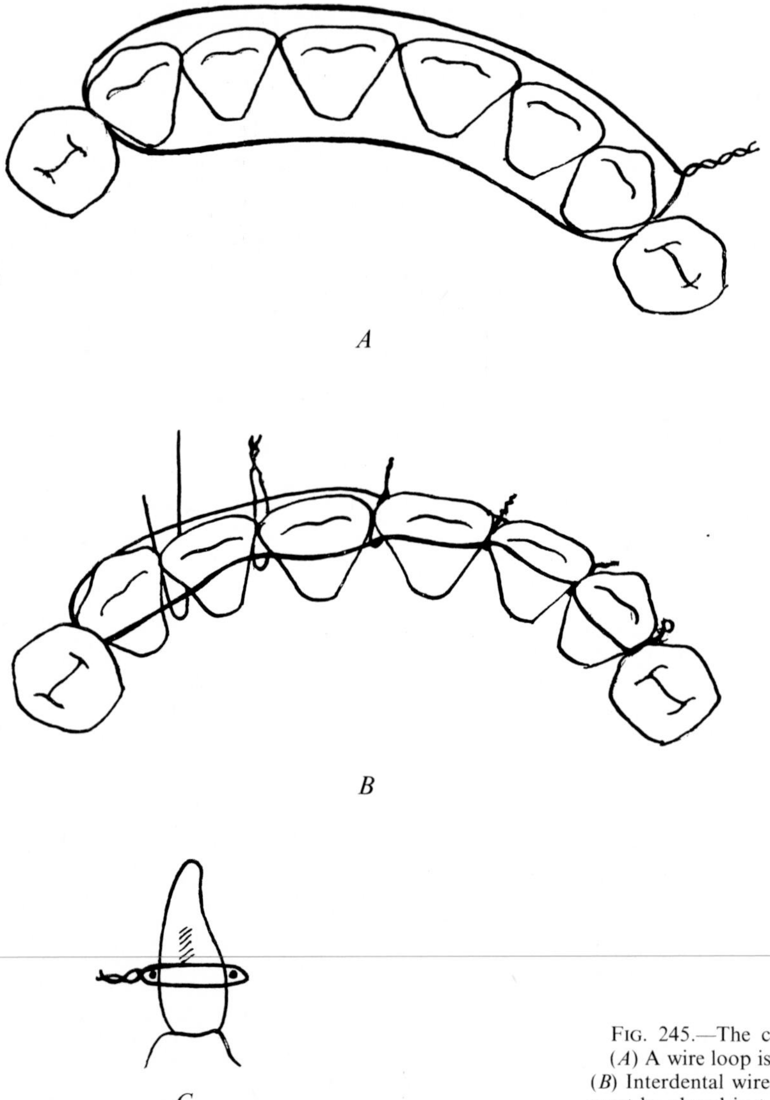

FIG. 245.—The construction of a wire and acrylic splint. (*A*) A wire loop is placed around all the teeth to be splinted. (*B*) Interdental wires are placed and tightened. (*C*) The splint must be placed just apical to the contact point.

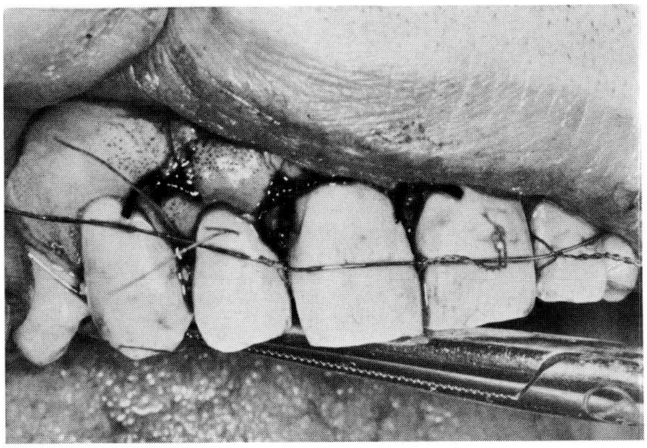

A

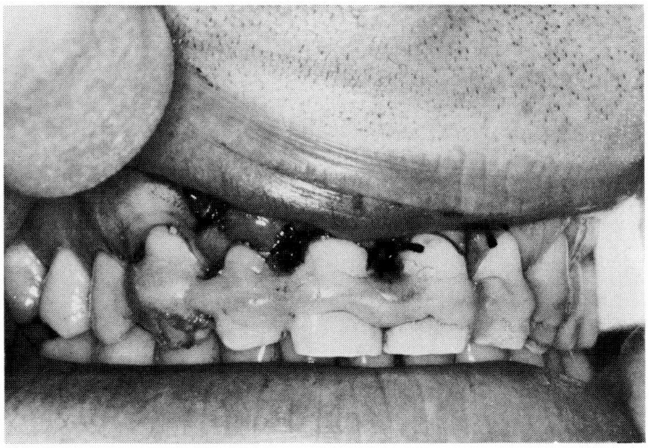

B

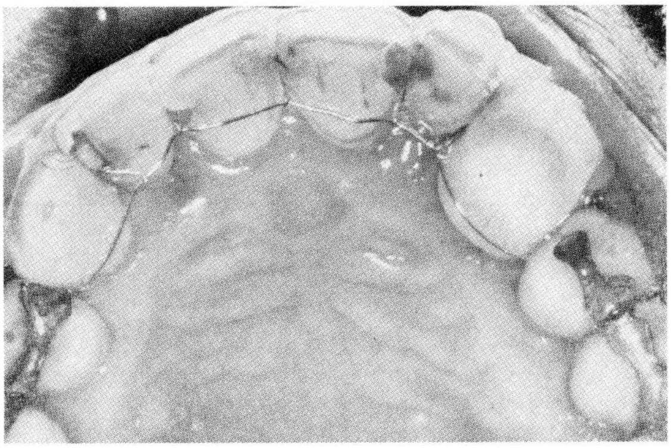

C

FIG. 246.—A temporary splint being applied at the time of a flap operation.

(*A*) Interdental wires being placed. (*B*) The wire covered in acrylic prior to polishing. (*C*) Wire seen from palatal aspect.

just below the contact points (Figs 245*C*). When tightening the wires it helps to twist them all the same way, either clockwise or anti-clockwise. The ends of the wires are then cut leaving 2–3 mm which can be tucked neatly between the teeth. The area is then dried and a thin mix of quick-set acrylic is run over the wire. Care is taken to ensure that the wire is evenly covered. The acrylic can be given a half-round contour as it is run on (Fig. 246).

When set, the shape is improved and the acrylic is trimmed so that the embrasures are free from acrylic at the cervical margins, and the bite is checked. In many cases it is impossible to cover the wire on the lingual aspect of the teeth, but this does not usually impair the efficiency of the splint. The acrylic is polished smooth so that it is easy to keep clean.

Another type of acrylic splint may be preformed on a model. This is a continuous collar of acrylic joined at either end by a wire. This is then cemented onto the teeth (Fig. 247). It does not provide the rigidity of the acrylic splint, but is useful for supporting molar teeth that have difficulty of access.

A temporary splint can also be made from orthodontic bands soldered together (Fig. 248), or from temporary acrylic crowns joined together (Fig. 249).

A temporary splint should be in place for no longer than six weeks. If tissue repair has not occurred in this time further retention of the splint will be useless. If teeth are still mobile after this time they must be permanently splinted or extracted.

PERMANENT SPLINTS

Indication

A permanent splint is indicated where the amount of supporting tissue remains insufficient to withstand normal functional stresses, as demonstrated by persistent mobility after all periodontal lesions have been treated and the occlusion adjusted.

Before applying a permanent splint all periodontal disease must be eliminated, and the occlusion should be adjusted so that stresses are evenly distributed. Splinting teeth without removing the disease is to be condemned unless there is a good reason for avoiding surgery. Teeth should

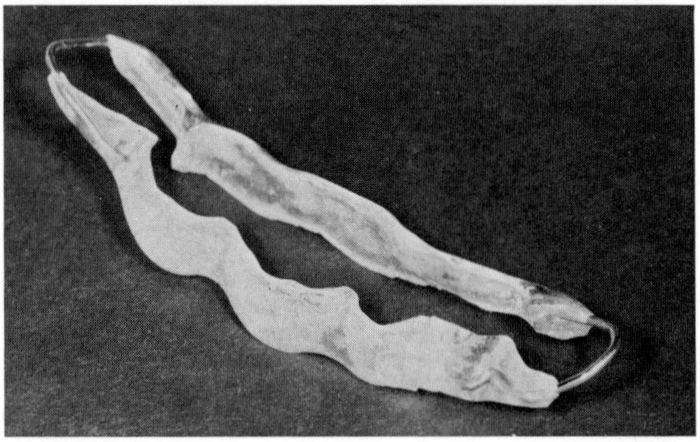

A

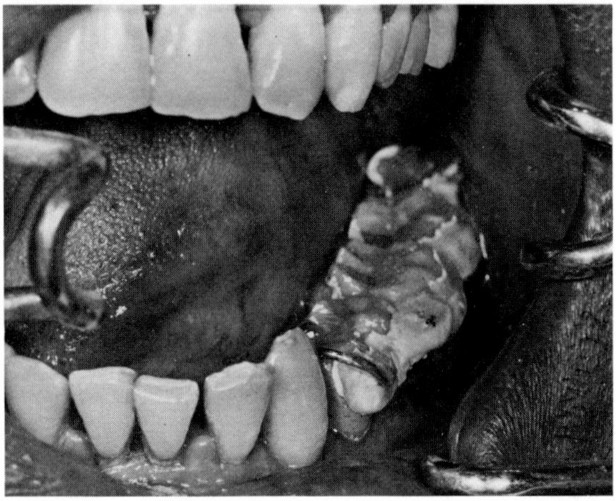

B

FIG. 247.—(*A*) Preformed acrylic collar. (*B*) Cemented in place.

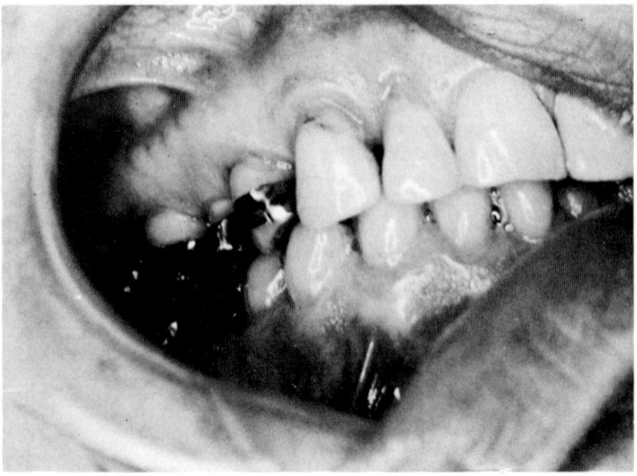

FIG. 248.—Posterior teeth splinted with orthodontic bands.

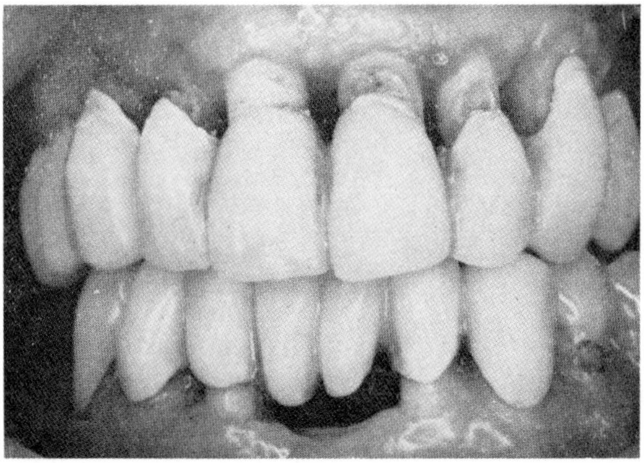

FIG. 249.—Splint of temporary acrylic crowns placed before gingivectomy which was subsequently carried out.

not be splinted if their retention will produce further loss of alveolar bone. Occasionally a patient insists that teeth be retained in some way, even though periodontal destruction is so far advanced that attempts to treat the disease are unjustified. The application of a permanent splint will frequently prolong the life of such teeth (Fig. 250), but in this case the patient should be informed of the limitations and the dangers of this treatment. If the occlusion is not adjusted prior to fitting a splint, an unnecessary handicap is imposed on the efficiency of the appliance.

Permanent splints are either removable or fixed.

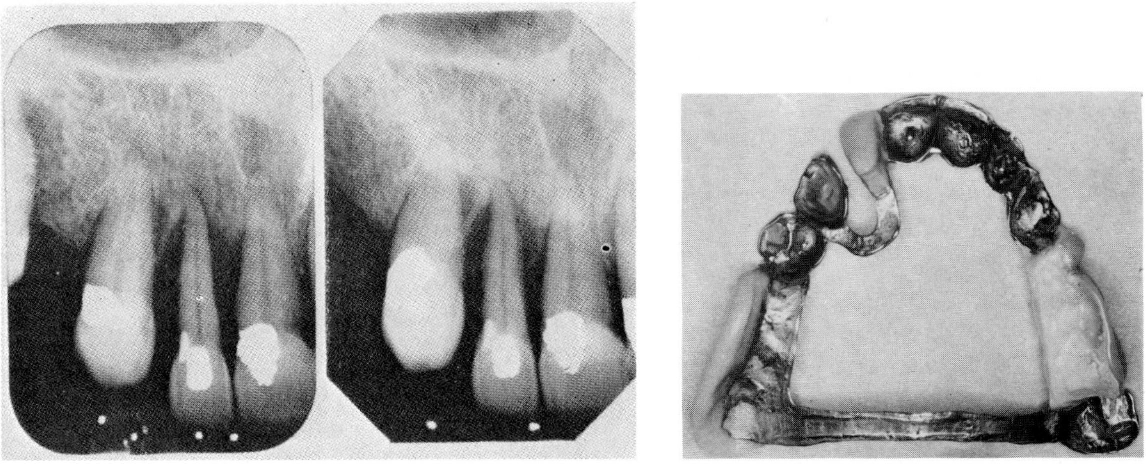

A *B* *C*

FIG. 250.—(*A*) Highly mobile teeth prior to splinting. (*B*) The same teeth eight years later after wearing the removable splint shown at (*C*).

REMOVABLE SPLINTS

Like all removable appliances the removable splint represents a potential source of irritation to the gingival margin. Nevertheless, with a carefully designed splint and a co-operative patient, such irritation can be reduced to a minimum. The removable splint is less difficult to construct than a fixed splint; it takes up little chairside time and can be altered, renewed, or even discarded. On the other hand it may provide less stability than a fixed splint.

The Continuous Clasp Splint

A continuous metal arch with multiple clasps and occlusal rests has been a commonly used form of splint where all or most of the teeth are present (Fig. 251). It is simple to construct and easy to keep clean. Maximum stability is obtained by designing the splint to embrace all the teeth in the arch. Great care must be taken to ensure that occlusal rests do not interfere with the occlusion. The use of this splint is restricted to the mandible, because the labial arch is seen in the front of the mouth.

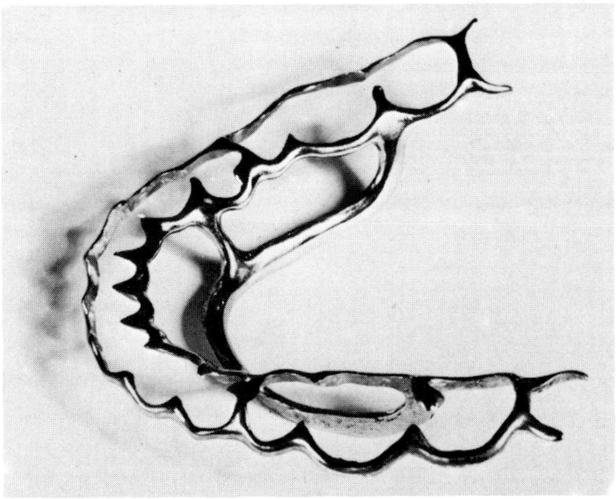

FIG. 251.—A continuous clasp splint.

The Simple Lingual Coverage Splint

This type of splint is essentially a metal partial denture with extensions covering the lingual surfaces of the teeth to be supported (Fig. 252). It is simple to construct, but because of the tissue coverage, is liable to cause gingival irritation, particularly if the patient's oral hygiene is not perfect. This splint tends to be bulky, and may interfere with the occlusion so that a certain amount of adjustment of opposing teeth may be necessary. If the splint is brought over the incisal edge of the anterior teeth to improve support the metal can be seen. Where spaces are present between the anterior teeth the splint has to be cut back out of sight. In doing this it is sometimes difficult to make the distance between the margin of the metal and the gingival margin sufficiently great to avoid gingival irritation (Fig. 253).

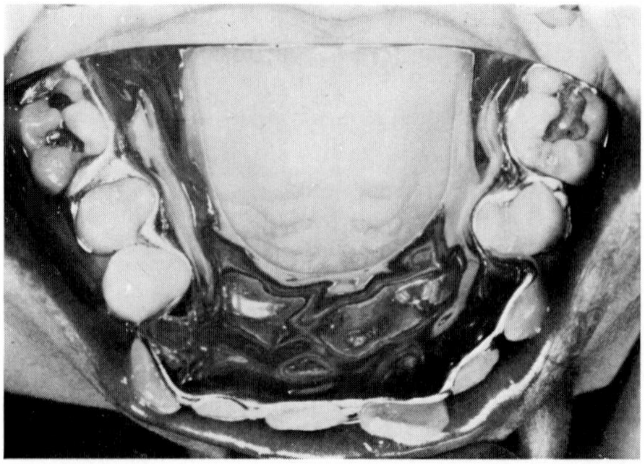

A

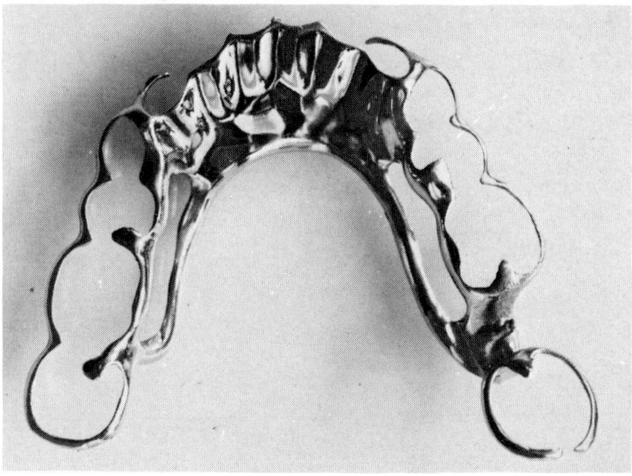

B

FIG. 252.—(*A*) Lingual coverage splint supporting upper anterior teeth. (*B*) A combination of lingual coverage and continuous clasp splint.

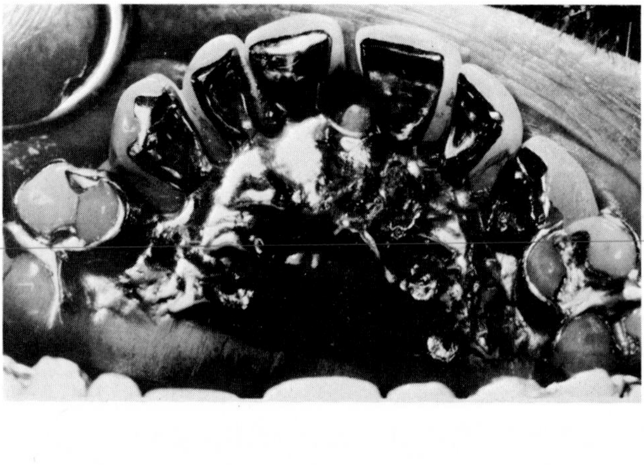

FIG. 253.—Splint designed so that it is not seen between spaced teeth.

The Weissenfluh Splint

By combining features of both removable and fixed appliances this device overcomes some of the problems of the lingual coverage splint. Special thimbles are cemented into small cavities prepared in parallel in the cingulae of the teeth to be splinted. A chrome-cobalt skeleton prosthesis is made with pins which fit into the thimbles (Fig. 254). This splint is comparatively easy to construct and is useful where a partial denture is required. It has the advantages of supporting teeth with a minimum of intracoronal preparation so that the pulp is not irritated, and at the same time is unobtrusive and usually requires minimal occlusal adjustment (Fig. 254*C*). It is an excellent appliance for splinting teeth after orthodontic movement and may be used where spaces remain between the anterior teeth, but there is the disadvantage that caries may occur around the edges of the thimbles unless these are kept very clean. It is obtainable in a special kit and detailed instructions for its construction are supplied.

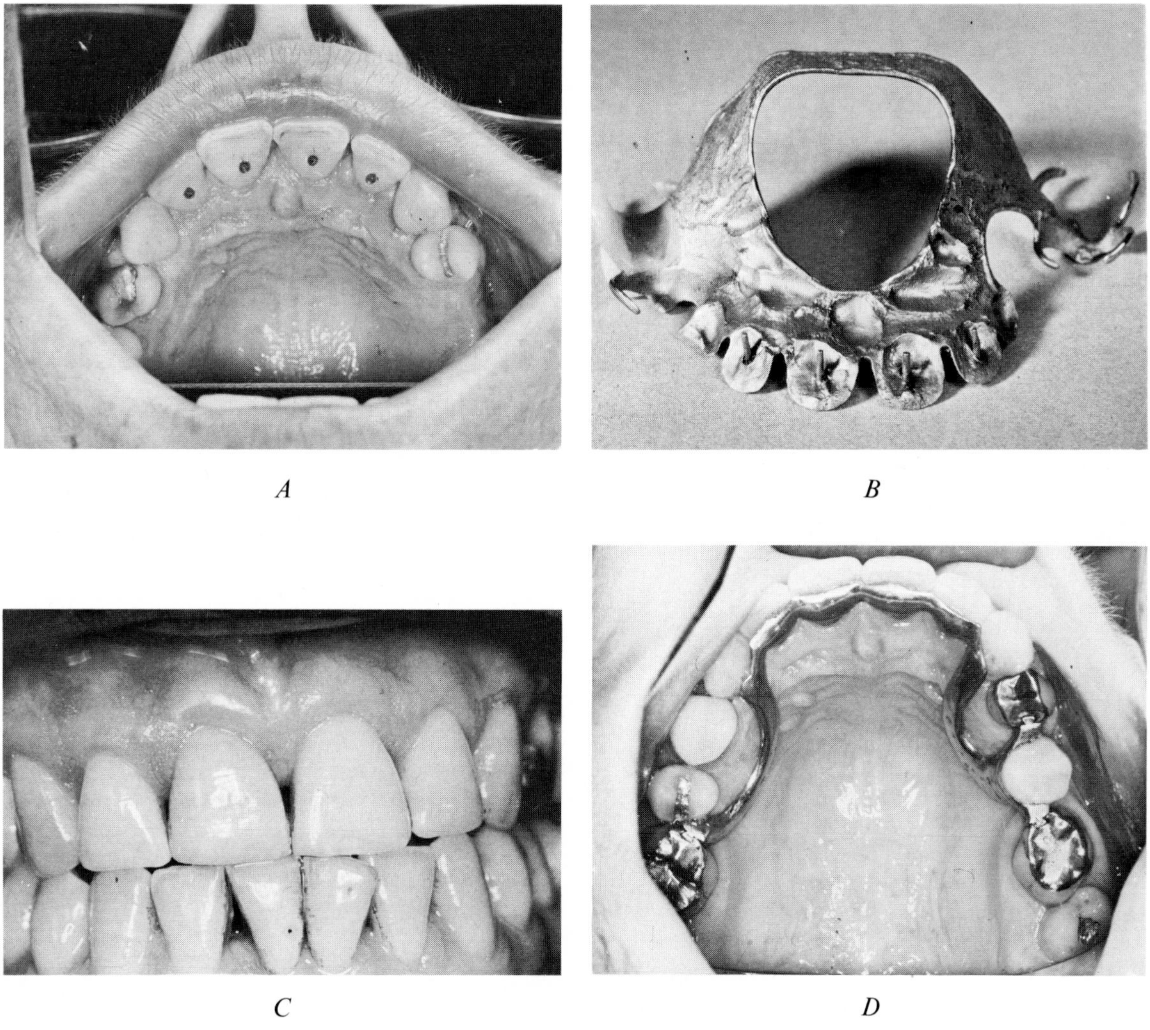

FIG. 254.—The Weissenfluh splint.

(*A*) Thimbles placed in the four anterior teeth to be splinted. (*B*) The splint with four parallel pins. (*C*) Teeth splinted after orthodontic movement. The splint is completely unobtrusive and does not interfere with the occlusion. (*D*) The same case with the splint reduced to a slim bar which is supported by dovetail attachments on fixed bridges replacing missing posterior teeth.

FIXED SPLINTS

These splints consist of linked intracoronal preparations. There are many types, some of which are relatively simple and make little demand on the operator, while others represent the most difficult form of advanced restoration. Generally the simpler forms must be regarded as only semi-permanent.

The Goal-Post (or Staple) Splint

Dovetail Class III preparations are made in the lingual surfaces of the teeth to be splinted. Pin-holes are sunk in the floor of the preparations and 0.8 mm stainless steel wire is bent into U-shaped staples (goal posts) so that the ends can be cemented into the pin-holes (Fig. 255). After cementation and cavity lining the cavities are filled with quick-set acrylic or composite material. The gingival aspect of the interproximal bridge is carefully shaped and polished so that efficient food shedding can take place. Usually used for anterior segments this splint can be constructed for six teeth in a visit of about one hour. It is economical and makes little demand on the operator. But there is the possibility of pulp damage and, as shrinkage or fracture of the filling material may take place with subsequent caries, it must be regarded as a semi-permanent appliance. These remarks also apply to the A-splint and to the continuous intracoronal bar.

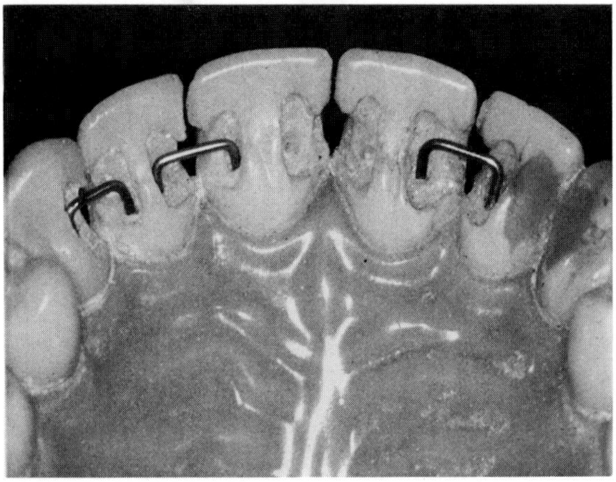

A

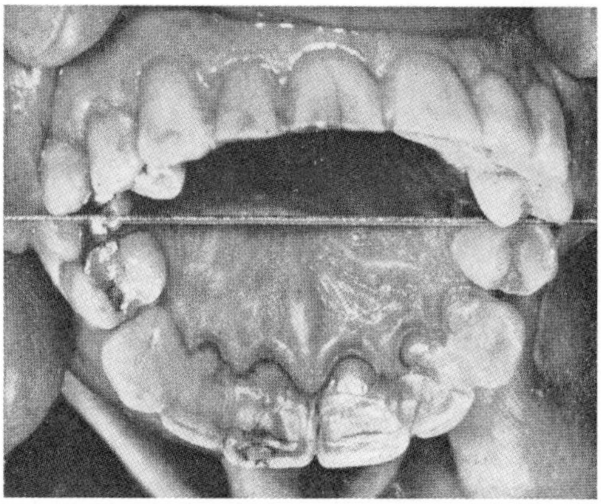

B

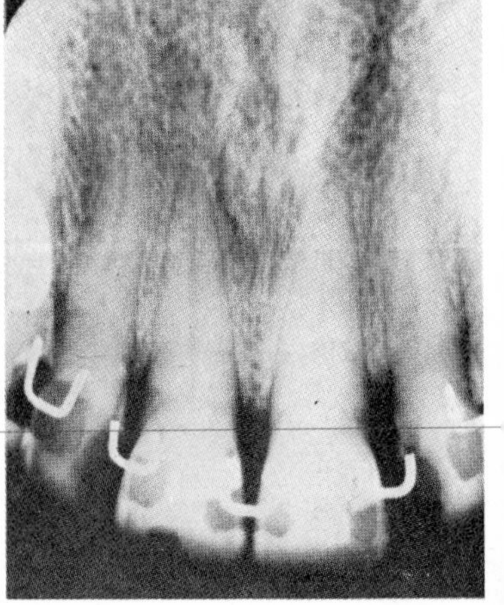

C

FIG. 255.—The Goal-Post (or Staple) splint.
(*A*) Model showing preparations with metal staples in place. (*B*) Mirror image of splint in place supporting upper anterior teeth from canine to canine. The splint had then been in place for two years. (*C*) Radiograph of the splint.

The A-Splint

Shallow rectilinear preparations are made in the lingual surface of teeth to be splinted, to the dimensions of 1 mm × 0.5 mm gold bar (17 ct platinized). The cavities are slightly undercut and lined, and the gold bar is cemented in with self-curing acrylic or composite materials (Fig. 256): Dentatus pin wire can be used instead of gold bar. As the cavity must be shallow retention is relatively poor, and where occlusal stresses tend to push splinted anterior teeth labially the gold bar may be dislodged. This type of splint has the considerable advantages of being simple and quick to construct; six teeth may be splinted within one hour, and dislodged gold bars are easily replaced.

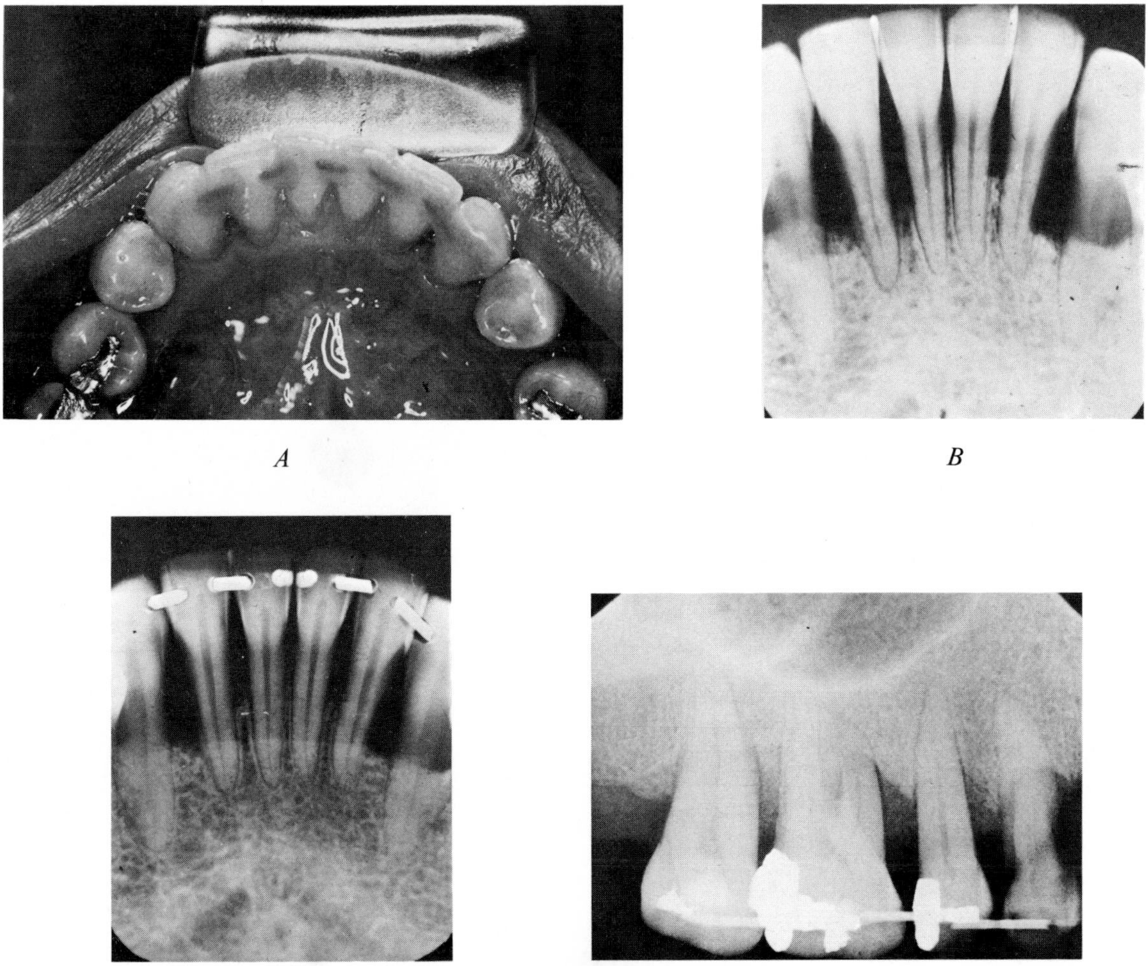

A *B* *C* *D*

FIG. 256.—The A-Splint.

(*A*) Splint in place in lower anterior teeth of a 26-year-old woman. (*B*) Radiograph of lower teeth just before splinting and gingivectomy. (*C*) Three years later showing gold bars in position. The bar between the central incisors has just been dislodged and temporary fillings inserted in its place. Note the slight condensation of interdental bone. While it cannot be said that there is a marked improvement in the condition, there has been no deterioration of a condition in which the periodontal tissues had previously been rapidly breaking down. (*D*) Modification of A-splint supporting posterior teeth as a temporary measure.

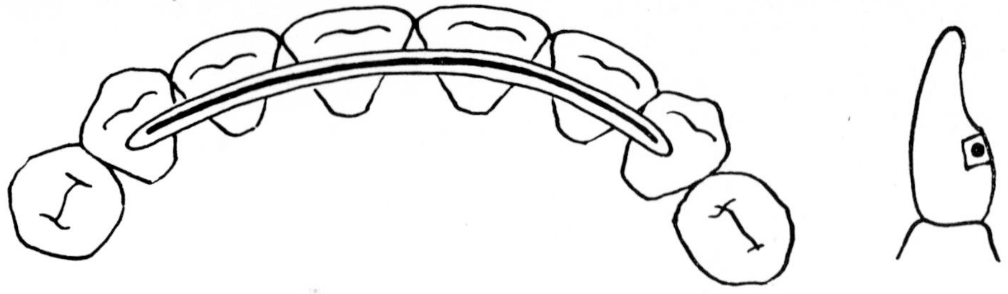

FIG. 257.—(*A*) and (*B*). The construction of a continuous intracoronal bar.

The Continuous Intracoronal Bar

A transverse groove, 2–3 mm wide, is cut in the lingual surface of anterior teeth coronal to the cingulum, or in the occlusal surface of posterior teeth. The groove is made about 1.5 mm deep and slightly undercut. A stainless steel wire is bent to fit the groove which is filled with self-curing acrylic and the wire quickly pressed home. After the acrylic has set it is shaped and polished (Fig. 257).

Alternatively, a gold bar may be cast to fit the preparation and cemented in place. As occlusal pressures may push anterior teeth away from the bar it is advisable to improve retention by making pin-hole preparations in the base of the groove, but even with this added retention it is not advisable to splint upper anterior teeth in this way. The horizontal-pin splint (Fig. 258) represents a

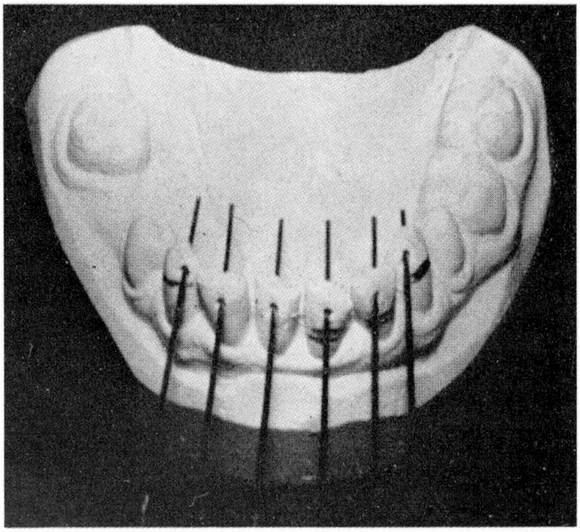

A

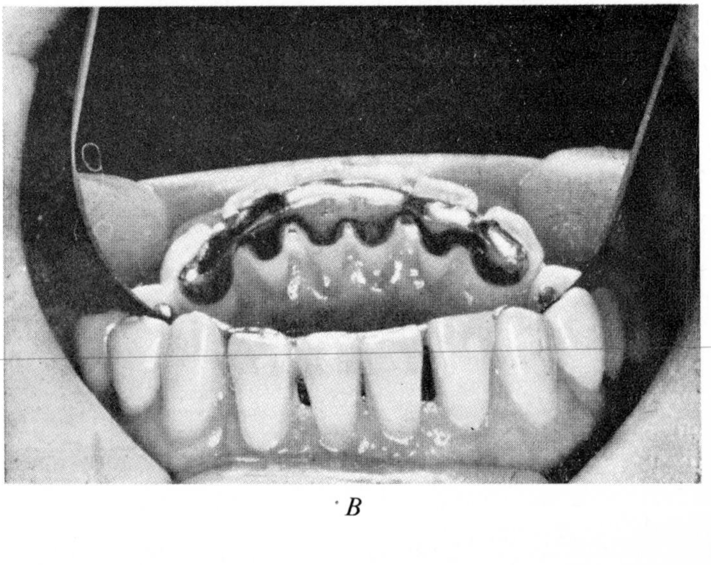

B

FIG. 258.—Horizontal-pin splint.
(*A*) Horizontal pins being placed in parallel in preparations in model of the case. (*B*) Finished splint in place. The labial face of the pin-hole is filled with silicate cement.

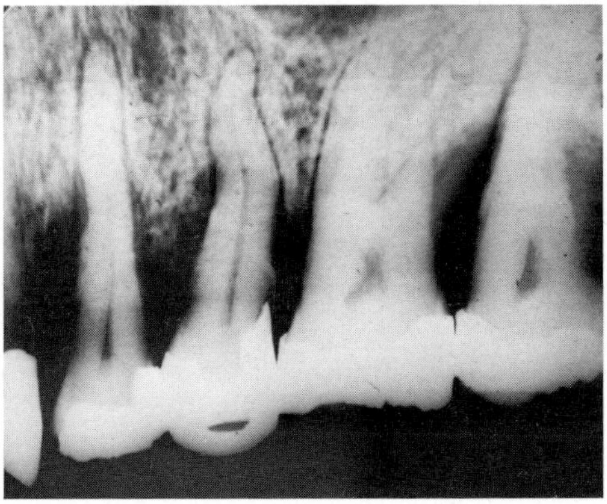

A

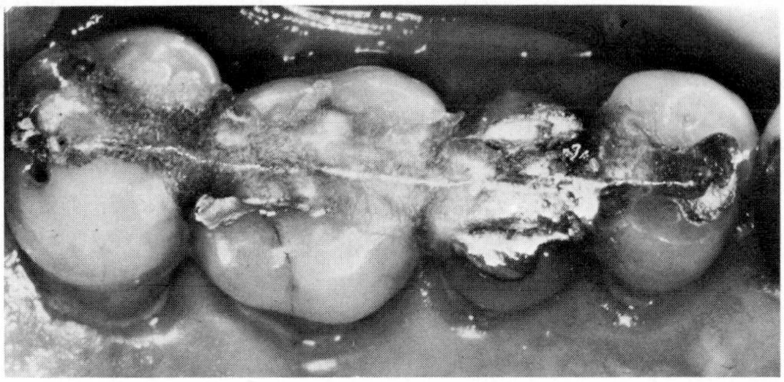

B

FIG. 259.—Amalgam splint. (*A*) X-ray showing bone destruction and widened periodontal spaces around teeth which have just been linked. (*B*) Occlusal surfaces showing metal wire shining through acrylic in slots cut in restorations.

variation of the continuous intracoronal bar. It is strong and well retained but can be used only where some pulp recession has taken place.

A form of continuous intracoronal bar which is used to stabilize a posterior segment consists of M.O.D. amalgam fillings placed in the teeth to be stabilized, and then subsequently linked by a bar cemented with acrylic into a channel cut through the amalgams (Fig. 259).

Linked Inlays

These are self-descriptive. Inlays which fit into dovetail preparations in the lingual surfaces of anterior teeth may be displaced if an excessive anterior force is exerted on any individual tooth. In the posterior region a series of linked M.O.D. inlays can make a satisfactory and permanent splint (Fig. 260).

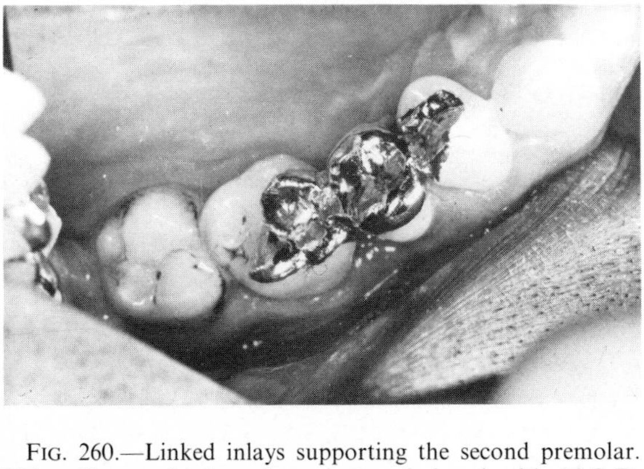

FIG. 260.—Linked inlays supporting the second premolar. This splint would have been better designed with M.O.D. inlays or 3/4 crowns in the first premolar and first molar.

Linked Crowns

The most reliable form of immobilization and support is provided by a fixed splint of linked crowns of various types (Fig. 261). This splint is extremely strong, holds the teeth rigidly and is the most aesthetically satisfying and unobtrusive type of splint. If teeth are missing the multiple abutment fixed bridge may be used to replace these teeth and to stabilize a segment or a complete arch. This type of splint allows one to modify the form of the teeth, and in fact provides one of the most satisfactory methods of occlusal rehabilitation.

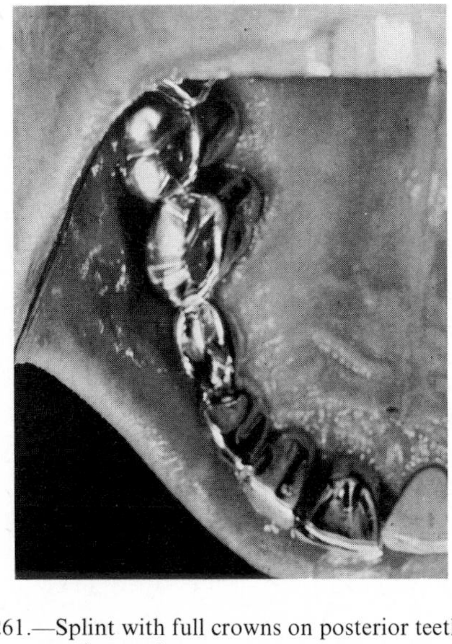

FIG. 261.—Splint with full crowns on posterior teeth and 3/4 crowns on anterior teeth.

It can be designed to cover roots exposed by surgery – and therefore improves appearance, covers sensitive root and should reduce the chances of cervical caries.

This form of splint is more difficult to make than a removable appliance and requires a great deal of chairside time and skill, although the introduction of accurate elastic impression materials has markedly simplified the technique. Considerable tooth preparation is necessary and there is often the possibility of pulpal involvement. Alternatively, telescope crowns soldered together may be used. These are fitted over gold copings which are cemented onto the teeth. The telescope superstructure may be fixed with temporary cement so that it may be removed periodically for inspection and cleaning.

If the periodontal lesion can be eradicated completely, the caries rate is low, and the patient is sufficiently conscientious to reduce the chances of disease recurrence to a minimum, the provision of this type of splint is justified.

One modification of the linked crown splint is the multiple pinlay splint which reduces tooth-tissue loss to a minimum. Three parallel pin-holes are made in each tooth to be splinted. Usually six teeth are incorporated into the splint and paralleling eighteen pin-holes presents some difficulty. Pin retention is not as good as that provided by inlay or crown, therefore this appliance can only be used with success where functional forces are not acting to separate the appliance from the tooth, as they might be where upper incisors are under some occlusal stress. This factor restricts the application of the pinlay splint to the lower incisors.

The Endodontic Splint

This form of splinting uses a metal pin which is inserted through the root canal into the alveolar bone (Fig. 262). The implant lengthens the root of the tooth artificially thus improving the crown-root ratio, 'nailing' the tooth to the bone and therefore stabilizing the tooth (Castagnola and Orlay, 1952).

The procedure is described in detail by Orlay (1965) and in summary is as follows:

1. Endodontic procedures are carried out in the usual way except that the root canal has to be enlarged to take the metal implant.
2. The apical foramen is induced and using special reamers a tunnel is drilled into the bone for a predetermined length.
3. A chrome-cobalt post is inserted through the tooth and into the bone, and its position checked by X-ray.
4. When the correct length is reached the pin is cemented in place, great care being taken that the cement is not introduced into the bone.

The advantages of this form of splinting are:

(i) No other tooth is involved except the one to be stabilized.

(ii) It is an 'internal' procedure in which the implant is sealed by the tooth against the oral environment.

However this form of splinting has several disadvantages:

(i) It is not a particularly easy procedure, especially for the inexperienced, to carry out.

(ii) There is danger of injuring anatomical features, *e.g.* maxillary antrum, inferior dental nerves, unless great care is taken through radiological examination to determine the exact relationship of the implant to these structures and to the cortical plates of bone.

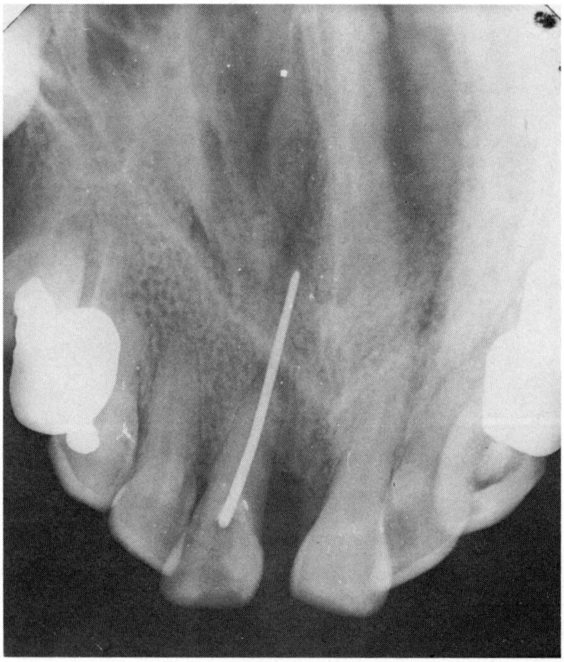

FIG. 262.—Endodontic splint in upper central incisor. (By courtesy of Dr H. G. Orlay.)

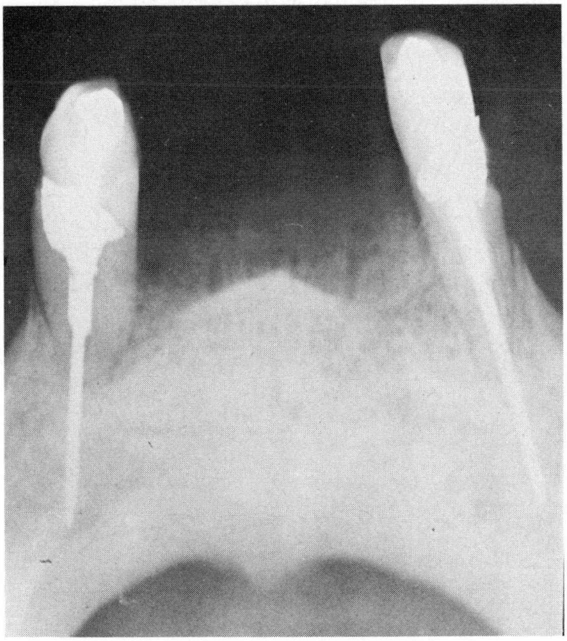

FIG. 263.—Endodontic splints in lower canines to provide abutments in otherwise edentulous mandible. (By courtesy of Dr H. G. Orlay.)

(iii) As with all implants there is danger of infection and rejection.

(iv) Mechanically it is an inefficient stabilizing system when compared with crown fixation which reduces the load on the tooth (Picton *et al.*, 1974).

Despite the limitations endodontic splinting has a place in the conservation of teeth in the appropriate case, as for example where a single incisor is fractured or involved in advanced periodontal destruction (Fig. 262) and its loss would mean complex restorative work or reliance on unreliable neighbouring teeth. It is also a valuable form of stabilization for mobile lower canines when they are the sole abutments for an otherwise difficult lower dentine (Fig. 263).

It should go without saying that the patient should be healthy and all periodontal disease treated prior to splinting.

CHOICE OF PERMANENT SPLINT

Several factors must be taken into consideration in determining the type of splint to be used in a given situation:

1. The prognosis. A fixed permanent splint is indicated if bone loss is not too great, is horizontal and appears to have progressed slowly, and if the patient is fully co-operative in maintaining good oral hygiene.
2. If there is considerable bone loss, or the patient is not completely co-operative, a fixed semi-permanent splint, *e.g.* A-splint, should be used.
3. If teeth are missing, the distribution of missing teeth represents a factor to be taken into account. Where the spaces are small a fixed bridge with multiple abutments may be ideal but, where many teeth are missing, a Weissenfluh or simple lingual coverage splint is indicated.
4. If upper incisor teeth have been retracted they may be retained by a Weissenfluh splint, of by a fixed appliance.
5. Where alteration of tooth form is necessary to improve occlusal relationship or food shedding, a fixed appliance is necessary. In the posterior region M.O.D. inlays, three-quarter or full crowns are used. Jacket crowns are used in the anterior region, as they must be where the appearance is to be improved.
6. Many forms of splints are complex, difficult to execute well and costly. In many cases it is necessary to compromise on this account, and to use a semi-permanent form of splint, such as the A-splint, which can be renewed every few years.

REFERENCES

CASTAGNOLA, L. and ORLAY, H. G. (1952). Treatment of gangrene of the pulp by the Walkhoff method. *Brit. dent. J.*, **93**, 93.

FRIEDMAN, N. (1953). Temporary splinting – an adjunct in periodontal therapy. *J. Periodont.*, **24**, 229.

ORLAY, H. G. (1965). Stabilization with endodontic implants. *J. oral Implant Transplant. Surg.*, **11**, 44.

PICTON, D. C. A., JOHNS, R. B., WILLS, D. J. and DAVIES, W. I. R. (1974). The relationship between the mechanisms of tooth and implant support. *Oral Sci. Rev.*, **5**, 3.

ADDITIONAL READING

GLICKMAN, I., STEIN, R. S. and SMULOW, J. B. (1961). The effect of increased functional forces upon the periodontium of splinted and non-splinted teeth. *J. Periodont.*, **32**, 290.

16. The Practical Management of Chronic Periodontal Disease

While the management of chronic periodontal disease takes the classical form of case history, examination, diagnosis and treatment, successful periodontal treatment depends upon more than merely making a diagnosis and applying a set formula of treatment procedures. If the disease is to be controlled, predisposing factors, initiating factors and aggravating factors must be recognized and their mode of action understood. The practitioner must also take into consideration the patient's attitudes, habits and health. Only then can a treatment plan be devised which has a chance of producing a permanent result. The following outline represents a reliable programme for the management of the periodontal patient.

1. The present complaint.
2. Past dental history.
3. Medical history.
4. Family history.
5. Patient examination.
6. Oral examination.
   (i) Oral mucosa.
   (ii) Oral hygiene state.
   (iii) Teeth.
   (iv) Gingivae.
   (v) Occlusion.
   (vi) Appliances.
7. Radiographic examination.
8. Special tests.
9. Diagnosis.
10. Prognosis.
11. Patient selection.
12. Treatment plan.
    (i) Emergency treatment.
    (ii) Plaque control.
    (iii) Extraction where necessary.
    (iv) Correction of aetiological factors.
    (v) Occlusal correction.
    (vi) Surgical treatment.
    (vii) Post-operative procedures.
13. Maintenance.

THE CASE HISTORY

The case history must be comprehensive but relevant. Therefore, it should take a well-defined, systematic form, the dentist directing the enquiry carefully but not too narrowly. Much can be missed by chivvying the patient along a preconceived path.

The Present Complaint

The condition the patient presents to the dentist is not necessarily the chief problem, but it represents the best starting point of enquiry. The present complaint, its character, location, timing, aggravating and relieving factors, are described as well as treatment received, the response to that treatment, and any other relevant factors.

Past Dental History

Items to be included in this section are:

1. Frequency of visits for routine restorative work and the amount of work usually required.
2. Date of last scaling; history of any gum treatment.
3. Date of and reason for last extraction.
4. History of bleeding after extraction.
5. Details of other oral lesions, recurrent ulcers, swellings, pains, or trouble in or about the mouth.
6. Details of any habits such as bruxism, smoking, etc.
7. Frequency of tooth-brushing (usually a useless piece of information, but the patient expects to be asked).

The regularity (or irregularity) of receiving dental attention, including scaling, reveals the patient's attitude to his mouth, and his likely attitude to periodontal treatment. At the same time it has to be remembered that most people have had little dental education and the condition of their mouths is partly the product of ignorance. An intelligent explanation of his problem may alter the patient's attitude completely (see Chapter 6.).

The Medical History

In most cases a medical history is more relevant to the form of the treatment than to the aetiology of the disease. The periodontal tissues may be healthy in a sick person and few general diseases have specific periodontal symptoms.

Rather than allow the patient the opportunity for a medical travelogue, or for restricting his story to what he thinks the dentist should know, specific questions must be asked:

1. Do you attend a physician now? If so why, and what treatment do you receive? Who is your physician?
2. Do you take any medicines or pills (drugs is a pejorative word)?
3. Do you feel fit? Can you climb stairs without trouble?
4. What serious illnesses have you had in the past?
5. Have you had rheumatic fever?
6. Do you ever bleed excessively?
7. Are you allergic to anything? Do you have asthma, hay-fever or eczema? Have you had penicillin or any other antibiotic? If so did you have a bad reaction?
8. Do you have a well balanced diet? Do you eat fresh fruit and vegetables?
9. Have you reached the menopause? (For female patients.)

If the patient is reluctant to give information he should be informed that his general health affects the course of treatment, and that if necessary his physician may have to be consulted.

Family History

Information about parents or siblings is usually irrelevant, except in revealing factors that must condition the patient's attitude to his own teeth. If everyone else in the family has worn full dentures from an early age with satisfaction the patient may be only too anxious to share the 'benefits' of the edentulous state.

Patient Examination

While taking the history a general appraisal of the patient should be made. The colour of skin, eyes, posture, breathing and general behaviour may be valuable clues to the patient's general health.

Oral Examination

This should be a comprehensive examination of both soft and hard tissues. Tissue changes in the initial stages of periodontal disease are subtle and any deviation from normal must be noted. The ideal morphology should always be kept in mind (Fig. 264).

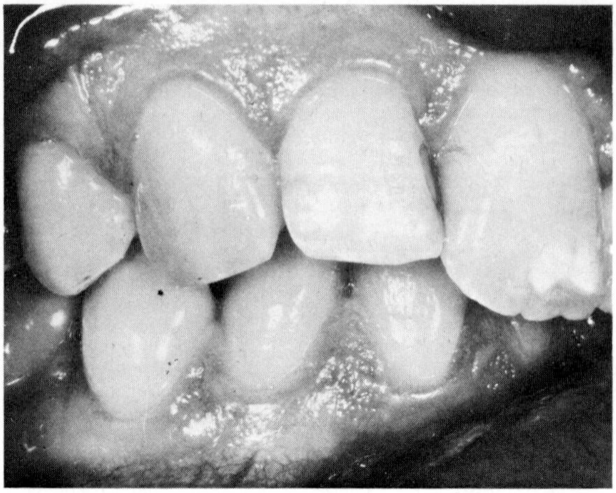

FIG. 264.—Healthy gingivae in a 20-year-old woman.

1. **Oral mucosa**
   Cheeks, lips, tongue, floor of mouth and palate can be examined for ulcers, swellings and white patches.
2. **State of oral hygiene**
   Examine for plaque (which may be demonstrated with a disclosing solution or tablet), supragingival and subgingival calculus, food debris and materia alba. Record the location of these irritants; their presence in places other than the usual sites (lingual to lower incisors and buccal to upper molars) should point to predisposing factors. It is common, although by no means the rule, to find more plaque, and therefore gingival inflammation, on the right side in right-handed individuals because they clean the left side more easily (Fig. 265).
3. **Teeth**
   (a) *Chart teeth* present and missing, cavities and restorations. Particularly note poor restorations for overhanging edges, poor contour and contact points; note arch irregularity.

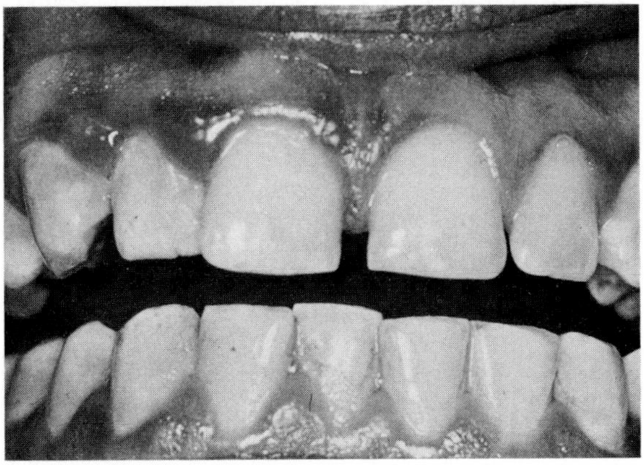

FIG. 265.—Gingival inflammation and plaque accumulation on the right side in a right-handed individual.

(b) *Percuss teeth for sensitivity.* Although nothing can be diagnosed from a false note it should lead one to examine the tooth more closely.

(c) *Assess tooth mobility.* It is important to note whether any teeth show abnormal mobility and according to a rough index, the degree of that mobility; thus Degree I – discernible mobility. Degree II – up to 1 mm of movement from the long axis. Degree III – movement of 1 mm and over.

More critical assessment is academic. Mobility is caused by breakdown of periodontal fibres which may come about with loss of bone, or with inflammation and little or no loss of bone. Where there is acute inflammation the tooth may be very loose and the prognosis may be excellent; on the other hand, there may be gross bone loss, little mobility and a poor prognosis.

(d) **Examine tooth-wear.**

(i) *Attrition.* The degree and pattern of occlusal wear is a useful guide to habits. It also may indicate the quality of the periodontal tissues. Generalized attrition rarely occurs unless the periodontal tissues are strong enough to withstand an assault capable of wearing the hard tooth substance. Generalized attrition is, therefore a pointer to a favourable prognosis. Severe generalized attrition in a relatively young individual points to tooth grinding, uneven tooth wear indicates that some teeth are taking more than their share of the occlusal load.

(ii) *Abrasion* is usually associated with gingival recession and indicates faulty tooth-brushing habits (Fig. 266). In the right-handed individual the teeth of the left side, particularly the maxillary canines and first premolar, are subject to the severest wear. Of course, one rarely finds plaque in areas of abrasion.

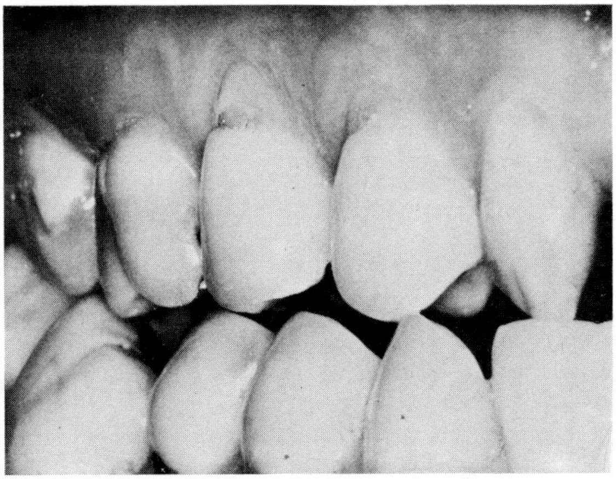

FIG. 266.—Toothbrush abrasion and gingival recession.

(e) Determine tooth vitality. When a differential diagnosis must be made between a periodontal (lateral) abscess and a periapical abscess, tooth vitality has to be assessed. It is doubtful whether the special pulp-testing appliances currently available give more reliable evidence than the application of a pledget of cotton wool soaked in ethyl chloride.

4. **Gingivae**

The colour, shape, size and consistency, any special surface characteristics, and the presence of recession should be noted. Ideally, pockets both mesial and distal to the tooth and on the lingual and buccal aspects should be measured, although in practice so many readings will not always be necessary. Measurements are made with a pocket measuring probe held parallel to the axis of the tooth and inserted gently into the pocket (Fig. 267). If the probe is held firmly against the tooth surface it may catch on subgingival calculus and give an incorrect measurement.

5. **Occlusion**
The initial examination of the occlusion can be cursory. Tooth relations in centric occlusion, and in lateral and protrusive positions are noted. The patient is asked to open and close so that any deviation from the normal path of closure is disclosed.

The occlusion should be examined more closely where:
(i) Teeth are mobile.
(ii) Radiographs show a widened periodontal space.
(iii) A tooth is sensitive to percussion.
(iv) There has been tooth migration.
(v) There are unevenly distributed wear facets.
(vi) There is facial or temporomandibular joint discomfort. In these instances models of both jaws are required and the techniques described in Chapter 14 should be applied.

6. **Prosthetic Appliances**
All appliances must be examined for (a) fit and design; (b) cleanliness; (c) their relationship to area of food stagnation, gingival inflammation and pocketing; and (d) relationship to mobile teeth and bone destruction.

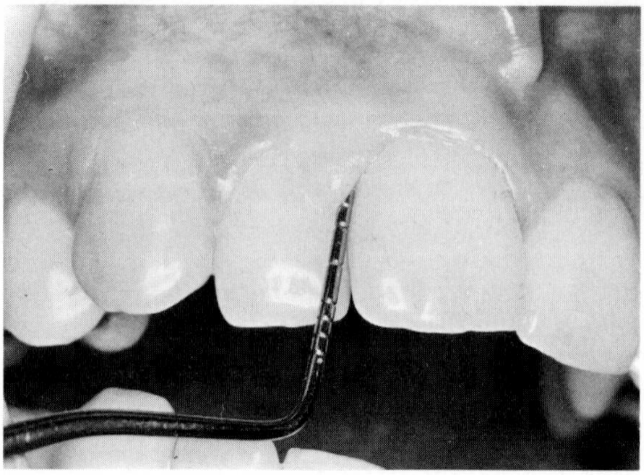

FIG. 267.—Pocket measuring probe (Williams) in shallow pocket.

Radiographic Examination

The counsel of perfection is full mouth radiographs for every patient, but this is unnecessary unless pocketing and tooth mobility indicate generalized bone loss. Bite-wing radiographs of the posterior teeth are essential; apart from interproximal caries they show:

1. The integrity of the marginal bone about the posterior teeth in both jaws. Because the angulation of the beam is correct this information is reliable unless there is gross bone destruction.
2. Faulty edges of restorations.
3. Interproximal calculus.

Bite-wing radiographs showing marked crestal bone loss must be followed by periapical films.

When periapical radiographs are taken, careful angulation of the beam is essential. If the radiographic evidence is equivocal further radiographs should be taken with the angulation of the beam altered. The 'long-cone' technique is very useful for obtaining reliable information about the position of the bone margin.

If there is doubt about the presence of an infrabony defect or the position of the bone margin, the radiograph should be taken with a gutta percha or silver point placed in the pocket (Fig. 268).

Special Tests

If periodontal breakdown appears to be out of proportion to the obvious local factors, or if the case history or general appraisal of the patient suggests that a systemic disease may be present, this may be confirmed by urine or blood analysis or by other special tests. Generally these are best carried out by the patient's physician. If a patient is already receiving medical treatment, consultation with the physician or hospital consultant should be arranged before anything but the simplest periodontal procedures are carried out.

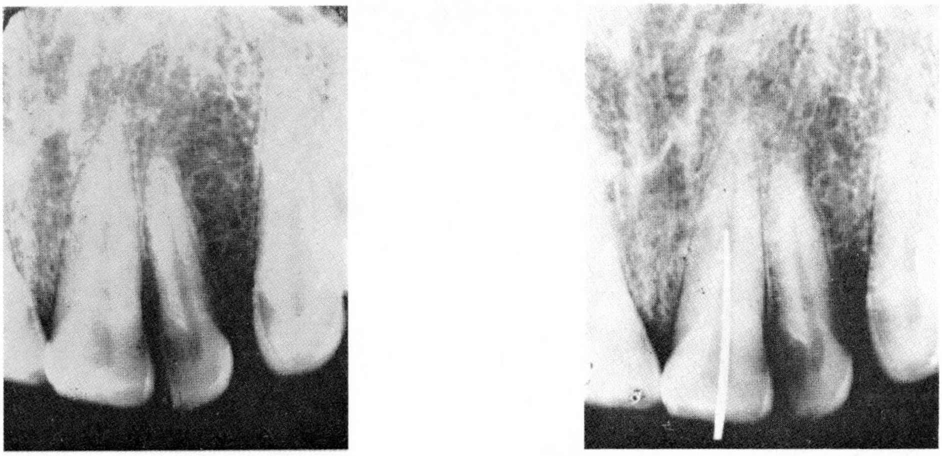

A *B*

FIG. 268.—(*A*) Radiograph of upper incisor gives no indication of the extent of bone loss on the palatal aspect. (*B*) Radiograph taken with silver point in place indicates the extent of palatal bone loss.

DIAGNOSIS

It is not very difficult to make a diagnosis of a periodontal disease, either chronic gingivitis or chronic periodontitis, or of one of the few diseases in which the periodontal tissues can be involved. But it is not enough to attach a name to the clinical features under examination. In the examination of the patient an attempt must be made to relate the condition of the tissues to aetiological factors. Thus 'chronic marginal gingivitis' may be an accurate name for a chronic inflammation restricted to the gingival margin but 'chronic marginal gingivitis due to poor oral hygiene and faulty restorations with poor contour and overhanging margins' is a much more valuable statement of the condition. The aim of treatment is not merely to relieve symptoms but to eliminate or control all aetiological factors, predisposing, initiating and aggravating, so that a permanent cure may be effected. To this end all aetiological factors must be defined if possible.

PROGNOSIS

Before deciding on the exact form of treatment an attempt has to be made to predict the outcome of treatment. This prognosis of the way the tissues will respond to treatment involves, amongst other things, an appreciation of the way the tissues have behaved under the burden of disease-producing factors. The prognosis is probably good if the tissues have resisted a combination of powerful and persistent irritants; if the tissues have succumbed rapidly to an apparently minor irritant the prognosis is almost certainly poor.

In arriving at a prognosis the following factors must be taken into account and only experience allows the operator to give proper weight to each factor.

1. Age of Patient

The older the patient the better the prognosis for any given degree of periodontal destruction; this is in spite of the fact that young tissues generally have a better power of reparation. The amount of bone destruction apparent on the radiograph, when considered with the age of the patient, gives some indication of the rapidity of tissue destruction. A better prognosis is indicated in a man of fifty who has a fifty per cent bone loss brought about by a combination of gross calculus, ill-fitting partial dentures and bruxism than the same condition in a man of forty. The prognosis for periodontosis, in which tissue destruction is advanced by the age of twenty, is very poor indeed.

The age of the patient must also be taken into account because the elimination of periodontal disease often entails trouble and even pain. In dealing with a patient whose life expectancy is only a few years the complete elimination of disease is usually unjustified. While surgical treatment of 5 mm pockets may be justified in a patient of fifty who is anxious to conserve his teeth and is likely to be co-operative, the same condition in a patient of seventy would be better treated by regular scaling. In the older individual the powers of tissue repair may be diminished and, while a gingivectomy wound will usually heal rapidly and uneventfully, bone surgery is followed by a very prolonged and uncomfortable healing period. To attempt re-attachment in an older individual may be foolhardy.

2. General Health

Although certain specific systemic conditions affect the reaction of the periodontal tissues to irritation (as described in Chapter 17), the effect of general health on the progress of periodontal disease is largely undefined. Certainly the reparative powers of tissues of a sick individual are impaired, and the possibility of secondary infection is increased. But in general there appears to be little correlation between the rapidity of periodontal breakdown and general health; very rapid breakdown occurs in apparently completely healthy individuals, and little or no periodontal breakdown in individuals suffering prolonged and debilitating disease. On the other hand, if a systemic condition such as diabetes is diagnosed and then controlled, the prognosis for periodontal treatment will be much improved.

3. The Extent and Pattern of Bone Destruction

Obviously the greater the bone loss the poorer the prognosis. Generalized horizontal bone loss is more amenable to thorough treatment than is a case with much vertical bone loss. The three-walled infrabony defect is more favourable than a two-walled defect. The three-rooted molar has a much better prognosis than an incisor with the same degree of bone loss.

Pocket depth alone is not a reliable index of prognosis because gingival recession or swelling may markedly alter pocket depth without any change in height of alveolar bone; for example, a 7 mm pocket with swollen tissue may be associated with less bone loss than a 3 mm pocket where there is recession.

4. The Possibility of Removing Aetiological Factors

If any of the many factors involved cannot be removed or controlled the prognosis is less hopeful. Thus cosmetic consideration may make complete pocket elimination around upper incisors impossible; bifurcation or trifurcation involvement make perfect cleanliness very difficult to achieve; incomplete lip seal or bruxism may be impossible to control. All these factors must affect the prognosis.

Patient co-operation is essential to the complete control of aetiological factors, and so much may be demanded of the patient, particularly when the disease is advanced, that he may well take the attitude of 'so far and no further'. He may be willing to have gingival surgery and to keep his mouth clean yet draw the line at orthodontic treatment or the more complex forms of rehabilitation. He may want to keep his old partial denture ('fits like a glove') and thereby make nonsense of surgery. It is impractical not to take such factors into account before drawing up a treatment plan.

5. The Number and Position of Teeth Present

This will determine the load taken by each tooth, whether a prosthesis is necessary, and if so the type of appliance. The presence of teeth on only one side of the mouth makes a much less favourable situation than if teeth are placed symmetrically.

6. Tooth Mobility and Gingival Inflammation

Tooth mobility is related to the degree of inflammation and the amount of bone loss. The inflammation reflects the presence of local irritants that can be removed, therefore, other things being equal, mobility in the presence of inflammation indicates a better prognosis than mobility without inflammation.

PATIENT SELECTION

Patient co-operation is essential to the success of

periodontal treatment. Only those individuals who can and will co-operate should receive treatment. Before embarking on anything other than emergency treatment it is important to present the patient with a simple account of his periodontal problem and the treatment involved. An informed patient is much more likely to be co-operative; one who is not sufficiently concerned about his mouth may decide not to submit to treatment. Unfortunately, too many cases of periodontal disease are diagnosed only when gross destruction has taken place. In many cases it is impossible to produce a permanent result and, if the patient is anxious to conserve his teeth for a few years, compromises have to be made. In such cases it is essential that the patient be informed of the poor prognosis at the outset. Disappointment and even ill-feeling can thus be avoided.

If systemic disease is present, this should receive proper attention at this stage and the patient's physician should be informed of the necessity for periodontal treatment. Delay in attending to a systemic disease may only complicate treatment and cause the patient unnecessary suffering. Periodontal treatment should not be imposed on patients who are physically or psychologically ill.

If a patient has a history of excessive bleeding after injury, tooth extractions or other surgery a comprehensive blood examination is essential. Haemolytic disorders may be due to abnormalities of blood clotting, of platelets or capillary fragility, therefore screening tests must include bleeding time, clotting time, capillary fragility tests, platelet counts and any other test indicated.

THE TREATMENT PLAN

The treatment plan is not an inventory of separate mechanical operations; it should be a system of integrated procedures that represents a realistic attempt to conserve the dentition as an efficiently functioning unit. Each patient presents with individual problems, therefore one cannot prescribe a rigid formula of treatment, but the following outline represents the general form of treatment plan. In many cases only one or two of the following measures are necessary to achieve a good result; in others all available resources must be employed to the full.

1. Emergency Treatment

The relief of pain and the elimination of acute infection must be the first step in treatment. This may involve antibiotic therapy, draining abscesses, extracting teeth or inserting dressings in carious cavities.

If a patient suffers valvular heart lesions or gives a history of rheumatic fever the heart lesion must be protected from the bacteraemias which accompany surgical procedures including scaling. To achieve this a bactericidal agent (not merely bacteriostatic) must be present in adequate concentrations in the blood stream at the time of the procedure. Several routines are prescribed: all now avoid early dosage with antibiotics which might give time for resistant strains to develop. Recommended regimes are as follows (Kay, 1972):

1. Benzylpenicillin 600 mg i.m. not more than 1 hour before the dental procedure, followed 4 hours after treatment by phenoxymethylpenicillin 250–500 mg orally q.d.s. for 2 days.
2. Erythromycin 500 mg orally 2 hours before the procedure, followed by erythromycin 250 mg orally q.d.s. for 3 days.

2. Plaque Control

The first clinical procedures after emergency treatment must be scaling and instruction in oral hygiene. This may be the only treatment required, but where periodontal surgery is necessary a preliminary scaling will reduce oral sepsis, reduce inflammation, and prepare the patient psychologically for further treatment. Scaling can be a very useful tool in patient selection; the patient who does not maintain a good standard of oral hygiene after the preliminary scaling will not benefit much from any other form of treatment.

3. Extraction of Teeth with a Poor Prognosis

The preservation of individual teeth is not the primary objective of periodontal treatment. If the retention of a tooth jeopardizes the health of the dentition it should be extracted, therefore the decision whether to extract or conserve a tooth must be made on the basis of its effect on the dentition as a whole. To this end one must consider not only the amount, the pattern, and the rapidity of bone loss about the tooth but the effect of the tooth's absence, and of the probable methods of replacement.

It is not possible to apply mechanical rules such

as 'if half the bone is lost, extract'. An upper molar with half its supporting bone destroyed may be an excellent abutment for a fixed appliance if the bone loss has occurred slowly and the remaining bone is dense, and if the pocketing can be eliminated so that the gingival margin can be kept free of debris. The loss of half the bone support about an upper lateral may justify extraction if complete elimination of the pocket will create a cosmetic problem and any compromise treatment jeopardize the neighbouring teeth, particularly if the canine and central incisor can act as adequate bridge abutments.

Vertical bone loss on one aspect of an upper incisor should justify an attempt at re-attachment, but the same condition involving all the upper incisors may indicate extraction.

Extractions must be carried out prior to or at the same time as periodontal surgery.

4. Immediate Correction of Aetiological Factors

The stage at which irritating factors are corrected has to be assessed in each case, and frequently some correction of these factors can be carried out with advantage before surgery. For example, a badly designed partial denture replacing anterior teeth cannot be discarded immediately after periodontal surgery, nor can a new denture be made until treatment of the periodontal lesion has been completed. Therefore a compromise has to be made. The margin of most dentures can be cut back to reduce gingival irritation without making them unwearable and a filling with a gross cervical overhang can be replaced by a dressing until periodontal treatment is complete. In many cases it is advantageous to dovetail the periodontal treatment with the restorative and prosthetic work, particularly as periodontal treatment may be prolonged.

5. Occlusal Correction

Repair of the tissues about teeth under excessive stress may be delayed or prevented. Rest is essential to the first stage of tissue repair. This is particularly the case where infrabony defects are to be treated.

It is therefore essential at this stage to (a) eliminate harmful habits (by the provision of a bite-guard, if necessary); (b) eliminate obvious occlusal disharmonies; (c) carry out minor tooth movement; and (d) apply a temporary splint where teeth are very mobile.

6. Surgical Treatment of the Periodontal Lesion

A variety of lesions may be present in any one section of the mouth. Thus in just one segment there may be suprabony pockets, thickened and cratered bone margins and an infrabony defect. With adequate preparation it should be possible to integrate the various surgical procedures and to treat all the lesions in this segment at one operation. All techniques in periodontal surgery have two basic aims, to eliminate the periodontal lesion and to produce a functionally efficient tissue architecture.

The mouth may be treated by quadrant or segment, but sometimes it is expedient to treat half or even the complete mouth at one time under general anaesthesia. The patient's needs and the operator's facilities dictate the management of the surgical phase.

7. Post-operative Procedures

There should be as little delay as possible in the correction of any aetiological factor after periodontal surgery is complete.

1. Check oral hygiene technique. There may be a tendency for the patient to avoid thorough brushing in the immediate post-operative phase yet this is the period in which good oral hygiene is essential.
2. Correct or replace faulty restorations. It is unwise to insert any permanent restoration involving the cervical margin before the completion of periodontal surgery. This is particularly the case when crowns are to be constructed (Figs. 269 and 270).
3. Check occlusion for minor occlusal disharmonies; teeth often move after surgery.
4. Remove temporary splints if they have been in place for six weeks.
5. Construct permanent splints, or other necessary prostheses (Fig. 271).
6. Recheck patient's oral hygiene techniques.

Maintenance

The patient should attend at three-monthly intervals for about a year to have the periodontal condition and oral hygiene checked. Subsequently six-monthly inspections and scaling are usually adequate, but the interval between inspections must be determined by the individual's need and not according to some rigid formula. Where oral hygiene is difficult to maintain, examination and scaling at three- or four-monthly intervals may be required.

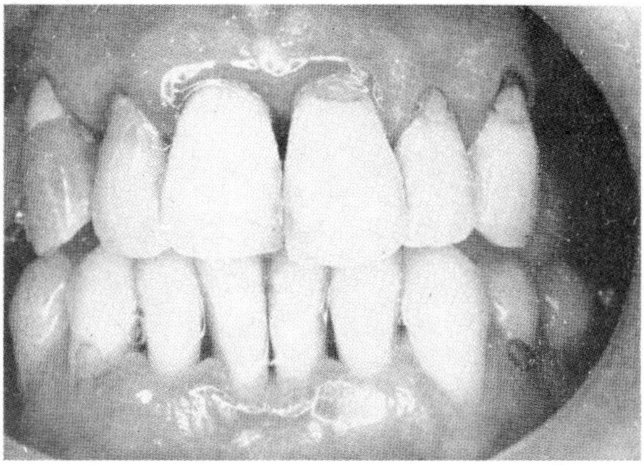

A

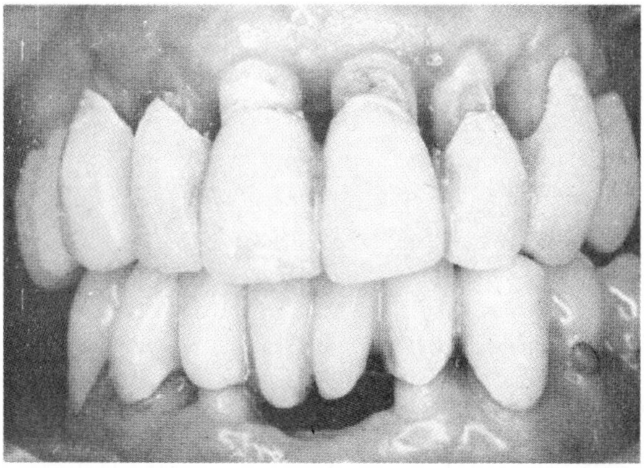

B

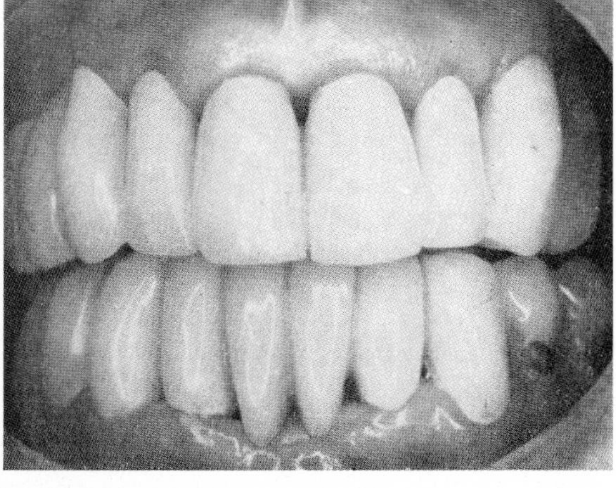

C

FIG. 269.—(*A*) Pre-operative appearance in a 41-year-old woman. There are generalized 5 mm pockets and gross bone loss at 1|1. (*B*) Post-surgical appearance. Gingivectomy and extractions were carried out in the lower jaw, and an apically-repositioned flap procedure in the upper jaw. Before periodontal surgery temporary splints made of connected acrylic crowns were placed. The edge of the acrylic marks the pre-operative gingival position. (*C*) Permanent crowns constituting a fixed splint have been made to the new gingival margin.

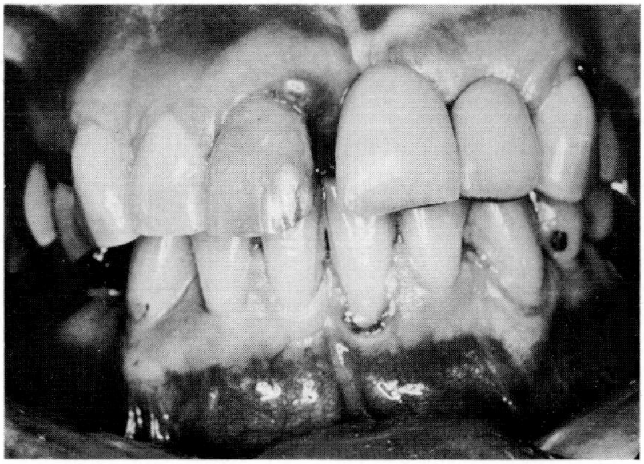

A

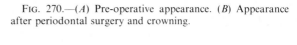

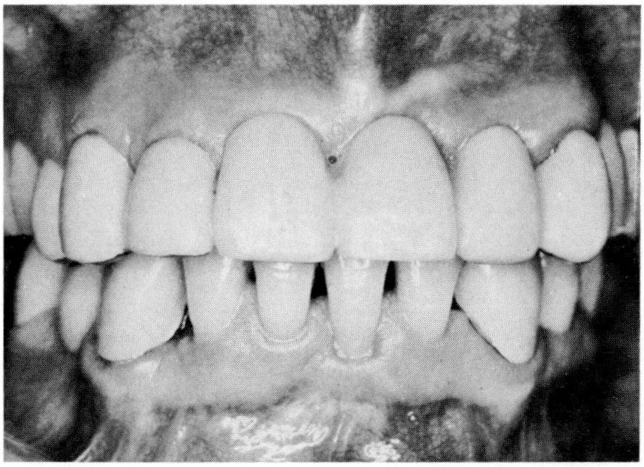

B

FIG. 270.—(*A*) Pre-operative appearance. (*B*) Appearance after periodontal surgery and crowning.

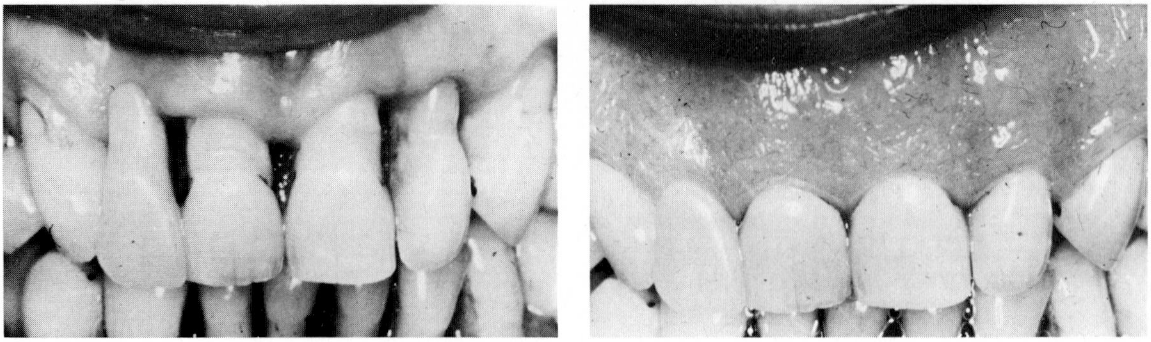

A B

FIG. 271.—(*A*) Gross gingival deformity after radical gingivectomy. The patient was anxious to conserve her teeth, but there was considerable bone loss and 2| had to be extracted. (*B*) Pink acrylic veneer in place.

REFERENCE

KAY, L. W. (1972). Drugs in dentistry, 2nd ed. John Wright, Bristol, p. 89.

RECOMMENDED READING

CROSS, W. G. (1953). Periodontal diagnostic instruments. *Brit. dent. J.*, **94**, 187.
GREENE, A. H. (1962). Study of the characteristics of stippling and its relation to gingival health. *J. Periodont.*, **33**, 176.
HIRSCHFELD, L. (1953). Calibrated silver points for periodontal diagnosis and recording. *J. Periodont.*, **24**, 94.
HIRT, H. A. and MÜHLEMANN, H. R. (1956). Diagnosis of bruxism by measurement of the tooth mobility. *Dent. Abstr.*, **1**, 356.
PRICHARD, J. F. (1961). Role of the roentgenogram in the diagnosis and prognosis and periodontal disease. *Oral Surg.*, **14**, 182.
TROTT, J. R. and WADE, A. B. (1959). Clinical examination of the periodontium. *Dent. Practit.* **4**, 345.

17. The Management of the Special Patient

Many forms of dental treatment can be carried out satisfactorily without much regard to the general condition of the patient. If periodontal treatment is to be carried out successfully and the periodontal condition brought under control the general health of the patient, both physical and emotional, must be considered, its influence understood and its implications taken into account in treatment.

Two general situations exist which indicate that special care is required in the management of the case.

1. As described in Chapter 4 the tissue changes in periodontal disease may be conditioned by a variety of systemic factors, hormonal, haematological, dietary, etc., an understanding of which is essential to the control of the periodontal condition.
2. Periodontal treatment may be necessary in patients who also suffer a disease unrelated to the periodontal condition but which must influence the management of treatment, *e.g.* cardiac or respiratory disease.

HORMONAL DISTURBANCE

Alteration in the balance of sex hormones produces changes in gingival tissue reaction. These alterations are most commonly manifested in puberty, menstruation, pregnancy and menopause. The other hormonal disturbance of significance in periodontal disease is diabetes.

Puberty

An exaggerated response to gingival irritation is frequently found in puberty. A small amount of plaque that might otherwise not produce an obvious tissue reaction may, in puberty, produce a striking inflammation. The gingivae become red, soft and swollen particularly in areas of food stagnation (Fig. 272). They bleed on toothbrushing and the patient then brushes less vigorously and therefore less effectively, so that debris accumulates and the gingivitis is exacerbated.

When puberty is complete there is a definite remission of symptoms but the gingivitis does not disappear. A chronic inflammation persists and may progress to a chronic periodontitis unless timely treatment is carried out.

Treatment

This consists of thorough scaling and instruction in oral hygiene. It is rarely necessary to perform any gingival surgery; indeed surgery during puberty is often unrewarding as granulation tissue tends to form in response to the slightest irritation. If it seems evident that a poor gingival contour will persist after thorough scaling it is advisable to delay surgery for a year or two.

The adolescent patient is impressionable and responds well to suggestions that inflamed gums spoil an otherwise attractive smile. The demonstration of plaque by disclosing solution is usually received with rewarding expressions of astonishment, and makes motivation to a good oral hygiene regimen easier to achieve.

Menstruation

The monthly period is not generally associated with any specific oral manifestation, but a number of women do complain of either slight soreness or bleeding of the gingivae a day or two before the onset of menstruation. These symptoms do not appear to occur in the absence of some local irritant, however slight.

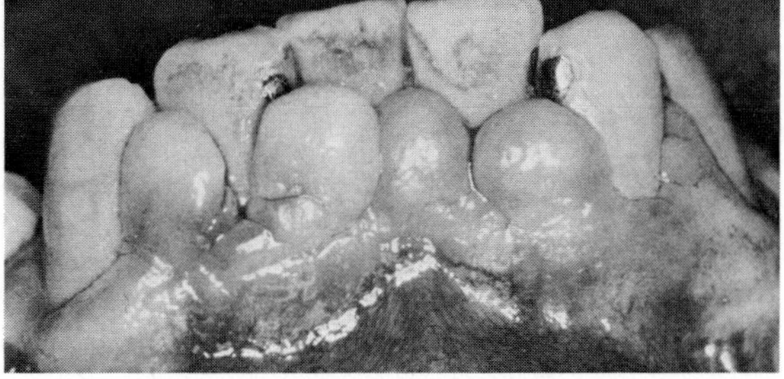

FIG. 272.—Chronic hyperplastic gingivitis in a 15-year-old boy. Multiple aetiological factors are poor oral hygiene, malaligned teeth and lack of lip seal.

Treatment

It is as well to postpone treatment until after menstruation. Reassurance and a warm water mouthwash (glycerine and thymol flavoured) is the immediate treatment. Scaling and instruction in oral hygiene technique can be carried out a few days later.

Pregnancy

Gingivitis is complained of so frequently in pregnancy that it is the general belief that pregnancy causes gingivitis. This is not the case (Fig. 273); the altered tissue response in pregnancy, *i.e.* an exaggerated production of inflammatory tissue in response to the slightest irritation, produces an obvious tissue reaction to local irritants that previously elicited no gingival symptoms and therefore went unnoticed.

Bleeding is the most common complaint. The gingivitis varies from the mild case in which only the interdental papillae are swollen and red to more severe cases where there is a generalized enlargement of the gingivae which are dark red or plum-coloured (Fig. 274). The inflammation usually increases in severity to about the eighth month when the condition begins to improve. After parturition the inflammatory changes diminish and a less spectacular chronic gingivitis remains.

The 'pregnancy tumour' is a localized manifestation of this tendency to produce inflammatory tissue (Fig. 275). It is distinguished from a pyogenic granuloma only by the fact that the patient is pregnant (Fig. 276). It may be scarcely more than an enlarged interdental papilla; occasionally it presents as a dark-red pedunculated swelling

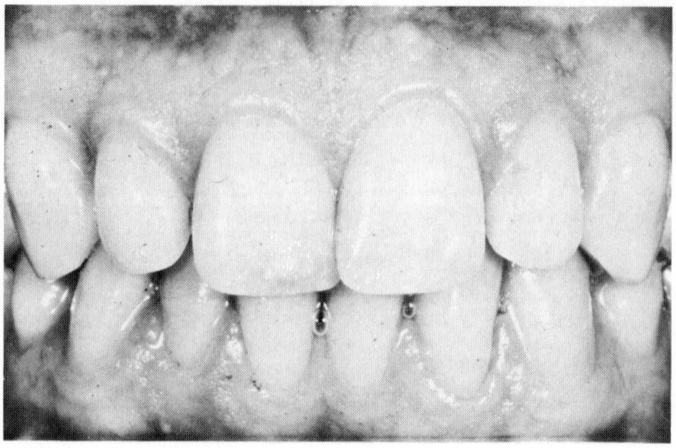

FIG. 273.—Gingivae of a 36-year-old pregnant woman. The gingivae in the maxilla are healthy; in the lower jaw a slight chronic gingivitis is associated with plaque deposits.

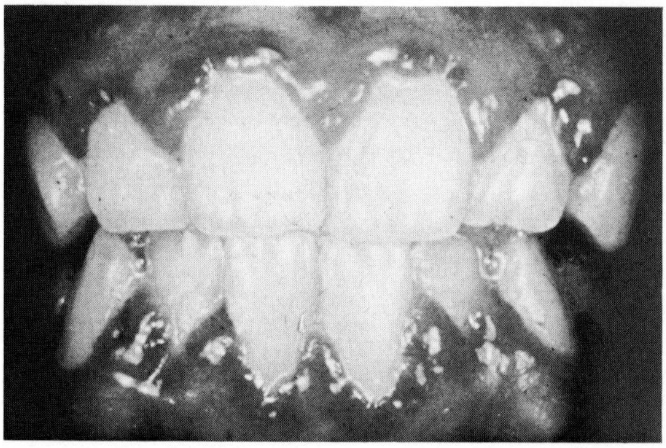

FIG. 274.—Chronic gingivitis in a 21-year-old pregnant woman.

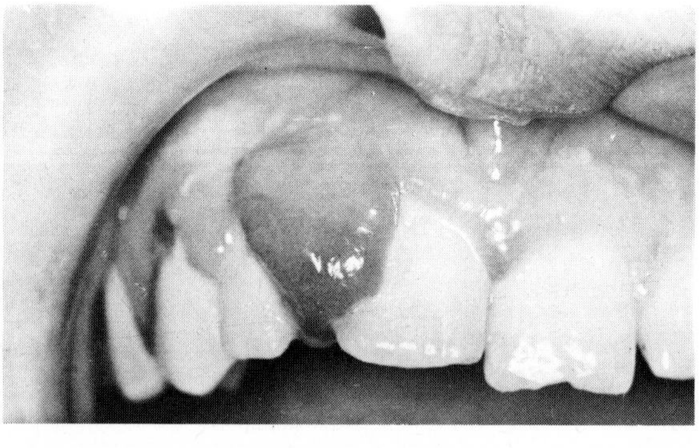

FIG. 275.—A 'pregnancy tumour'; pyogenic granuloma in a pregnant woman.

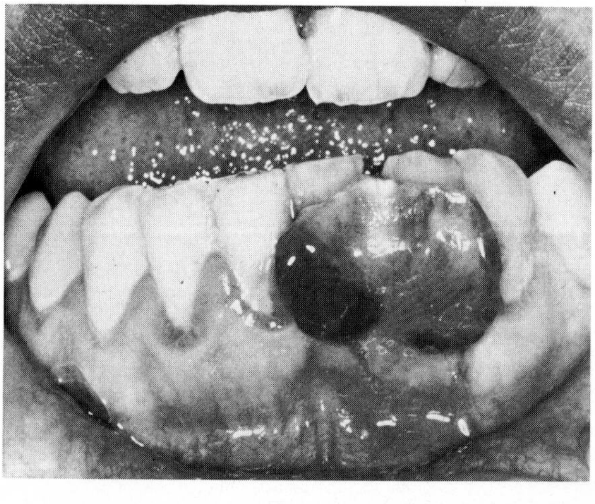

FIG. 276.—A pyogenic granuloma in a 26-year-old woman.

more than a centimetre in diameter, which bleeds readily and causes the patient considerable alarm. It is frequently associated with irritation from calculus, an overhanging filling or a partial denture.

Treatment

Tissue response and patient co-operation vary so considerably in pregnancy that it is best to approach each case empirically. Unless there are medical reasons for doing so it is unnecessary to defer treatment until the pregnancy is terminated. The removal of local irritants is essential, therefore scaling and instruction in oral hygiene techniques should be started immediately. It is wise to explain to the patient that in pregnancy the tissues are extra-sensitive to irritation and therefore her co-operation is essential for success. Other local factors should be corrected as well as possible; the replacement of an ill-fitting denture should be delayed until sound gingival health is established.

If gingival surgery is indicated this may be carried out, but it is advisable to confer first with the patient's physician. The presence of a pregnancy tumour may be the cause of considerable concern and even interfere with eating. Reassurance as to its benign nature is essential. If removal is necessary it can be removed by incision or, with advantage, by electro-surgery. It is essential to incise well below the tumour and remove it entirely, otherwise the lesion will flourish rapidly. Bleeding may be copious but is easily controlled by pressure and a periodontal dressing.

It is essential to identify and correct any aggravating local factor, *e.g.* the overhanging margin of a restoration or a poor contact point causing food impaction. Some factor of this sort is almost always present and failure to identify and correct it is likely to lead to recurrence of the lesion.

Menopause

Several oral symptoms appear to be associated with the hormonal changes which take place at menopause. These are frequently of a rather indefinite nature; abnormal tastes, dryness of the mouth and burning sensations in the oral mucosa including the gingivae, are common complaints.

Desquamative Gingivitis

The term 'desquamative gingivitis' is a rag-bag term applied to erosive gingival lesions which probably reflect a variety of systemic disturbances, of which hormonal imbalance may be the most frequent. Although not confined to women or to the climacteric, desquamative gingivitis is most often seen at menopause and occasionally following hysterectomy in young women.

The disease is characterized by degeneration of the gingival epithelium with exposure and inflammation of the underlying connective tissue. Clinically the disease is seen as a diffuse erythema of the gingivae. Tiny vesicles are formed which

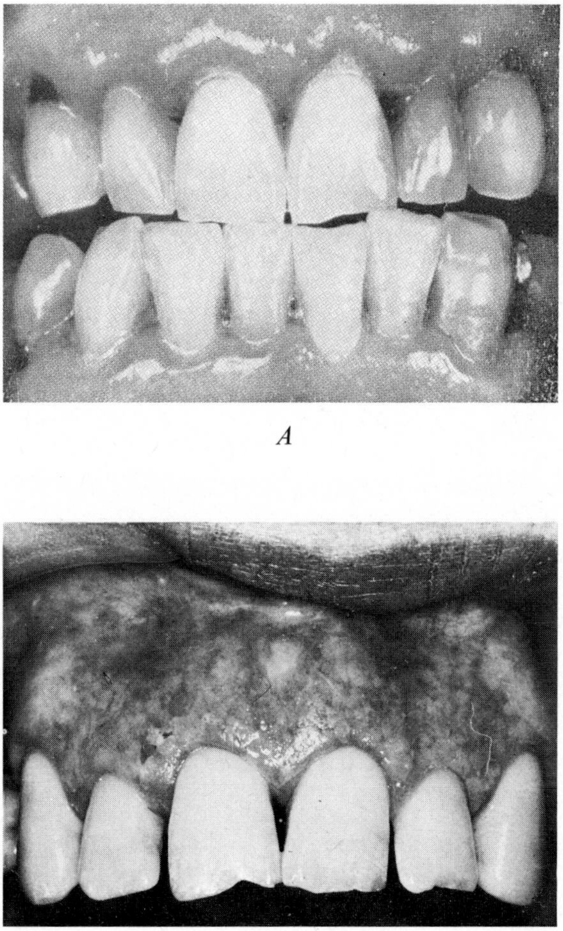

A

B

FIG. 277.—(*A*) Desquamative gingivitis in a 44-year-old woman. The gingivae are smooth, red and sensitive. (*B*) Typical mottled appearance of atrophic tissue in desquamative gingivitis.

rupture to form small and irregular red patches with a grey margin of desquamated epithelium. In some cases extensive areas of the gingivae are smooth and red (Fig. 277). These areas are very sensitive and the patient complains of soreness aggravated by spicy foods. The sore patches may persist for many weeks and then slowly disappear before further patches appear; recurrent episodes may occur for several years.

The lesions of desquamative gingivitis are similar to and indeed may be manifestations of benign mucous membrane pemphigoid and erosive lichen planus (Fig. 278), which are diseases requiring special attention. Therefore an attempt at a differential diagnosis is essential. If the lesions are very painful and persistent, if oral mucosa other than the gingivae is involved, or if there are skin or ocular lesions, the patient should be referred for specialist treatment.

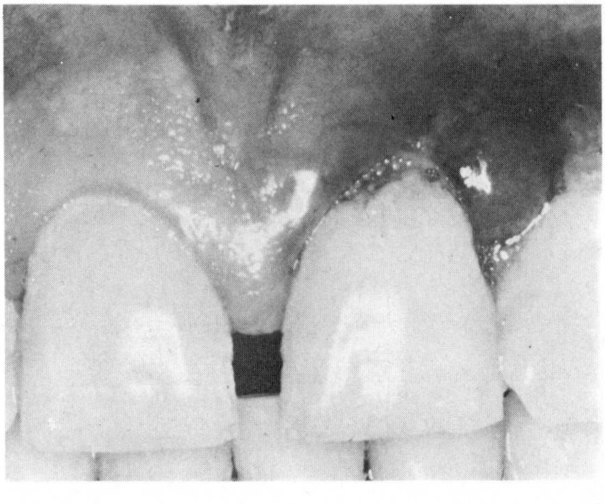

FIG. 278.—Benign mucous membrane pemphigoid. Right side, healthy gingivae; left side, erosion around swollen interdented papilla. (By courtesy of Dr F. F. Nally.)

Treatment

It is tempting to treat the menopausal patient as neurotic because she may appear to be unduly concerned about symptoms which are difficult to define and may seem trivial, but it is important to reassure her that the complaint is minor, localized and most likely transient. Oral hygiene standards should be high, irritant mouthwashes such as strong hydrogen peroxide solutions should be avoided, and the diet must be well-balanced.

The present local treatment of desquamative gingivitis is unsatisfactory. Topical application of oestrogens or corticosteroids in an adhesive base have been recommended, but the adhesive base (Orabase) alone seems to be equally as effective or ineffective. The administration of systemic corticosteroids may control the condition, but this form of treatment should be instituted by the patient's physician.

If periodontal surgery is indicated an attempt should be made to keep this to a minimum. When surgery is essential as in the treatment of a periodontal abscess care should be taken in the handling of the tissue (the closed wound produced by flap procedures is preferred to the open wound of gingivectomy) and the procedure should be carried out under antibiotic cover.

DIABETES

In patients with inadequately controlled diabetes it is common to find severe gingival inflammation, rapid bone loss and a tendency for periodontal abscesses to form. For many years this periodontal breakdown was interpreted as a symptom of diabetes. This is not so. In uncontrolled or incompletely controlled diabetes tissue resistance is low and healing is poor, but periodontal breakdown does not occur if there is no local irritant. In patients with controlled diabetes tissue reaction and healing is normal.

Management of the diabetic patient

A patient with uncontrolled diabetes may attend with acute pain frequently associated with a periodontal abscess. He may or may not know that he is diabetic. If he complains of recurrent periodontal abscesses, if the gingivae are very swollen and inflamed and rapid bone breakdown is evident, a pointed case history must be taken. Frequent urination and thirst, loss of weight, recurrent boils. general malaise and a family history of the disease indicate diabetes, and the patient must be referred to his physician for immediate haematological and urine-sugar tests.

In emergencies, antibiotics should be administered (*e.g.* 500,000 units of crystalline penicillin in intramuscular injection, followed by 250 mg capsules penicillin V-4 capsules a day for 5 days). If a fluctuant abscess is present this should be incised and hot salt water mouthwashes prescribed.

Once the diabetes is controlled routine periodontal therapy can be instituted. If minor surgical procedures are necessary they should be organized so that the patient's dietary regime is not disturbed. It is advisable to premedicate with antibiotics, although in other respects the patient may be treated as a healthy individual. If the patient is on insulin and extensive surgery is required hospitalization may be advisable and the management of the treatment worked out with the patient's physician.

A satisfactory regime for the diabetic patient undergoing prolonged general anaesthesia is as follows:

1. Preferably operate in the morning.
2. No insulin is given on the morning of the operation.
3. 5% Dextrose drip is started after induction.
4. 1/4-hourly blood sugar estimates with Dextrostix are plotted on a graph.

Any trend out of an acceptable range of blood sugar may be corrected by:

(a) varying the speed of the drip.
(b) intravenous injection of 25% glucose into the drip.
(c) injection of small amounts of insulin (say 10 units) into the drip.

The patient should be returned to his usual routine at the earliest opportunity, and frequent post-operative urine examinations must be carried out.

If operation is in the afternoon half the usual insulin allowance is given and a normal breakfast is taken a minimum of 4 hours before operation. The management is then as above.

The diabetic patient must be made aware of his special condition and therefore of his special responsibilities. His oral hygiene should be meticulous; regular inspection and scaling are essential.

VITAMIN DEFICIENCIES

While a deficiency of any nutrient item must impair tissue resistance and healing, the only deficiency clearly manifested in the periodontal tissues is that of ascorbic acid (vitamin C).

A frank scurvy is a rare condition in most developed countries. It is found only in food-faddists or in old people living at subsistence level, and then the oral manifestations, *i.e.* swollen, red and bleeding gingivae, form a part, often only a minor part, of a general syndrome. The more common condition is a vitamin deficiency insufficiently great to produce clinical features (*i.e.* a subclinical scurvy) that comes to light when inflamed gingivae fail to respond to apparently adequate treatment, and where healing is obviously retarded.

Treatment

The diagnosis of a vitamin C deficiency should be made only after thorough questioning about the patient's diet has revealed a probable deficiency, and this diagnosis should be confirmed by tests for blood-ascorbic acid levels. Vitamin C is too frequently prescribed without any evidence that there is a deficiency. The presence of an intractable gingivitis is more likely to indicate the presence of undetected plaque than a vitamin deficiency. If a patient is found to have an ascorbic acid deficiency the vitamin should be prescribed; dosage, two 100 mg tablets to be taken three times a day for a period of three months. During this time the patient's diet should be improved and oral hygiene techniques taught.

BLOOD DISEASES

Blood diseases do not cause periodontal disease, but may manifest themselves by changes in the oral mucosa and in an altered gingival response to local irritants, plaque, calculus and food debris. As these irritants are so commonly present gingival changes may well be the first obvious sign of blood disease, and the dentist must be ever watchful of tissue changes that seem out of proportion to the local irritant.

Leukaemia

The blood diseases most commonly manifested by gingival changes are the acute forms of monocytic, myelogenous and lymphatic leukaemia. The chronic forms of these diseases may not be accompanied by any pronounced gingival changes until an acute phase develops.

Acute Leukaemia

Ulcerative lesions may be present anywhere in oral mucosa and petechia may be found on the palate. The gingivae are dark red, bleeding and sometimes very swollen. Echymoses occur easily and give the swollen gingivae a blue colour. The gingivae may also become ulcerated and in severe cases show extensive sloughing. Because the gingivae are sore the patient's oral hygiene is poor; food debris and gross calculus are often present and add to the oral sepsis. The patient is usually pale and feels unwell. Diagnosis must be made on the basis of blood examination; therefore, if an abnormal blood state is suspected the patient must be referred immediately to a physician or hospital for blood tests.

Management of the Leukaemic Patient

Acute leukaemias are fatal; therefore, if the disease has been confirmed by blood examination, the dentist's responsibility is limited to making the patient's mouth as comfortable as possible. Gingival ulceration and bleeding make eating difficult and unpleasant, and oral infection represents a further hazard to life. Dental treatment is complicated by the dangers of haemorrhage and infection, and extractions must be avoided. Treatment should be carried out only after consultation with the patient's physician.

Treatment

Treatment of the gingival condition should be limited to improving the patient's oral hygiene; antibiotic cover should be started the day before treatment is commenced. All local treatment must be carried out gently. As the mouth is usually very dirty, cotton-wool rolls soaked in 10 volume hydrogen peroxide are wiped over the teeth and gingivae. The removal of calculus must be undertaken with caution so that the instruments do not traumatize the tissue. Only a few teeth should be scaled at one time. Superficial scaling and the establishment of an improved oral hygiene regime usually brings about a marked improvement of the gingival condition, and, with reduced swelling, more thorough scaling may be carried out.

The patient with chronic leukaemia must also be treated with care, but in most cases routine dental treatment, except surgery, may be undertaken without special modification. If surgery is necessary it is wise to premedicate with antibiotics and hospitalize the patient.

Iron Deficiency Anaemia

The most common form of anaemia seen by the dentist is microcytic hyprochromic anaemia due to iron deficiency.

The patient, usually a young woman, is pale and may complain of weakness and fatigue. The oral mucosa is pale so that if a gingivitis is present the colour of the inflamed gingivae stands out in contrast to that of the rest of the mucosa. The tongue may be sore, smooth and glossy, particularly at the sides and the tip, as a result of atrophy of the filiform papillae.

Treatment

A suspected iron deficiency should be confirmed by blood examination. Medication with iron should be undertaken by the patient's physician and, because tissue healing is slow and easily retarded by irritation, it is advisable to have this started before any periodontal surgery is undertaken.

Dilantin (Epanutin) Hyperplasia

Dilantin Sodium is frequently used for the control of epilepsy, and many patients on Dilantin develop gingival enlargement. By no means all patients taking the drug develop a hyperplastic gingivitis, and a patient on Dilantin may develop a hyperplastic gingivitis which is unconnected with the medication. It is probable that in a true Dilantin hyperplasia the initial irritant is the ubiquitous plaque to which an exaggerated proliferation of fibrous tissue is induced by the drug.

The resulting firm pink gingival enlargement may almost cover the crowns of the teeth (Fig. 279). An inflammation may be superimposed on

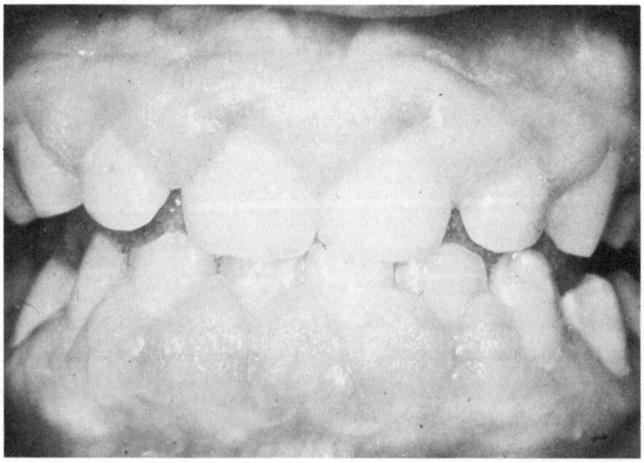

FIG. 279.—Firm, pink enlargement of gingivae in a 16-year-old girl on Dilantin.

the fibrous hyperplasia so that the gingival swelling becomes red, soft, and may bleed (Fig. 280).

The gingival enlargement is frequently so great that the patient's appearance suffers. He may be afraid to smile or even to talk. The condition may add to the very real social handicap the epileptic suffers, and make his integration into society more difficult.

Treatment

The amount of gingival enlargement does not seem to bear any quantitative relationship to the dosage of Dilantin, and reduction of the dose may have no effect on the gingival enlargement. If use of the drug is stopped the gingival enlargement may reduce. Other drugs are available for the control of epilepsy, but in many cases Dilantin is the most effective drug with fewest drawbacks, and it may be impossible for the patient to discontinue its use. This must be determined in consultation with the patient's physician. At the same time, thorough scaling and instruction in oral hygiene techniques should be started. The patient is usually young and, in the beginning, may not be very co-operative. Surgery is frequently required and the preliminary scaling period can be used to gain the patient's confidence. Surgery in this case has to be carried out in stages and the upper anterior segment should be operated on first. This produces the most obvious improvement in appearance, and therefore improved co-operation. Meticulous post-operative care is essential, and the electric toothbrush is valuable in these cases; three-monthly inspection and scaling is recommended. A great deal of patience may be required in the treatment of these cases, but the improvement in appearance and in the general well-being of the patient make the effort worthwhile.

IDIOPATHIC GINGIVAL FIBROMATOSIS

This is a rare condition of unknown aetiology seen in young people. The gingivae become enlarged and may almost cover the teeth. The enlargement is pink and firm and consists of hyperplastic fibrous connective tissue (Fig. 281). Hereditary hyperplasia has been reported, and the disease has been noted in association with hypertrichosis and congenital abnormalities of the fingers and toes.

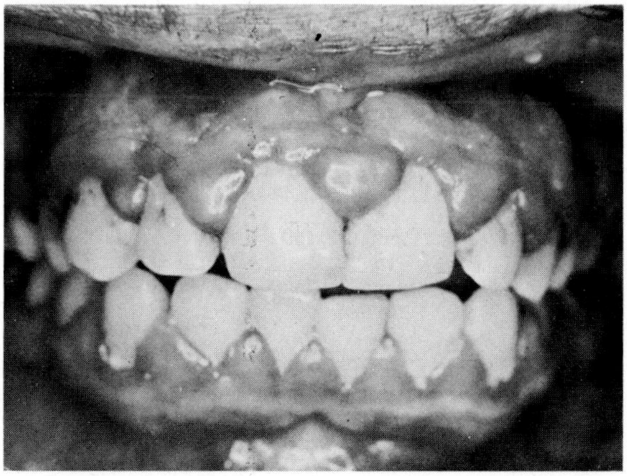

FIG. 280.—Inflammation superimposed on gingival enlargement in a patient on Dilantin.

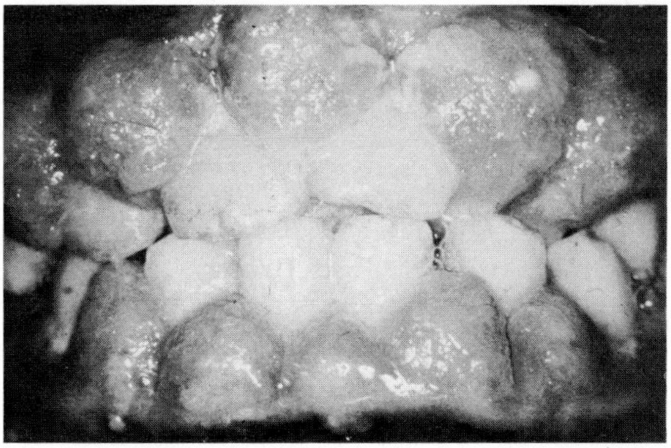

FIG. 281.—Gingival fibromatosis in a 17-year-old boy with a history of three gingivectomies.

Treatment

A strict regime of oral hygiene should be instituted so that any inflammation superimposed on the hyperplastic tissue is reduced to a minimum. Where the condition is unsightly and causing the patient distress gingivectomy is indicated, but recurrence is likely during childhood and adolescence.

In treating young people it is advisable to avoid surgery where possible. It is essential to insist on a good standard of oral hygiene and if surgery then appears necessary it can be carried out in the knowledge that the patient can maintain the tissues in good condition. If oral hygiene is poor then surgical treatment must fail, bringing disappointment to both operator and patient.

THE PATIENT UNDER MEDICAL TREATMENT

Cardiovascular Disease

Patients with a history of coronary disease, hypertension and angina pectoris are required to avoid excessive excitement and fatigue. The patient's doctor must be consulted prior to periodontal treatment and he may advise pre-operative sedation where needed.

There has been concern about the amount of vasoconstrictor used in local analgesia solutions and the New York Heart Association (1955) recommended a maximum dose equivalent to 10 ml of local analgesia solution containing 1:200,000 adrenaline. Providing a low concentration of adrenaline is used and only up to two cartridges of anaesthetic solution used slowly and carefully there would seem to be little risk to the ambulant patient with cardio-vascular disease (Kay, 1972). When the patient has rheumatic or congenital heart disease or a history of rheumatic fever prophylactic antibiotics need to be administered prior to scaling and surgical procedures (*e.g.* Cephaloridine lg i.m. 1/2 hr prior to procedure followed by Ampicillin 250 mg orally q.d.s. for 3 days). In order to avoid multiple doses of antibiotics treatment must be organized into as few stages as possible. Where multiple doses are unavoidable it is wise to change the antibiotic used to avoid developing resistant strains.

Anticoagulant Therapy

Excessive bleeding is not usual after minor oral surgery in the patient undergoing anticoagulant therapy but it is always essential to consult the patient's physician or haematologist. Certain drugs *e.g.* tetracyclines, aspirin, actually enhance the anticoagulant effect and therefore these drugs should not be prescribed. Surgery should be carried out in stages with care, and all wounds sutured. In the case of persistent haemorrhage synthetic Vitamin K (phytomenadione 10–20 mg) can be given i.m. or i.v. However such medication should have the approval of the patient's physician.

Patients on Corticosteroids

Corticosteroids are used for a variety of diseases and prolonged use leads to hypo-activity of the adrenals. The stress of oral surgery and post-operative pain may precipitate an adrenal crisis, therefore further corticosteroids need to be administered to patients either on steroids at the time of surgery or who have had steroid therapy during the previous twelve months. An acceptable regime is to administer 50–100 mg hydrocortisone hemisuccinate i.m. one hour prior to operation or 20 mg oral prednisone 2 hours prior to surgery when carried out under local analgesia. In major procedures it is necessary to repeat this dose 6–8 hours after surgery. If the patient is under steroid therapy the regime must be discussed with the physician.

Monoamine Oxidase Inhibitors

These drugs can produce a number of problems, *e.g.* hypertension when taken with general anaesthetics or the morphine type of narcotic analgesic such as pethidine. Abstinence from the monoamine oxidase inhibitor for three weeks and alternative medication where possible is advisable. However, for most dental procedures alternative analgesics are available. Barbiturate anaesthetics can be used only after test doses have been tried by the anaesthetist.

Tricyclic Antidepressants

These drugs can produce arrythmias with general anaesthetics and should be stopped twenty-four hours before a general anaesthetic is given.

Sickle Cell Anaemia

All negro patients must be screened for sickle cell anaemia prior to a general anaesthetic. Where there is latent or active sickle disease hospitalization is required for general anaesthesia and the necessary haematological precautions taken by the physician or anaesthetist.

REFERENCE

KAY, L. W. (1972). Drugs in dentistry, 2nd ed. John Wright, Bristol, p. 238.

ADDITIONAL READING

BENVENISTE, R., BIXLER, D. and CONNEALLY, P. M. (1967). Periodontal disease in diabetics. *J. Periodont.*, **38**, 271.
GLICKMAN, I. and SMULOW, J. B. (1964). Chronic desquamative gingivitis – its nature and treatment. *J. Periodont.*, **35**, 397.
KING, J. D. (1954). Experimental and clinical observations on gingival hyperplasia due to 'epanutin' (sodium diphenyl hydantoinate). *Brit. dent. J.*, **96**, 237.
LINDHE, J. and BYORN, A. L. (1967). Influence of hormonal contraceptives on the gingiva of women. *J. periodont. Res.*, **2**, 1.
LÖE, H. and SILNESS, J. (1963). Periodontal disease in pregnancy. I. Prevalence and severity. *Acta odont. scand.*, **21**, 532.
LYNCH, M. A. and SHIP, I. I. (1967). Initial oral manifestations of leukaemia. *J. Amer. dent. Ass.* **75**, 932.
MITTELMAN, G., BAKKE, B. F. and SCOPP, I. W. (1961). Alveolar bone changes in sickle cell anemia. *J. Periodont.*, **32**, 74.
PARFITT, G. J. and HAND, C. D. (1963). Reduced plasma ascorbic acid levels and gingival health. *J. Periodont.*, **34**, 347.
PELTIER, J. R. and OLIVER, R. M. (1961). Oral manifestations of idiopathic thrombocytopenic purpura. *Oral Surg.*, **19**, 130.
RUSHTON, M. A. (1957). Heredity or idiopathic hyperplasia of the gums. *Dent. Practit.*, **7**, 136.
SANDLER, H. C. and STAHL, S. S. (1960). Prevalence of periodontal disease in a hospitalized population. *J. dent. Res.*, **39**, 439.
SILNESS, J. and LÖE, H. (1963). Periodontal disease in pregnancy. II. Correlation between oral hygiene and periodontal condition. *Acta odont. scand.*, **22**, 121
STAFFORD, J. L. (1960). Oral manifestations of blood diseases. *Dent. Practit.*, **10**, 248.
WADE, A. B. and STAFFORD, J. L. (1963). Cyclical neutropenia. *Oral Surg.*, **16**, 1443.

18. Juvenile Periodontitis ('Periodontosis')

Chronic periodontitis is characterized by:

1. The presence of identifiable aetiological factors.
2. The slow rate of destruction of the periodontal tissues, so that the period of time which elapses between the onset of gingival inflammation and tooth loss may be of the order of 20–40 years.

Occasionally one encounters an adolescent or young adult with very advanced bone destruction around several teeth where neither local nor systemic aetiological factors can be identified to account for the severity of tissue destruction.

The disease has been described as diffuse alveolar atrophy by Gottlieb (1923) who ascribed the condition to failure of the cementum to deposit continuously (Gottlieb, 1946). Orban and Weinmann (1942) coined the term 'periodontosis' believing that the condition represented a degeneration of the periodontal ligament. However, there is no evidence for that belief and the term 'juvenile periodontitis' has been adopted because it indicates the clinical features of the disease and does not suggest any particular aetiological agent of pathological process.

The aetiology and pathogenesis of the disease have been something of a mystery but there is evidence that it represents a selective cell-mediated immuno-deficiency disease in which a selective impairment of DNA synthesis of lymphocyte to plaque and some Gram-negative organisms is associated with an intact macrophage migration inhibition mechanism (Lehner *et al.*, 1974).

There is little doubt that juvenile periodontitis (periodontosis) is a clinical entity (Baer, 1971) which possesses the following characteristics:

(a) Age of Onset. The patient is usually under 25 years old on examination. A reliable history is rarely available. Unfortunately gingival bleeding is frequently not taken seriously and even tooth mobility and drifting may go unremarked. Therefore it is possible that the onset is several years earlier than the age at which symptoms provoke the patient to seek attention. Baer (1971) reports occasional onset during the circumpubertal period, *i.e.* between 11–13 years of age.

(b) Clinical Manifestations. Drifting and mobility of teeth, usually the incisors, is the most frequent complaint. Occasionally an acute periodontal abscess may develop and on subsequent radiological examination the full extent of the bone destruction is disclosed.

(c) Bone Destruction. In the classical case there is advanced bone destruction localized to the incisors and first molars (Fig. 282). Deep infrabony defects mesial to the first molars are characteristic. The left and right sides may be almost mirror images. Frequently the second molars and second premolars are also involved. In a small proportion of cases alveolar bone loss is diffuse and affects almost all the teeth.

(d) Sex. Orban and Weinmann (1942) reported occurrence in more women than men. Benjamin and Baer (1967) report a ratio of 3 females to one male.

(e) Race. Several epidemiological studies report a greater severity of periodontal destruction in periodontal disease in non-European populations and there is some evidence that in Britain the incidence of juvenile periodontitis is much greater in West Indians (Manson and Lehner, 1974).

(f) Familial Tendency. Most studies of 'periodontosis' suggest that a familial tendency does exist and one which follows the maternal line (Benjamin and Baer, 1967). This fact together with the mirror-image pattern of bone destruction suggests a form of genetic involvement (Kaslick and Chasens, 1968).

(g) General Health. There appears to be no relationship between the periodontal state and general health. Cases have been reported in which the Papillon-Lefevre syndrome occurs with advanced periodontal destruction in a child but this is rare and not characteristic of juvenile periodontitis in which the patient is otherwise healthy. The blood picture is normal but there is some evidence of a greater prevalence of the disease in individuals with blood group B (Kaslick *et al.*, 1971).

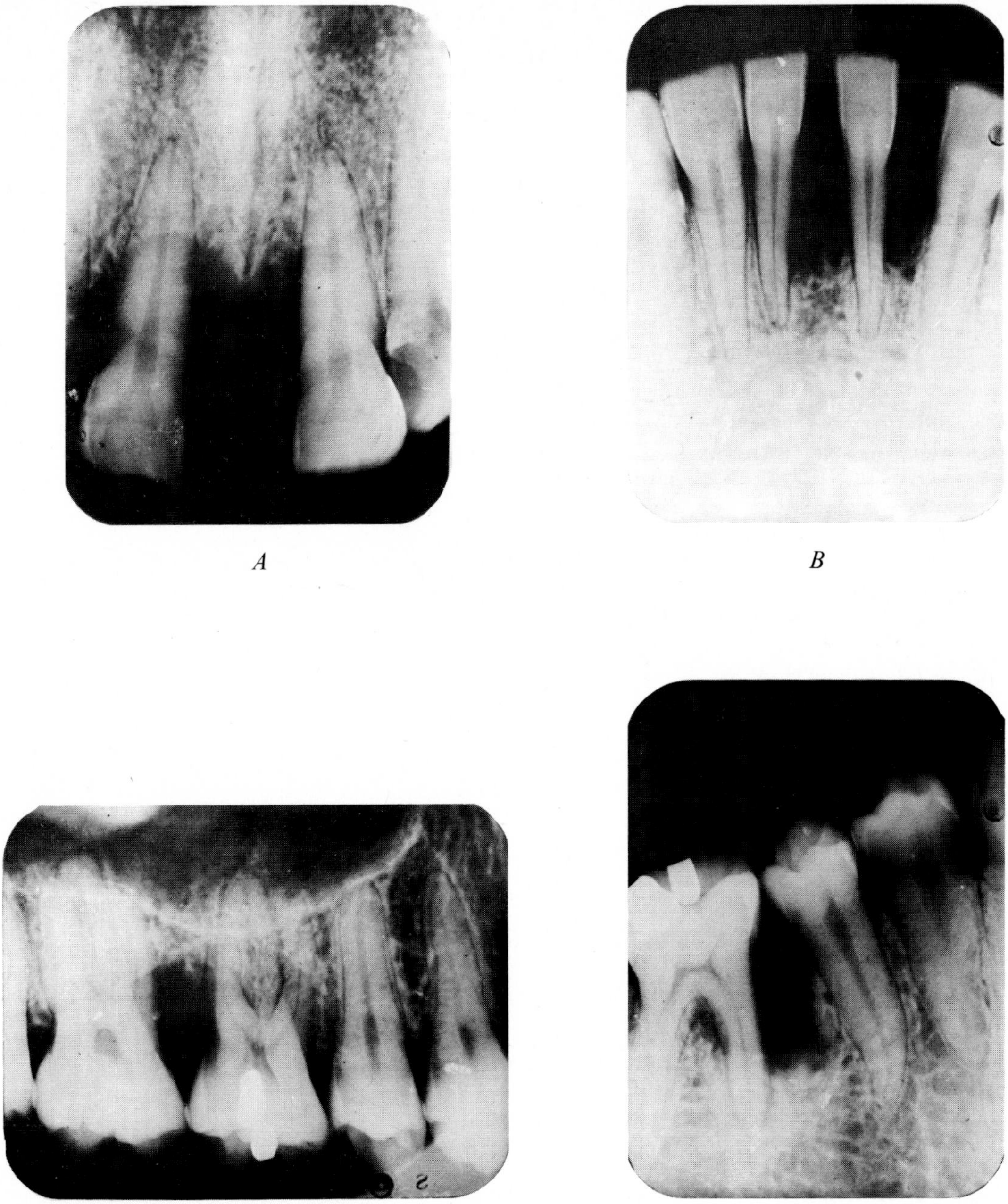

FIG. 282.—Juvenile periodontitis in West Indian adolescent boy. (*A*) and (*B*). Typical bone loss and spreading of incisors. (*C*) and (*D*). Typical crescentic bone destruction around molars.

Treatment

The idea that all the teeth should be extracted before further loss of bone reduces the amount of denture-bearing tissue rests on the untenable assumption that a denture does not stimulate resorption of alveolar bone. If the loss of alveolar bone is rapid in periodontal disease it is likely to be just as rapid under a denture. Therefore it is completely unjustified to condemn a young person to wearing full dentures for the rest of his life.

Although the treatment of periodontosis may only be symptomatic, it is always essential to investigate thoroughly both local and systemic aetiological factors before treatment. Local factors such as poor oral hygiene, food impaction, traumatic occlusion (possibly with bruxism) must be identified, and, if present, corrected. Blood and urine analysis and some form of diet analysis should be undertaken. If these tests indicate a systemic abnormality this must be treated prior to the treatment of the periodontal disease.

In almost all cases no abnormal systemic factors are evident, and the treatment takes the following form:

1. Scaling and instruction in oral hygiene techniques. If patient co-operation is poor any further periodontal treatment will be a waste of time.
2. Extract teeth with poor bone support.
3. Adjust occlusion so that multiple contacts are made in all positions and excursions (Chapter 14).
4. Splint teeth which have drifted and are mobile but where bone support is still fairly good.
5. Provide a bite-guard for wear at night if there is a possibility of bruxism.
6. Treat pocketing as one would routinely; close supervision during the post-operative period is essential.
7. Provide correctly designed partial dentures.
8. Ensure a regular three-monthly recall and closely supervize the case with emphasis on assiduous attention to good oral hygiene.

Everett and Baer (1964) have recommended systematic and repeated grinding of the occlusal surfaces to permit eruption of involved teeth. They suggest that this might stimulate cementum deposition at the apex of the tooth and bone deposition at the alveolar crest which could compensate for tissue lost. It is difficult to assess the effectiveness of any procedure as the tissue destruction appears to be intermittent and may come to a halt.

REFERENCES

BAER, P. N. (1971). The case for periodontosis as a clinical entity. *J. Periodont.*, **42**, 516.

BENJAMIN, S. D. and BAER, P. N. (1967). Familial patterns of advanced alveolar bone loss in adolescence (periodontosis). *Periodontics*, **5**, 82.

EVERETT, F. G. and BAER, P. N. (1964). Preliminary report on the treatment of the osseous defect in periodontosis. *J. Periodont.*, **35**, 429.

GOTTLIEB, B. (1923). Die diffuse atrophie des Alveolarknochens. *Z. Stomat.*, **21**, 195.

GOTTLIEB, B. (1946). The new concept of periodontoclasia. *J. Periodont.*, **17**, 7.

KASLICK, R. S. and CHASENS, A. I. (1968). Periodontosis with periodontitis: a study involving young adult males. II. Clinical, medical and histopathologic studies. *Oral Surg.*, **25**, 327.

KASLICK, R. S., CHASENS, A. I., TUCKMAN, M. A. *et al.* (1971). Investigations of periodontosis with periodontitis: literature survey and findings based on ABO blood groups. *J. Periodontol.*, **42**, 420.

LEHNER, T., WILTON, J. M. A., IVANYI, L. and MANSON, J. D. (1974). Immunological aspects of juvenile periodontitis (periodontosis). *J. Periodont. Res.*, **9**, 261.

MANSON, J. D. and LEHNER, T. (1974). A clinical study of juvenile periodontitis (periodontosis). *J. Periodont.*, **45**, 630.

ORBAN, B. and WEINMANN, J. P. (1942). Diffuse atrophy of the alveolar bone (periodontosis). *J. Periodont.*, **13**, 31.

19. Acute Gingivitis

By definition an acute gingivitis is of sudden onset, of limited duration and has well defined symptoms. Acute inflammation of the gingivae may be caused by a variety of physical and chemical agents, by specific micro-organisms, or by non-specific members of the oral flora.

Theoretically a large variety of problems can involve the gingivae, *e.g.* the snail track ulcer of secondary syphilis, but in this chapter only the following relatively common conditions will be described.

1. Chemical and physical trauma.
2. Acute ulcerative gingivitis.
3. Acute herpetic gingivo-stomatitis.
4. Candidiasis.
5. Streptococcal gingivitis.
6. Drug sensitivity reaction.
7. Pericoronitis.
8. Gingival abscess.
9. Aphthous ulceration.

PHYSICAL AND CHEMICAL TRAUMA

A great many physical and chemical agents can injure the gingivae. The most common of these are:

1. Any hot food or drink taken injudiciously.
2. Escharotic drugs such as silver nitrate, phenol, even hydrogen peroxide used at strong dilutions and too frequently.
3. Aspirin burns resulting from a misguided attempt to eradicate toothache by resting an aspirin on the gingiva.
4. Toothbrush bristle or a woodstick lacerating the gingiva.
5. Tobacco burns.

Usually there is no doubt about the diagnosis. The patient may suffer fairly severe pain for a short time after which the affected area is sore and extremely sensitive to any further irritation. A localized patch of inflammation or a vesicle may form. As vesicles in the mouth remain intact for only a short time the wound is usually seen as a bright red area denuded of epithelium and with a ragged edge of loose necrotic tissue that can be felt by the tongue. The healing wound takes on a sheen as it is quickly covered by a thin layer of epithelium. Sensitivity lasts for several days until the wound is completely covered. In a debilitated individual secondary infection may occur, in which case pain continues and beads of pus form over the wound. This may also be accompanied by lymph gland enlargement and malaise.

Treatment

The wound usually heals without active interference, providing secondary infection does not occur. The patient must avoid hot and spicy foods and will probably do this automatically. Drinking cold water or any cold bland fluids will soothe. Troches containing a local anaesthetic may be prescribed, and a mouthwash of glycerine and thymol may be advised for the patient anxious to have more active treatment. Analgesics should be given if the pain is marked. Triamcinolone in Orabase will control the inflammatory reaction, diminish symptoms and shorten the healing time, but the use of corticosteroids should be restricted to those cases in which injury is fairly extensive or the pain is severe. If there is secondary infection a systemic antibiotic should be prescribed: Caps. penicillin V.-250 mg, 4 caps. per day for 5 days. Hot salt water mouthwashes may be irritant and should not be prescribed.

ACUTE ULCERATIVE GINGIVITIS

(Syn: Vincent's disease, acute necrotizing gingivitis, trench-mouth.)

Aetiology

The exact cause of this common disease has not yet been defined. The disease is associated with the presence of specific micro-organisms, B. Fusiformis and Borrelia Vincentii as well as Treponema microdentium and other organisms (Fig. 283), but the evidence seems to indicate that these micro-organisms are not the primary cause

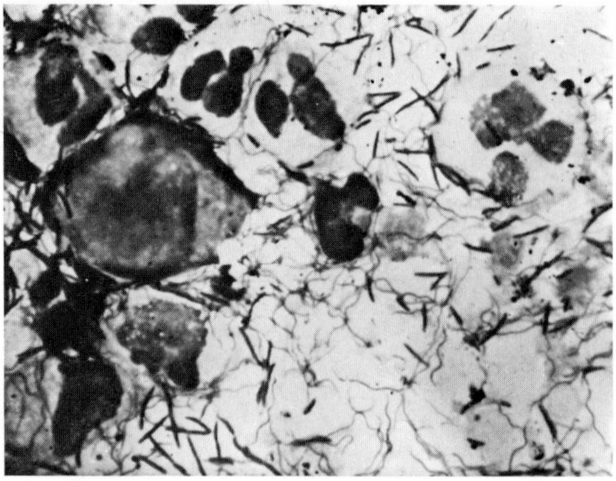

A

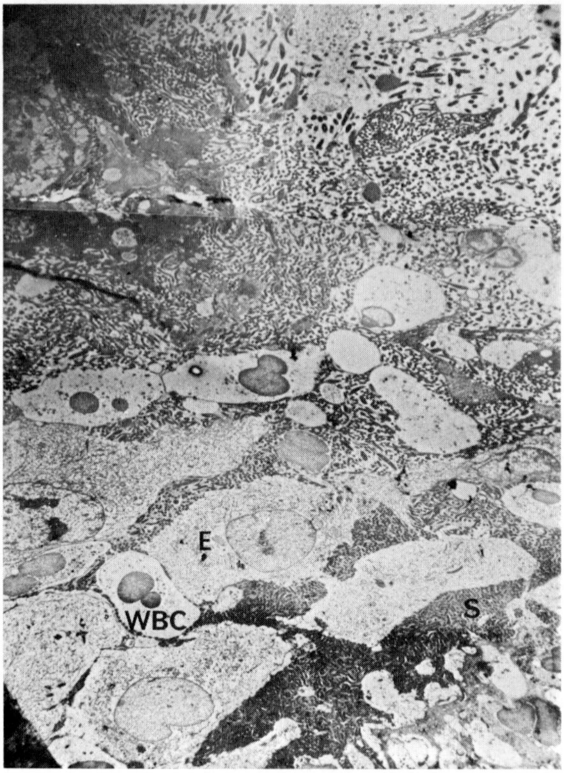

B

FIG. 283.—Flora in acute ulcerative gingivitis.

(*A*) Direct smear to show *Treponema Vincenti* and *B. Fusiformis*. (By courtesy of Dr G. C. Blake.)

(*B*) Electron micrograph of organism penetrating gingival tissue. Epithelial cell (E): polymorphonuclear leucocyte (WBC): spiral organism (S) possibly *Treponema* (X 3,080). (By courtesy of Dr R. Taylor-Heylings.)

of the disease. Whatever the direct cause there frequently seems to be a conditioning of the tissues by stress of work, worry, fatigue and smoking, and once an individual has suffered the disease there is a definite tendency for recurrence to take place as though the tissues have become sensitized to some local agent (Goldhaber and Giddon, 1964).

Although the disease is associated with bacterial infection there is no positive evidence that it is contagious. The fact that many people within a group may be affected appears to be due to shared predisposing factors (*e.g.* the stress of living conditions, as in the armed forces) rather than the infection of one individual from another (Pindborg, 1956).

Clinical Features

The disease occurs about equally in both sexes, the majority of patients being between 18–26 years old. It appears to occur most commonly in spring and autumn. Fairly frequently one finds a subacute form superimposed on a chronic gingivitis or chronic periodontitis in older individuals, but it is rare to find the disease in a child under twelve except in underdeveloped countries such as West Africa, where the incidence of the disease in children is high (Emslie, 1963).

Patients complain of gingival soreness and sometimes of considerable pain. There may be spontaneous gingival bleeding and an objectionable taste. Tooth-brushing is painful and food debris is allowed to collect. There may be halitosis, but this is not always present or as characteristic as is often stated.

In the early stages the gingival margins are bright red and the tips of the papillae show the typical punched-out grey ulcer (Fig. 284). This ulceration spreads along the gingival margins so that an extensive area of gingiva is involved (Fig. 285). If the false membrane of necrotic tissue covering the ulcer is wiped away a raw bleeding

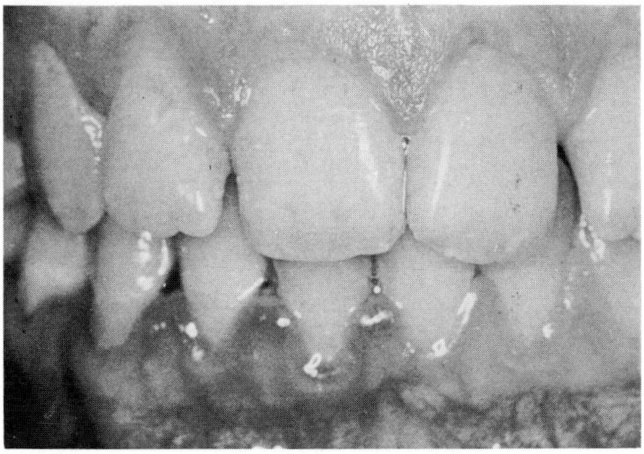

FIG. 284.—Typical early lesion of Vincent's disease.

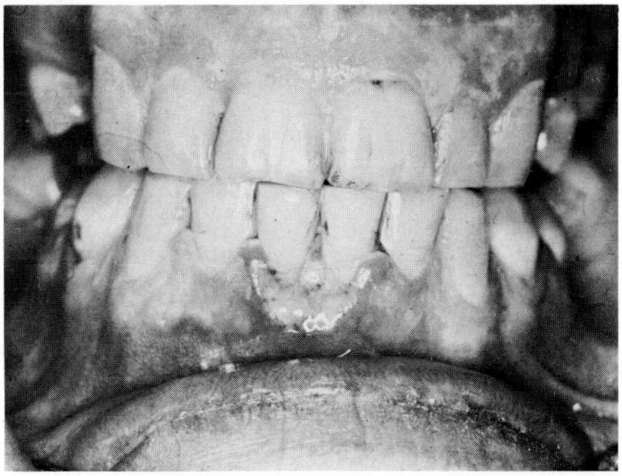

A

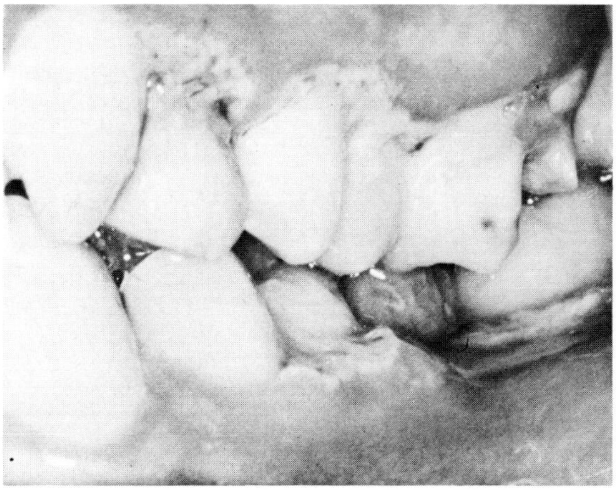

B

FIG. 285.—(*A*) Spread of ulceration along the gingival margin. Note the ulcerated tips of the papillae mesial to the lower lateral incisors. (*B*) Extensive ulceration of the gingival margin about upper and lower teeth.

area is left. The ulceration may be localized to one region, commonly the lower incisor region, or may involve the whole mouth. The localization appears to be associated with the collection of food debris and calculus, food impaction, overhanging margins, partially erupted teeth, and occasionally with the impingement of lower incisors on palatal tissue in cases of deep overbite; indeed the ulceration may be associated with any local factor that might cause tissue irritation and debility (Manson and Rand, 1961). This is not always the case; occasionally one encounters a severe infection in a clean, carefully tended mouth, and it is in these cases that an underlying emotional factor appears to be most obvious. In severe cases ulceration may occur on the palate, tongue and fauces (Vincent's angina).

Secondary infection may occur with an elevated temperature, submaxillary and cervical lymph gland enlargement and general malaise. In some cases with prolonged temperature elevation a primary herpetic infection is present with Vincent's disease, and it seems possible that the Vincent's infection is superimposed on the debilitated tissue involved in the virus disease.

Even without treatment spontaneous remission of the acute phase occurs; the symptoms subside but do not disappear entirely. Careful examina- often reveals persistent slight ulceration at the tip of the papillae (Fig. 286).

The destruction of the papilla and the proliferation of repair tissue which thickens the margin of the lesion creates the typical saucer-shaped deformity of Vincent's disease. Food debris, plaque and calculus collect in this interdental defect, gingival irritation is perpetuated, and recurrence of an acute episode may take place after days, weeks or months. With each acute episode the gingival deformity worsens and without adequate treatment the resultant persistent chronic inflammation develops into a chronic periodontitis. In time these bouts of acute

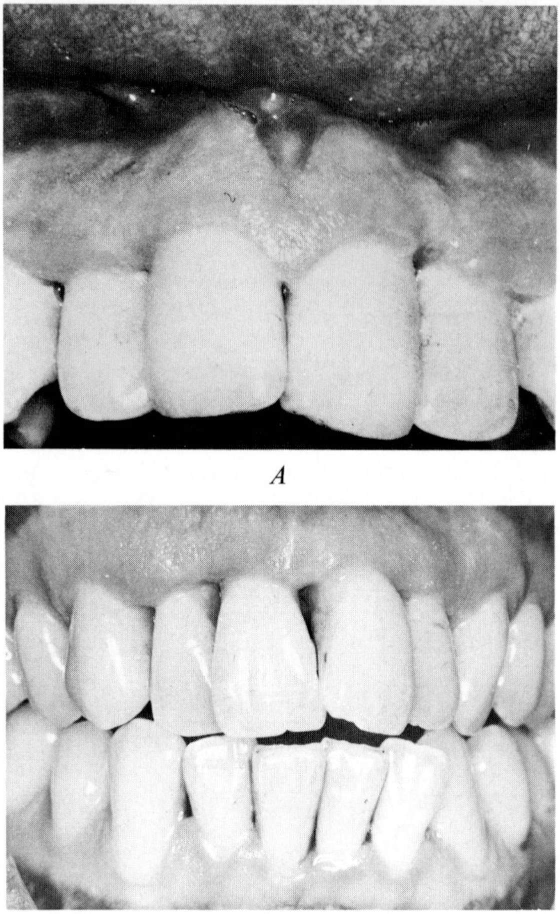

A

B

FIG. 286.—(*A*) Gingival deformity resulting from Vincent's disease. Very slight ulceration persists at |2. (*B*) More severe gingival deformity resulting from recurrent episodes of Vincent's disease.

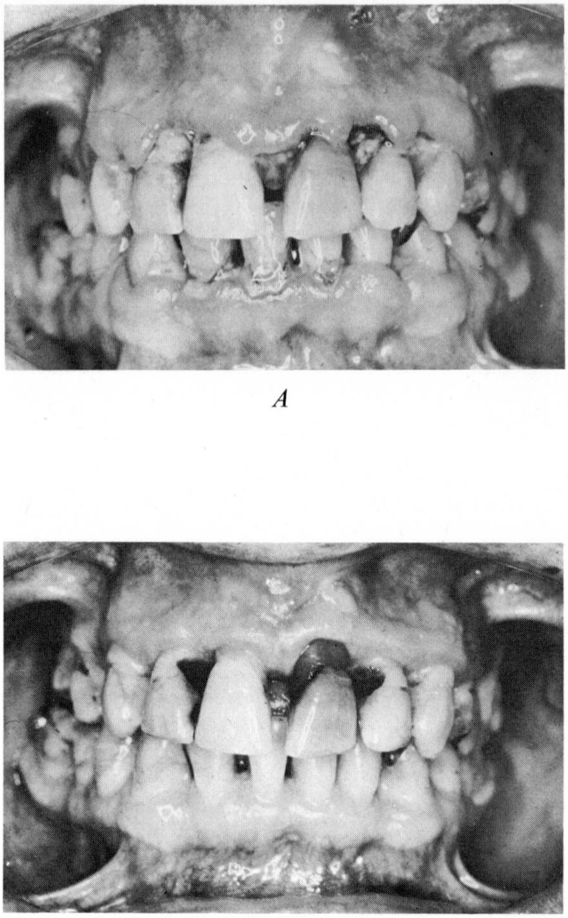

A

B

FIG. 287.—(*A*) Gross gingival deformity after many episodes of acute ulceration. A chronic periodontitis is also present. (*B*) After gingivectomy. Sound restorative work can now be undertaken.

gingivitis become less severe, but occasional episodes of sub-acute ulceration may be superimposed even on advanced periodontal disease in the older individual. The permanent gingival deformity is so characteristic that a previous episode of Vincent's disease can be diagnosed in a middle-aged individual who has not suffered an acute episode for many years (Fig. 287).

Treatment

The treatment of ulcerative gingivitis may be divided into (1) control of the acute phase and (2) treatment of the residual condition.

Principles of Control of the Acute Phase

A large variety of procedures and medicaments have been advocated and discarded. Present treatments consist of a three-pronged attack on the disease:

1. Clean the area by irrigation with warm water and gentle scaling and debridement.
2. Apply oxygenating agents to depress the anaerobic organisms. The most commonly used oxygenating agent is a hydrogen peroxide mouthwash at 5 volumes strength or a buffered sodium peroxyborate mouthwash (Bocasan) which is essentially hydrogen

peroxide in a form which allows long-term storage. The effervescence of these solutions may also act to remove debris.

When the symptoms are mild these two measures are adequate to control the condition without resort to:

3. Use an antibacterial agent. Penicillin has been the most effective and frequently used antibiotic, usually prescribed in oral form as phenoxymethyl penicillin (dose 250 mg q.d.s. for 5 days). Tetracycline may also be used in the same dosage. An effective alternative is metronidazole (Flagyl) which is also used for trichomonal vaginitis (Shinn, Squires and McFadzean, 1965). It is prescribed in 200 mg tablets taken three times a day for 3–5 days. This is a generally safe substitute for penicillin especially where there is a history of penicillin sensitivity, but it must not be prescribed in early pregnancy or to patients who drink heavily. Indeed alcohol should be avoided during treatment. Prescription of metronidazole is also contraindicated where there is a blood dyscrasia. Side effects of the drug are not usual when the drug is used for short periods, but include nausea, headaches, a metallic taste and tachycardia.

Recommended Regime

(a) Without systemic manifestations

First Day

1. Thoroughly irrigate with warm water and gently remove with a curette gross debris, necrotic material and as much supragingival calculus as possible. Pain diminishes markedly after this procedure. Where the mouth is very dirty, sponging with cotton wool soaked in 10 vol. hydrogen peroxide is effective in removing loose debris. If the gingivae are not too sensitive, careful use of the ultrasonic scaler removes debris rapidly and efficiently.
2. Instruct the patient to use copious and frequent mouth-washes of warm water or dilute hydrogen peroxide. A dessert-spoonful of 10 vol. hydrogen peroxide in a half tumblerful of warm water should be used every hour if possible and this should be vigorously sucked between the teeth.
3. If oral symptoms are severe prescribe metronidazole 200 mg t.d.s. for 3 days.

Fifth Day

By this time the tissue response is usually good enough for a fine scaling and removal of all subgingival calculus. Instruction in oral hygiene must be given at this stage, and aggravating factors such as overhanging fillings and pericoronal flaps should be corrected (with extraction of the third molar if necessary).

(b) With systemic manifestations

Where the patient has a temperature, malaise and lymph gland enlargement, 250 mg capsules of penicillin V should be prescribed, one capsule to be taken four times a day for five days. If the patient has a history of abnormal reaction to penicillin or suffers from asthma, hay-fever or eczema, alternative antibiotics such as tetracycline should be prescribed in the same dosage and the patient is then ordered to rest for a couple of days. Mouthwashes must be used as described. Antibiotic therapy does not rule out the need for local measures. Usually by the fifth day the patient is well, and a meticulous scaling can be carried out.

Management of the Residual Condition

After the acute phase has passed and predisposing causes such as partially erupted teeth, overhanging fillings and so on have been corrected, an attempt must be made to correct any gingival deformity and to restore all teeth to normal function.

Gingivoplasty is required in a large proportion of these cases. If gingival deformity is not corrected, food impaction and stagnation in the interdental space continue and recurrence is likely. Plaque stagnation occurs readily about unused teeth which often form the site of disease recurrence. Removable or fixed prostheses must be constructed to bring these teeth into efficient function.

Subsequently regular inspection and scaling to ensure that a high standard of oral hygiene is maintained is essential.

As the chances of recurrence are high, Vincent's patients should be kept under observation for at least six months. Also systemic disease, particularly blood dyscrasias, may predispose the patient to acute ulcerative gingivitis. Patients suffering unexplained recurrent attacks should undergo blood examination.

ACUTE HERPETIC GINGIVO-STOMATITIS

Primary infection by the herpes simplex virus usually takes place in very young children (1–3 years), and almost every adult harbours the virus in the tissues about the mouth and nose. Primary infection may occur in adults who have escaped earlier infection, but the herpes lesion (cold-sore) generally seen in the adult represents a recurrence of virus activity.

Symptoms of primary infection appear abruptly with pain in the mouth, produce salivation and halitosis. The child is very irritable and refuses to eat even before oral lesions have become apparent. Temperature may be raised to as high as 103°F, lymph glands are enlarged and there is general malaise.

The early vesicular lesions are rarely seen. They quickly rupture to form a grey-yellow membrane surrounded by bright red mucosa. Every part of the mouth may be involved, and the gingivae, tongue and cheeks are characteristically covered in the necrotic membrane (Fig. 288).

The acute phase lasts about a week and complete healing of the ulcers takes a few days longer. Prolonged fever indicates secondary infection.

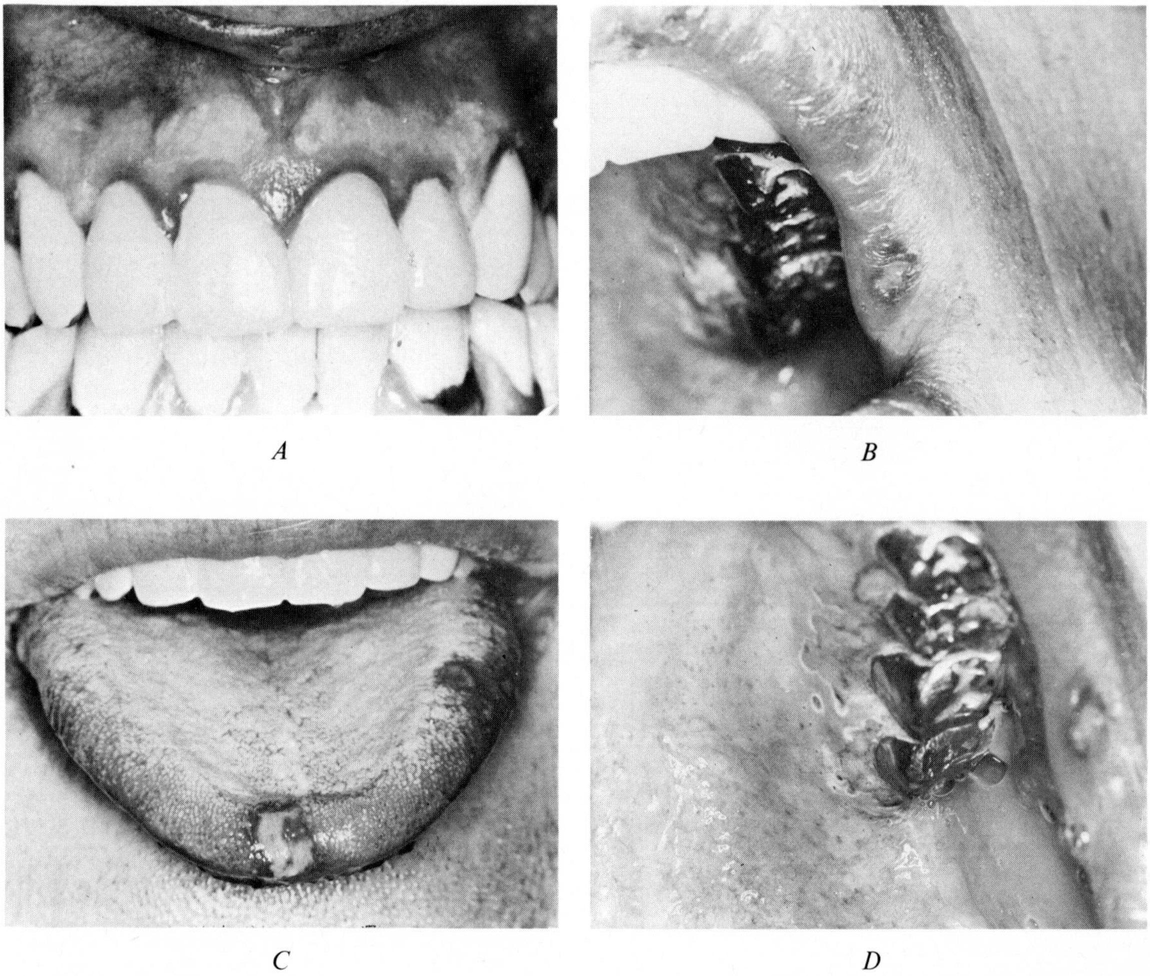

FIG. 288.—Primary herpetic lesions in an adult male.
(*A*) Bright red gingival margin plus grey slough. (*B*) Broken vesicle on lip. (*C*) Tongue lesions. (*D*) Lesions in palatal gingivae.

Treatment
No drug at present available is known to combat the virus, therefore treatment is symptomatic and supportive, *i.e.* bed rest, cool soft foods, plenty of fluids. Milk of Magnesia are 0.5 per cent Dequadin paint gently applied to the gingivae may have a soothing effect while Benzocaine lozenges can be prescribed for the older child.

Analgesic antipyretics should be prescribed to alleviate pain and reduce the temperature and an elixir of Phenergan is a useful sedative. Systemic antibiotics (*e.g.* tetracycline) may be prescribed to combat severe secondary infection, but should not be prescribed as routine treatment.

To lessen the risk of monilial infection after the use of a broad-spectrum antibiotic a combination of tetracycline (250 mg) and nystatin (250,000 I.U.) or Mysteclin has been recommended. For children Mysteclin syrup is more palatable: it can be rolled around the mouth for 3 minutes, the procedure being repeated three times a day for 3 days.

The anti-viral agent 5-iodo-2 deoxyuridine, although toxic, has been used with success in primary herpetic stomatitis. It can be used as a 0.1% aqueous solution and applied with a brush to the lesions several times a day (1 hourly on the first day, 2 hourly on the second day, 3 hourly on the third day and then 4 times a day for the next two days) (Jaffe and Lehner, 1968).

CANDIDIASIS

Candida albicans is normally found in the mouth as a saprophyte until tissue resistance is lowered by disease or poor diet. Candidiasis is common in pregnancy and the infant may be infected from the vagina. Infection may also develop where broad-spectrum antibiotic treatment has suppressed the normal oral flora and allowed Candida to flourish. Corticosteroid treatment also appears to be an important predisposing factor.

Infection may be present in the mouth in several forms; acute pseudomembranous candidiasis or thrush, acute atrophic candidiasis, chronic atrophic candidiasis or denture sore-mouth, and a more rare chronic hyperplastic form called candida leukoplakia (Lehner, 1967).

Acute Pseudomembranous Candidiasis (Thrush)
This is found in infants and debilitated adults. Lesions occur in the gingivae, tongue, cheeks and in the throat, and is a superficial, creamy-white slightly elevated patch which is easily wiped away leaving a red and raw base (Fig. 289*A*). There may be no pain or other symptoms but occasionally the patient will complain of soreness and dryness of the mouth and throat. The lesion is self-limiting in the healthy individual but can spread rapidly in the debilitated patient to the skin and oesophagus.

Diagnosis may be confirmed by microscopic examination of a scraping in which the yeast appears (Fig. 289*B*).

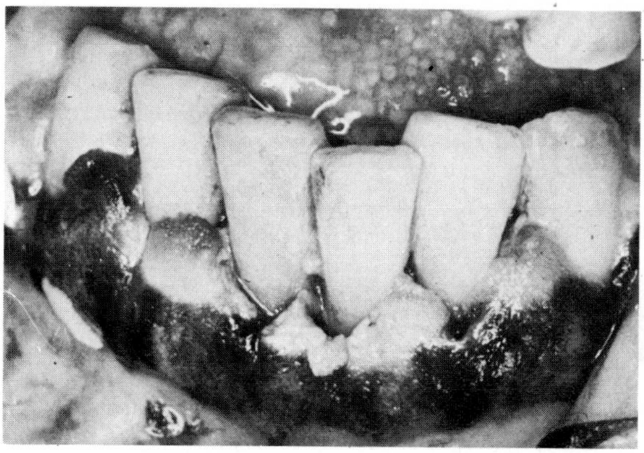

A

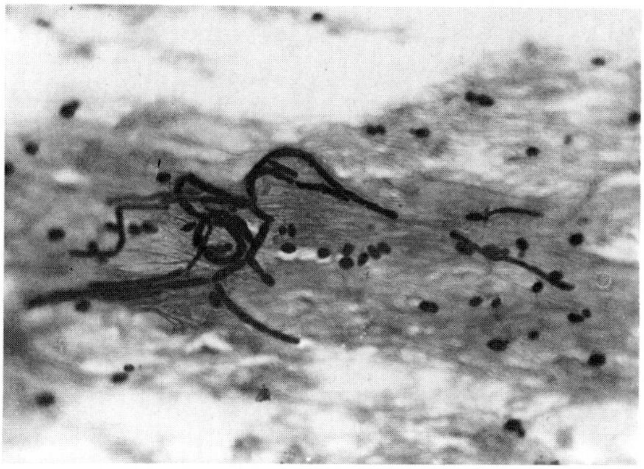

B

FIG. 289.—(*A*) Gingival lesion of candidiasis. (By courtesy of Dr T. Lehner.) (*B*) Typical appearance of yeast forms in a scraping from an oral lesion of candidiasis.

Treatment

In infants a suspension of nystatin (100,000 U/ml) can be painted on the lesions 2 or 3 times a day.

In adults nystatin lozenges (500,000 i.u.) or amphotericin B lozenges (10 mg) which has a more acceptable taste, can be sucked 3 or 4 times a day.

A medical examination of the patient is advisable.

Acute Atrophic Candidiasis

This form is usually associated with patients on prolonged steroid or antibiotic therapy. The mucosa is thin, fiery red and painful without membrane formation. Symptomatic treatment with nystatin or amphotericin B is given.

Chronic Atrophic Candidiasis (Denture Sore Mouth)

This is the result of secondary infection by candida of tissue irritated by a denture. Usually it occurs in the palate especially where the denture is worn day and night. The tissue is bright red and spongy, often delineating the denture-bearing area.

The candida organism is found to penetrate the atrophic layer of epithelium. Treatment includes the use of nystatin or amphotericin B plus re-designing a denture. A recommended regime is:

1. Advise the patient to leave out the denture when possible.
2. Immediately reline the denture with a tissue conditioner material, *e.g.* Tempo.
3. Instruct the patient to massage the denture-bearing area with a finger and amphotericin B cream for three minutes every evening.

Frequently associated with denture sore mouth is angular cheilitis where the wet folded angles of the mouth produced by overclosure become infected with candida albicans. Amphotericin B cream is used on the lesion but treatment should be aimed at adjusting the dentures so that the fold is eliminated.

STREPTOCOCCAL GINGIVITIS

Primary gingival infection by a specific micro-organism such as the haemolytic streptococcus is very rare. More commonly, secondary infection of the gingivae by haemolytic streptococci occurs in tissue that is already irritated and inflamed, *e.g.* around partially erupted teeth, or where some systemic condition such as a blood dyscrasia has lowered the tissue resistance (Fig. 290). It is possible that it is secondary to viral infection.

The gingivae and other oral tissues become intensely red and sensitive and the lymph glands enlarged. Because of the gingival soreness the mouth becomes very dirty and this aggravates the condition.

Treatment is symptomatic. The oral hygiene must be improved by constant bland mouth-washes, cool water or very dilute alkalis. Patients find ice soothing and cold foods acceptable. A 2% tetracycline mouthwash is very useful.

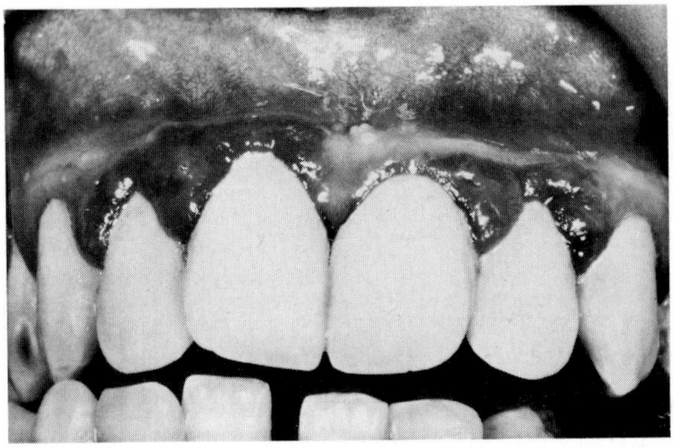

FIG. 290.—Streptococcal gingivitis in an 18-year-old youth with cyclical neutropenia.

DRUG SENSITIVITY

As the number of drugs in common use increase, manifestations of drug sensitivity become increasingly common. There is a wide range of sensitivity reactions, the most severe being fatal anaphylactic shock. This has been reported following the use of many drugs, including antibiotics and topical anaesthetics.

Many drugs in common use are responsible for allergic responses of skin and mucosa including oral manifestations.

Vesicles or bullae may form and rupture almost immediately, leaving sore ulcerated areas. Often the picture is complicated by secondary infection by streptococci or, if penicillin lozenges have been used, by candida.

If the oral manifestations are associated with skin eruptions, urticaria, or swollen painful joints, a prompt diagnosis may be possible, but in many cases the drug responsible is not identified until the patient has suffered several episodes.

Treatment consists of withdrawal of the drug if identified, frequent warm water mouthwashes to keep the area clean and reduce the possibility of secondary infection, and anaesthetic troches. If symptoms are severe prompt administration of systemic corticosteroids by the patient's physician is indicated. Antihistamines are most useful in cases of urticaria.

PERICORONITIS

Non-specific infection of the tissues associated with plaque stagnation around a partly erupted tooth is common. The lower third molar is the most frequently involved because it is often partially erupted and has a mucosal flap and pocketing which collects plaque. The inflamed and swollen tissue overlying the tooth is then traumatized by the opposing teeth.

The patient may complain only of soreness of the gum overlying the tooth. In more severe cases involving the lower third molar there may be considerable pain, difficulty in swallowing, trismus and facial swelling. The tissues over the tooth are red, swollen and tender. A slight amount of pus may exude from under the flap, and the patient may complain of a foul taste and halitosis. Submaxillary and cervical lymph glands may be enlarged, the temperature elevated and the patient may be definitely unwell. Quite frequently the flap is the site of a superimposed acute ulcerative gingivitis.

Treatment

If the inflammation is localized to the area of the tooth

1. Irrigate the area with hot salt water.
2. Very gently remove debris from beneath the flap with a curette or probe to allow drainage of pus from under the flap. This can be facilitated by the use of a shred of cotton wool soaked in trichloracetic acid and glycerine.
3. Grind the opposing tooth if it is traumatizing the tissue.
4. Prescribe salt water mouthwashes to be used very frequently.

If the inflammation has spread to surrounding tissues causing cellulitis, trismus or lymphadenopathy, systemic antibiotics should be prescribed. If urgently required an intramuscular injection of 500,000 units crystalline penicillin should be administered following by a course of penicillin V (phenoxymethyl penicillin) – 4 × 250 mg capsules each day for five days.

Once the acute inflammation has resolved it is essential to clean thoroughly any remaining pocket about the tooth. Where a flap remains and recurrence is likely, this should be removed by electrosurgery or with a scalpel. It is essential to remove the flap completely; incomplete removal results in recurrence of the trouble.

If the tooth is badly angulated so that food stagnation is inevitable it should be extracted. If the opposing tooth continues to irritate the tissue this may have to be extracted. This should not be undertaken lightly; the extraction of a third molar may result in distal drifting of the second molar and food impaction between the molars, particularly where a plunger cusp is active.

APHTHOUS ULCERATION
(Canker Sore)

'Aphthous ulcer' is the name given to mouth ulcers of as yet unknown aetiology and which are usually recurrent. It has been suggested that they are delayed hypersensitivity or auto-immune lesions, or associated with gastro-intestinal disorders, periods of lowered resistance, with allergies or as a psychosomatic manifestation (Ship, 1966).

Three forms of aphthous ulceration have been described. These are Mikulicz's recurrent aphthae, periadenitis mucosa necrotica recurrens and recurrent herpetiform ulcers (Kramer, 1967).

The Mikulicz's aphthae are the minor variety. One or a small number of ulcers occur on non-keratinized mucosa, especially the vestibule inside the lip and cheek and in the floor of the mouth (Fig. 291). They are shallow with little surrounding inflammation. They may be tender or scarcely noticed by the patient. They may appear at intervals of weeks or months or so frequently that the patient is rarely free from them. Their occurrence may be precipitated by tension or emotional trauma, minor trauma to the mucosa, eating certain foods or after injection with local

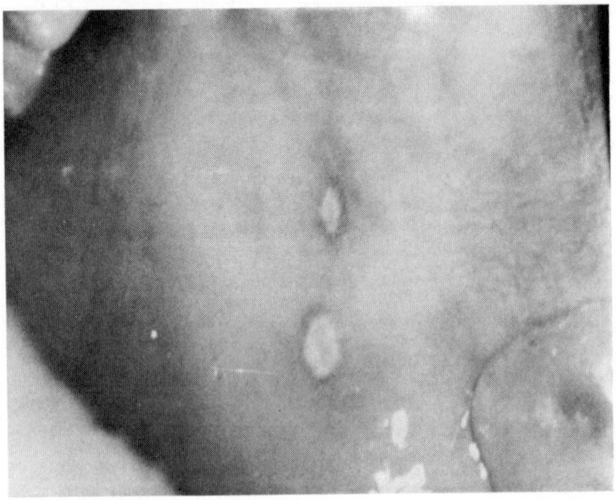

A

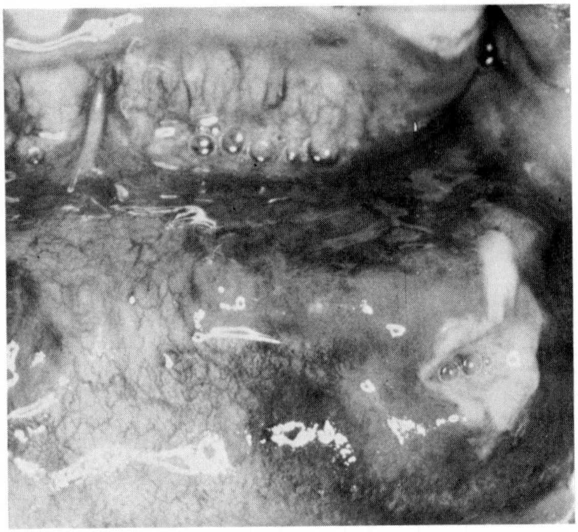

B

Fig. 291.—Aphthous ulcers in young female adults. (*A*) Minor or Mikulicz variety in left cheek. (*B*) Major variety which produces scarring in patient's vestibule. (By courtesy of Dr F. Nally.)

analgesic solution. They heal in 1–3 weeks and leave no scar.

In some women who suffer recurrent ulceration there appears to be a definite periodic rhythm, ulcers appearing at the same time in the menstrual cycle. The peak incidence has been found to be in the post-ovulation period. This may indicate a relationship between ulceration and the blood level of progesterone.

Periadenitis mucosa necrotica recurrens is the name given to the more severe form (major) of aphthous ulceration in which very painful ulcers, usually only one or two, last for weeks or months. They usually start as submucosal nodules which break down after 2–4 days to form a deep crater-like ulcer with considerable tissue destruction which heals with a scar.

Recurrent herpetiform ulcers (not related to herpes) are very small and form in large numbers in all parts of the oral mucosa (Fig. 292). They may coalesce to form a larger ulcer. They heal after about two weeks and leave no scar. They are common in Behcet's syndrome.

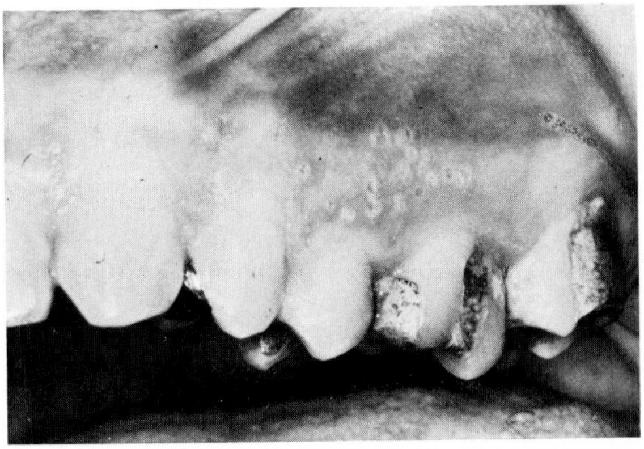

A

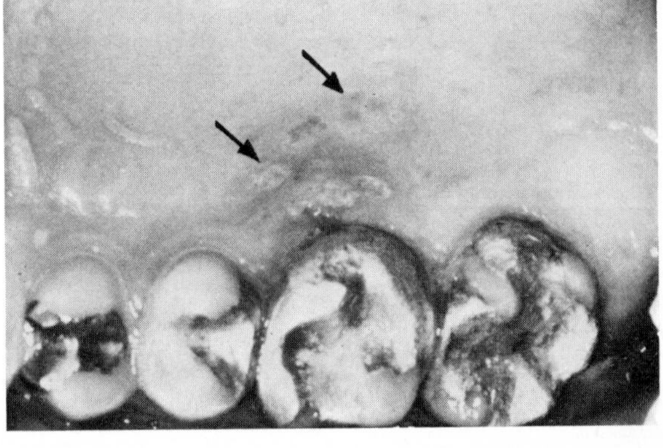

B

Fig. 292.—Herpetiform ulcers in young female during menstruation.

Treatment

Treatment is symptomatic. First the patient should be reassured about the innocence of the ulcers even though they may be painful. The commonly used applications of phenol and silver nitrate reduce the pain by destroying nerve endings, but may retard healing. Topical anaesthetics or Bonjela can be used. Frequent warm water or tetracycline mouthwashes also seem to relieve the pain temporarily and may aid healing by keeping the mouth clean. The corticosteroids are the treatment of choice for the major and minor forms of ulcer but not for the herpetiform type. A tetracycline mouthwash is advised for the latter form of ulceration (250 mg capsule emptied into a spoon of warm water and held in the mouth for two minutes, q.d.s.). No treatment is consistently successful. Two forms of corticosteroid may be used:

1. 5 mg tablets of hydrocortisone hemesuccinate (Corlan) allowed to dissolve against the lesions have occasional success; 4 tablets a day for three or four days are prescribed.
2. A cream of 0.1 per cent triamcinolone in Orabase applied frequently after drying the lesion reduces the pain and the inflammatory reaction, and shortens the healing time.

A non-steroid anti-inflammatory agent, carbenoxolone sodium used as a 2% gel (Bioral), has also proved to be effective in reducing symptoms and promoting healing in many cases.

GINGIVAL ABSCESS

This description is restricted to those abscesses which arise within the marginal tissue. It does not apply to the abscess in the deeper tissues – the periodontal abscess – which may also involve the marginal tissue.

Usually the gingival abscess is associated with physical damage to the gingival margin by such things as toothbrush bristles or fishbones, with subsequent infection of the wound. Incomplete elimination of a periodontal pocket by gingivectomy or curettage may result in an abscess which is localized to the marginal tissues.

Clinical Features

The abscess produces a localized, red and shining swelling of the gingival margin, often involving the interdental papilla. It is painful and associated teeth are sensitive to percussion. Untreated, the abscess may discharge after a day or two or, more rarely, spread into the underlying tissues to form a periodontal abscess.

Treatment

If the cause of the trouble is still present it should be removed. As the lesion is superficial drainage may be established by hot salt water mouthwashes used every two hours. If this is not effective the lesion should be incised under topical anaesthesia, ethyl chloride spray or infiltration anaesthesia.

A pocket often remains after the inflammation has subsided. If shallow this pocket may be eliminated by thorough scaling. If the pocket persists localized gingivectomy is necessary. This must be radical so that all flabby tissue is removed and a good contour achieved.

REFERENCES

EMSLIE, R. D. (1963). Cancrum oris. *Dent. Practit.*, **13**, 481.

GOLDHABER, P. and GIDDON, D. B. (1964). Present concepts concerning the etiology and treatment of acute necrotizing ulcerative gingivitis. *Int. Dent. J.*, **14**, 468.

JAFFE, E. C. and LEHNER, T. (1969). Treatment of herpetic stomatitis with iodoxuridine. *Brit. dent. J.*, **124**, 392.

KRAMER, I. R. H. (1967). Ulceration of the mouth in children. *Austr. dent. J.*, **12**, 83.

LEHNER, T. (1967). Oral candidosis. *Dent. Practit.*, **17**, 209.

MANSON, J. D. and RAND, H. (1961). Recurrent Vincent's disease. A survey of 61 cases. *Brit. dent. J.*, **110**, 386.

PINDBORG, J. J. (1956). The epidemiology of ulceromembranous gingivitis showing influence of service in the Armed Forces. *Paradontologie*, **10**, 114.

SHINN, D. L., SQUIRES, S. and MCFADZEAN, J. A. (1965). The treatment of Vincent's disease with metronidazole. *Dent. Practit.*, **15**, 275.

SHIP, I. I. (1966). Socioeconomic status and recurrent aphthous ulcers. *J. Amer. dent. Ass.*, **73**, 120.

20. Restorative and Prosthetic Procedures

Good restorative and prosthetic work is essential to the maintenance of the health of the periodontal tissues. Intelligently planned and skilfully executed restorative and prosthetic work is also required to augment periodontal procedures in the restoration to functional stability of the diseased and mutilated dentition.

No restorative or prosthetic procedure (apart from making full dentures) can be carried out without in some way effecting the periodontal tissues, and in practice this fact needs to be constantly borne in mind.

Two rules apply:

1. Avoid immediate and long-term gingival irritation. The possibility of immediate gingival damage exists at every stage of the construction of a restoration; tooth preparation, impression and restoration. Tooth form and tooth relationships act to protect the gingival margin, and the restoration of this form and relationship is important in avoiding long-term gingival irritation.
2. The occlusal load must be adjusted so that it can be absorbed by the tooth-supporting tissues in all mandibular positions and movements in normal function. Every effort must be made to reduce the total load taken by individual teeth and to ensure that the horizontal component of force, *i.e.* the torque-producing force, is minimal.

RESTORATIONS

Three aspects of restorations, whether filling, inlay or crown, must be considered in relation to periodontal health. These are the cervical margin, the crown form and the occlusion.

The Cervical Margin

In restoring a tooth with any plastic filling material accurately contoured and placed matrix bands stabilized by wedges are essential to avoid overhanging margins (Fig. 293). Firm condensation of the filling material is needed to give a surface density which will retain a high polish.

Unless the presence of caries dictates otherwise, in crown and inlay preparation the cervical margin may be placed in one of four positions – at the bottom of the crevice, between the bottom of the crevice and the gingival margin, level with the gingival margin or coronal to it (Fig. 294). *In any situation a well-defined finishing line is essential.* The advantages and disadvantages of each situation need to be considered in relation to the various stages of the restorative procedure.

1. Preparation of the margin at the bottom of the crevice is almost certainly associated with some gingival damage unless great care is taken. When copper rings are used for impression taking the periodontal fibres are certainly severed if the finishing line is to be adequately registered. Once the restoration is in position it is not possible to polish the margin. On the other hand the chances of plaque collecting around the edge are minimal providing the gingival margin has stayed healthy throughout the procedures, and the edge is hidden so that appearance should be good.
2. If the margin is prepared between the bottom of the crevice and the gingival margin a good finishing line can be prepared and registered

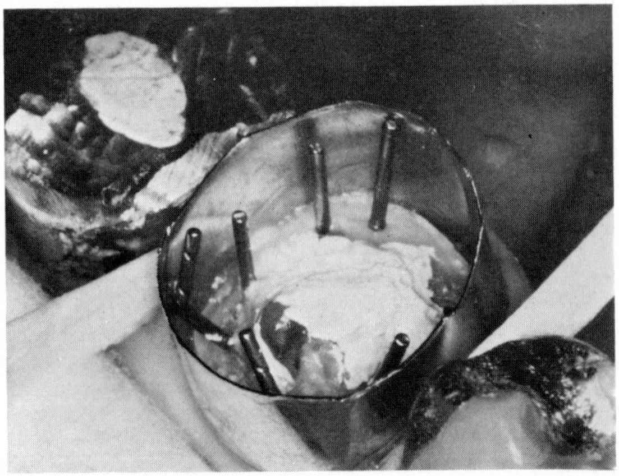

FIG. 293.—Copper ring plus wedges in position: a situation with potential for tissue damage if carelessly managed.

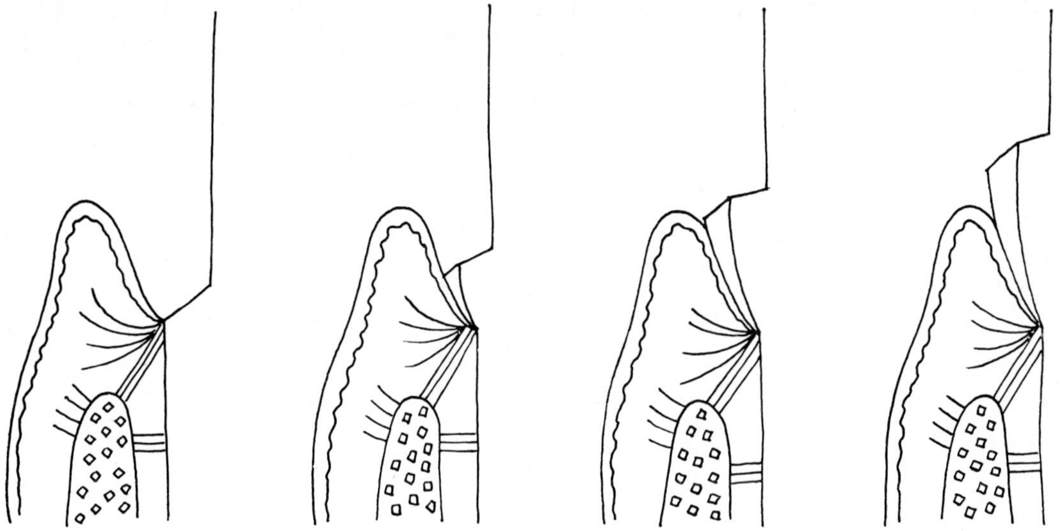

FIG. 294.—Alternative positions for margin of preparation in relation to gingiva.

even by copper-ring impression without damage to the gingiva if care is taken. The edge can be polished and although hidden by the gingival cuff is amenable to examination by a fine probe.

3. If the preparation margin is at the level of the gingival margin, preparation, impression and polishing can be easily carried out but the edge of the restoration will show and it is not protected from plaque accumulations.
4. With the margin of the restoration coronal to the gingival margin the appearance may be poor in the front of the mouth but technical procedures can be carried out with certain precision and the margin is in an area which is easy to keep clean (see Silness, 1970). If oral hygiene is poor and the patient is caries-prone, caries around the edge of the restoration is almost inevitable. However, permanent restorations of any complexity should not be placed in mouths where oral hygiene is poor and caries rampant.

It seems wise from the periodontal standpoint to use the coronally positioned margin except where appearance dictates otherwise (Fig. 295), in which case it is advisable to place the margin of the restoration between the bottom of the crevice and the gingival margin; 0.5 mm subgingival will suffice for most restorations (Johnston, Phillips and Dykema, 1971).

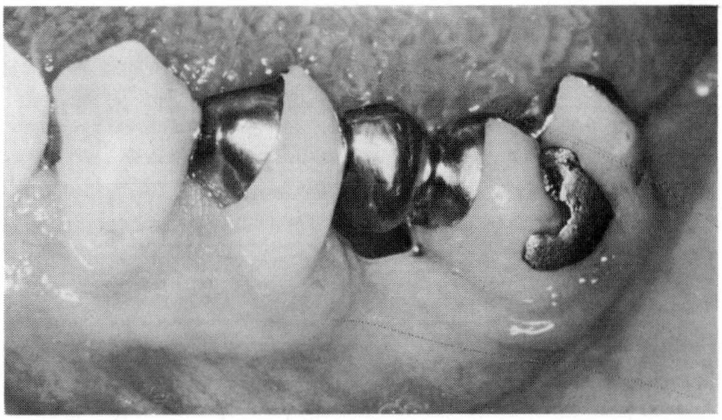

FIG. 295.—Preparation margin placed coronal to gingival margin in adult with excellent oral hygiene.

Gingival Retraction

In order to obtain an accurate impression of the cervical margin gingival retraction is frequently carried out using string or floss soaked in zinc chloride or adrenaline. In some cases several strands of string soaked in astringent are pressed into the crevice so that the tissue is separated from the tooth and the cervical margin of the preparation stands proud; it is possible that some damage can be done. Too much pressure and too strong an astringent must be avoided. If the gingival margin is healthy and not damaged by the preparation there should be little more needed than to dry the crevice. It is possible that where gingival retraction is necessary the gingival margin is not healthy and that either some inflammatory swelling or frank pocketing exists, in which case periodontal treatment should be carried out prior to the preparation and placing of a permanent restoration. If there is subgingival caries it may be necessary to carry out a localized gingivectomy prior to preparation.

Temporary Restorations

Temporary restorations are very frequently placed while permanent restorations are being constructed, or in order to sedate an inflamed pulp. Frequently little care is taken with the fit of such restorations with resulting gingival irritation and inflammation. If the temporary restoration is left in place for a few days no permanent damage may follow but where the restoration is to be left in place for some weeks it is necessary to make sure that the marginal fit is accurate. When restorations requiring complex technical work are to be carried out this should be scheduled beforehand.

Restoration of Crown Form

The facial and lingual tooth convexities protect the gingival margin in food-shedding. In carving restorations these surfaces may be under- or over-contoured. If the surfaces are under-contoured and flat the gingival margin is unprotected and will suffer constant minor irritation during mastication. If the surfaces are too bulbous a sheltered cervical area is created which may prove difficult to clean and become a repository for bacterial plaque. A balance between the two situations has to be achieved (Fig. 296), and it must be one which errs on the side of cleansability, *i.e. under-contour*.

Well-defined marginal ridges together with a carefully placed contact point are essential to protect the interdental area. A small but tight contact area between convex surfaces provides effectively self-cleansing contours and prevents food impaction. Broad flat contact areas which appear to provide considerable gingival protection rarely permit food shedding and frequently make effective patient cleansing almost impossible; food wedging is also more likely to occur. Open

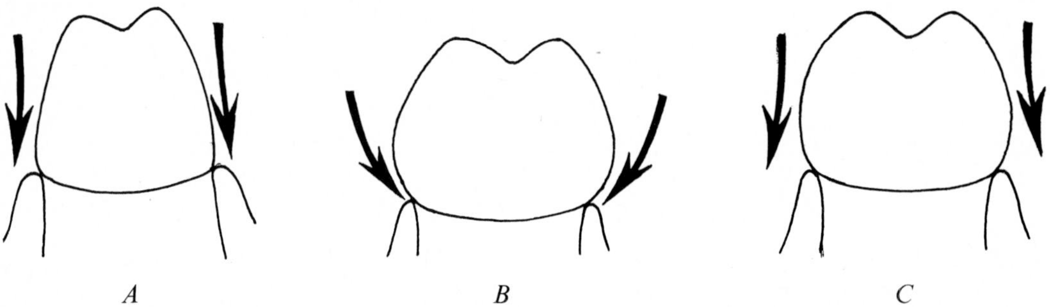

A *B* *C*

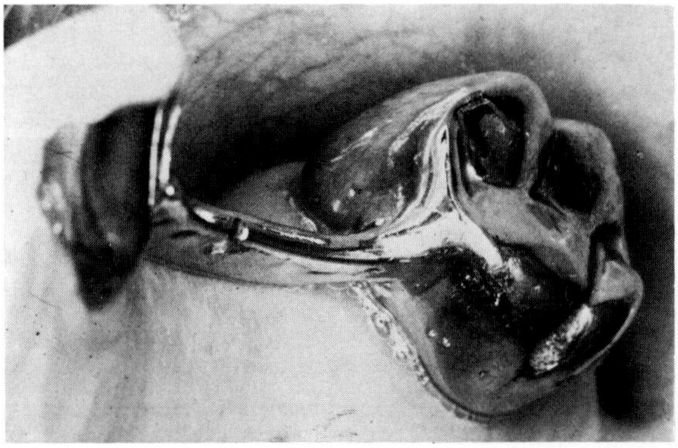

D

FIG. 296.—Crown morphology. (*A*) Under-contoured. (*B*) Over-contoured. (*C*) Acceptable morphology. (*D*) Well designed crown and well placed bar attachment.

contacts lead to food impaction. The space between two teeth has to be very wide before it becomes easy to keep clean, and cutting away interproximal surfaces is rarely successful in curing food impaction.

A common situation is one in which there is food impaction between say, first and second molars where neighbouring teeth, the third molar or second premolar or both, have been lost. No matter how tight or broad the contact is made wedging will occur followed by drifting apart of the teeth with subsequent food-packing. A solution is to link the two teeth with either crowns or inlays. In doing this the embrasure space beneath the contact needs to be made cleansable and any soldered joint must be highly polished.

The contact point is usually placed at the junction of the occlusal and middle third of the crown, but each individual situation needs to be assessed, taking into account tooth shape and its position in the arch. When malpositioned teeth are being restored the opportunity can be used to alter tooth form and contact in such a way that previously unprotected gingiva might benefit. Consideration of the final contour should not be left until the last stages of the restoration placement. Where a material needs to have a minimal thickness, *e.g.* porcelain, this must be taken into account at the time of tooth preparation otherwise the crown may be too thick and over-contoured. The width of the shoulder preparation should be 0.7–1.00 mm (Johnston, Mumford and Dykema, 1967). One of the most important and yet frequently neglected aspects of crown contour is the creation of a cleansable embrasure space. This should be big enough to receive at least the thin end of a dental woodstick (Fig. 297).

The Occlusal Surface

As described in Chapter 14 the occlusal surface of all restorations must be adjusted not only in centric occlusion but in functional excursions and positions so that disharmonies are avoided. In lateral excursions both working and balancing contacts must be scrutinized. As stated above it is advisable to examine these relationships during cavity preparation so that an adequate space for restorative material is left between the preparation and opposing teeth. In doing this it may be necessary to grind the occlusal surface of the opposing tooth. This should be carried out as part of the preparation of that part of the mouth and not as compensation for inadequate planning or preparation. The integrity of teeth as individual units or the 'sanctity' of enamel should not be allowed to interfere with the achievement of harmonious occlusal relationships. Marginal ridges and sluiceways which deflect food from the interproximal areas are essential.

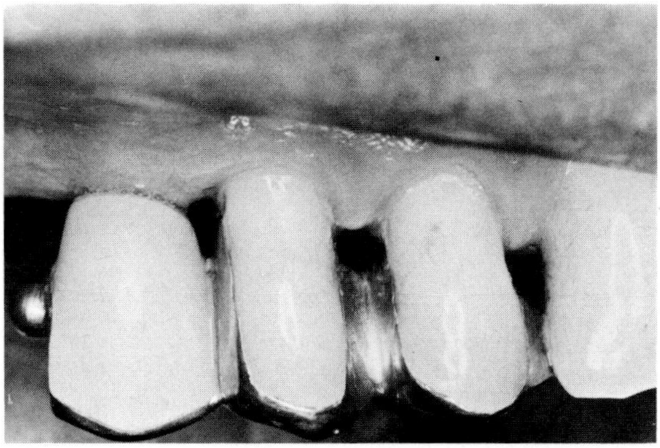

A

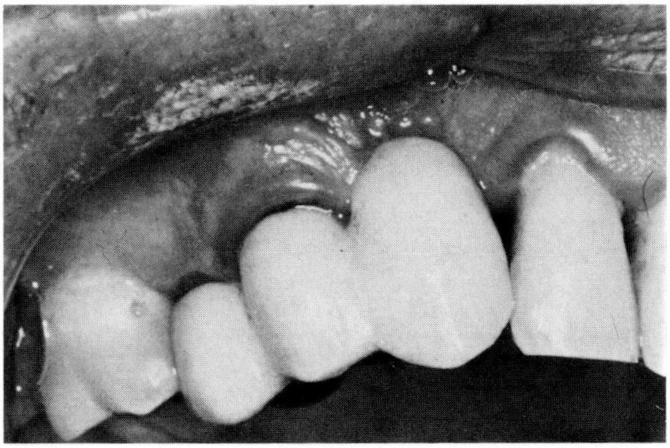

B

FIG. 297.—(*A*) Linked abutment teeth with adequate embrasure spaces. (*B*) Bridge with no embrasure spaces. Tissue damage is inevitable. (By courtesy of Dr L. Coppes.)

PROSTHESES

Provision of a prosthesis, either completely or partly tooth-borne, should not be dictated merely by the absence of teeth but by cosmetic and functional need. An appliance should improve functional efficiency by spreading the occlusal load and by helping to stabilize standing teeth. These aims apply where the supporting tissues are intact; where supporting tissue has been lost they become the main purpose of treatment.

Fixed Prostheses

Abutments

It is essential to have sufficient intact supporting tissue to bear the load of an appliance. The root surface area of the abutment teeth should be greater than that of the missing teeth. In practice this means that one should use about one and one-half abutment teeth for every tooth to be replaced. Thus a bridge to replace two teeth requires three abutment teeth.

In choosing abutment teeth the amount of bone support, the number and shape of the roots and the inclination of the roots has to be taken into account. An upper molar with three divergent roots and some bone loss (but free of pathology) may be a more effective abutment than a premolar with an intact periodontium.

In the construction of retainers, *i.e.* inlays or crowns, those points outlined above about crown shape, contacts and margins, must be observed. In designing the occlusal surfaces harmonious functional relations must be assured, and where possible the diameter of the occlusal table should be reduced to help to reduce the occlusal load and keep forces within the confines of the supporting root area.

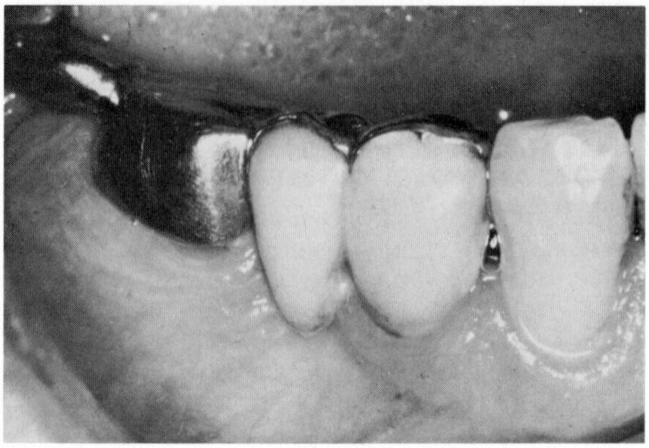

A

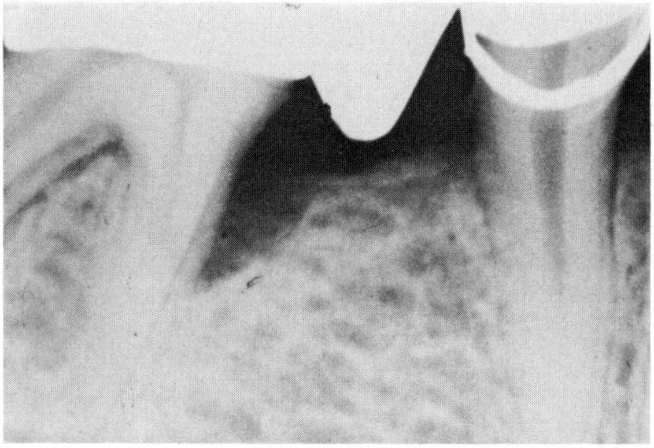

B

FIG. 298.—(*A*) Pontic impinges on gingival margin around abutment. (*B*) Resultant bone defect.

Pontics

Badly designed pontics are very frequently the cause of tissue damage, gingival inflammation, hyperplasia of the underlying mucosa and bone resorption.

Several factors may be involved (see Stein, 1966):

1. Contact with the gingival margin (Fig. 298).

   Pressure on the gingivae around abutment teeth together with the difficulty of cleaning where an adequate embrasure space is absent causes gingival inflammation and swelling which is perpetuated by consequent stagnation.
2. Excessive ridge coverage.

   A large area of ridge-lap is almost inevitable associated with some tissue irritation and hyperplasia (Fig. 299). It is a mistake to

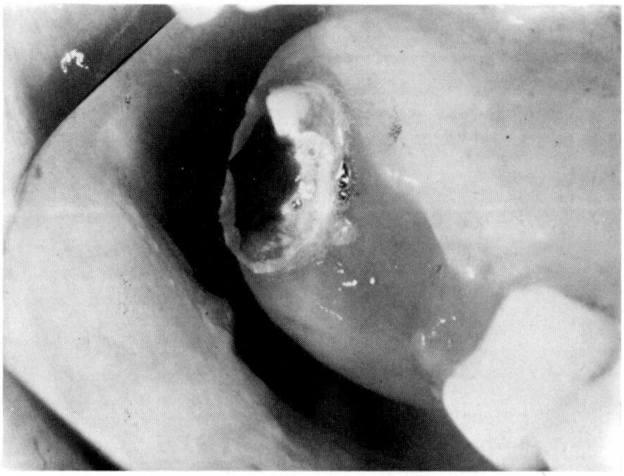

FIG. 299.—Inflamed tissue under bridge with excessive ridge-lap pontic. (By courtesy of Mr M. Saunders.)

trim the model so that the tight fit between pontic and tissue will prevent plaque accumulation. Pressure will cause underlying bone resorption and soft tissue hyperplasia around the neck of the pontic.

3. Failure to polish all surfaces.

   A rough under-surface will encourage plaque accumulation. The precise material of the pontic is not important providing it can be highly polished. The belief that acrylic is more of an irritant than porcelain derives from the failure to put as high a polish on the acrylic as the glaze confers on porcelain.

4. Inadequate food-shedding design.

   An occlusal table which is narrower than that of the abutments will act as a malposed tooth and may create a food trap behind the pontic. Also the facial and lingual sides of the occlusal tables should not be vertical but should have oblique or 'shunt' surfaces which act to deflect food.

5. Failure to eliminate periodontal disease around abutments or to remove hyperplastic mucosa over the edentulous ridge will ensure that the inflammatory process is accelerated once the prosthesis is in place.

Therefore in designing pontics the following requirements should be met:

1. All surfaces should be smooth, polished and convex. Soldered points must be polished.
2. Contact with the edentulous ridge should be minimal. Preferably there should be point contact and no pressure on the tissue (Fig. 300).
3. Embrasure spaces should be large enough to allow a wood stick or rubber tip to clean through (Fig. 297).
4. The occlusal table should be the same width as that of the abutment teeth, and food-shedding surfaces of the pontic in harmony with those of the abutments. Premature contacts must be avoided.

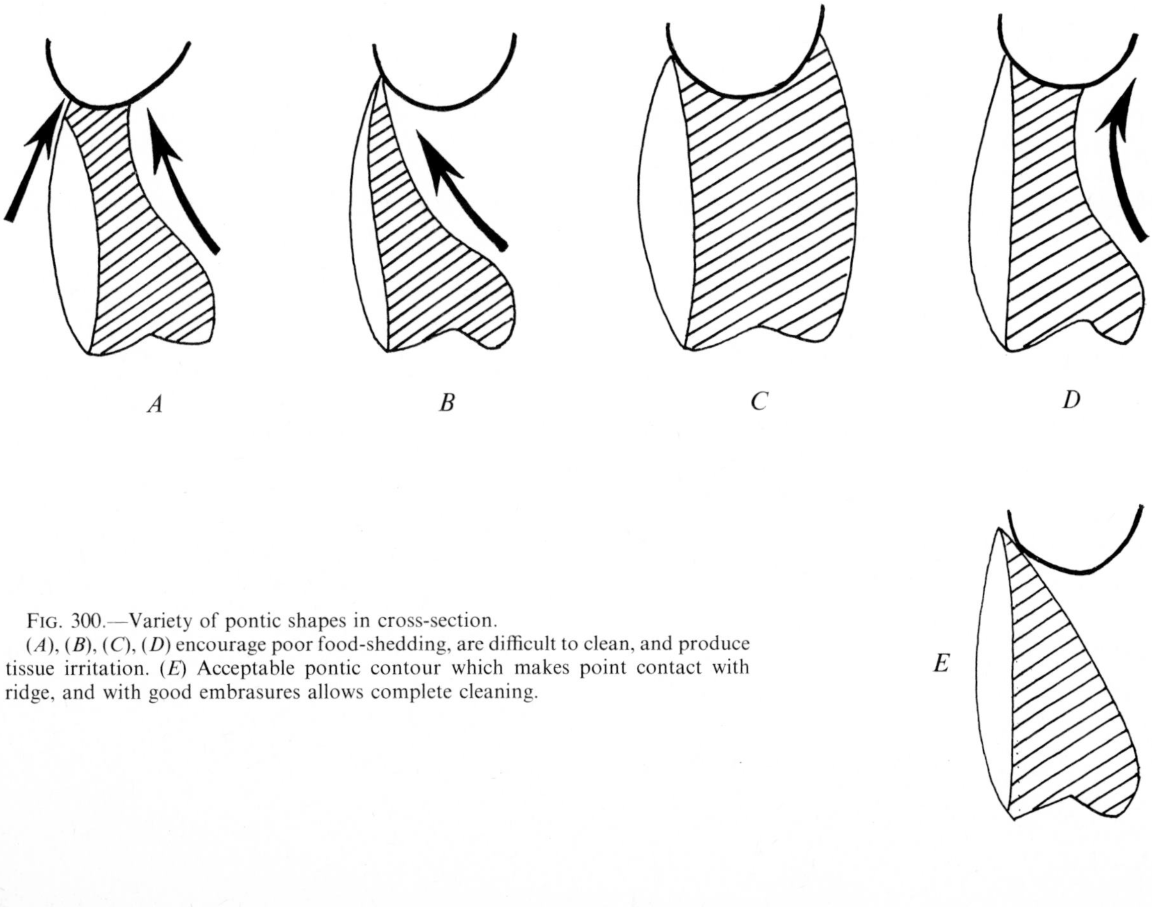

FIG. 300.—Variety of pontic shapes in cross-section.
(*A*), (*B*), (*C*), (*D*) encourage poor food-shedding, are difficult to clean, and produce tissue irritation. (*E*) Acceptable pontic contour which makes point contact with ridge, and with good embrasures allows complete cleaning.

5. All diseased tissue and enlarged fibrosed gingival margins should be removed prior to final preparation. Preparation of retainers and impressions should be made before a new gingival cuff has had time to mature. If temporary restorations are placed for any length of time these should be carefully designed so that tissue irritation does not recur. These conditions apply to both sanitary and full pontics: none of them need conflict with aesthetics. Where the vestibule is shallow sanitary pontics are essential.

Removable Prostheses

Functional stress stimulus is necessary for the health of the supporting tissues; but the line between what is an acceptable stress and overloading is difficult to define, therefore the rule must be to keep the load imposed by a prosthesis to a minimum. Attempts at the restoration of lost occlusal area should not be allowed to jeopardize the health of the periodontal tissues of remaining teeth.

A removable appliance may cause damage in several ways:

1. An inaccurate fit will result in unstable loading and therefore rocking of abutment teeth. Rocking is probably the most damaging of all forms of stress.
2. Interference on insertion and removal of the appliance frequently results from failure to survey models and establish parallelism. Stress is exerted on abutment teeth not only during insertion and removal but at all times, because the strains in the clasp and retentive arms are not balanced.
3. Pressure on or irritation to the gingival cuff of abutment teeth may be caused by the denture base or a connector arm. Inflammation and swelling occurs and if the irritant is not removed bone resorption and pocketing will follow. This also happens where a connector arm runs close to the gingival margin (Fig. 301). Any appliance in contact with the gingiva must be designed so that no pressure is exerted on the tissues, and placed so that plaque accumulation is avoided.

   Pressure on the soft tissue has two common causes: (i) carving the model – a completely unjustifiable procedure in any circumstances except for the provision of a posterior dam; and (ii) failure to use adequate occlusal rests. The soft tissues can be protected from pressure only if some part of the abutment teeth is used to take the load. The load is directed axially by carefully designed clasps and occlusal rests, and where necessary by tooth preparation. Sloping surfaces as on lower canines do not provide a stable surface and need to be prepared with a groove or ideally a restoration such as a three-quarter crown.
4. Tilting or torque-producing forces on abutment teeth may act in two planes. Mesiodistal tilting is caused most frequently where a free-end saddle denture is too short and has no posterior support from the ramus. Lateral tilting can be caused by unilateral appliances. Once tilting starts it continues with increasing rapidity. These stresses can be avoided by:
   (a) Using multiple abutment teeth.
   (b) Using abutment teeth with a wide root base, *e.g.* upper molar.
   (c) Taking the appliance around the arch.
   (d) Designing bilateral appliances (Fig. 302).
   (e) Reducing the bucco-lingual occlusal width.
   (f) Using a large basal coverage in the free-end saddle case.
   (g) Using some form of stress-breaker may reduce torque slightly but must transfer the load elsewhere, *i.e.* to soft tissue.

Precision Attachments

Precision attachments are being used increasingly and like other forms of attachment they possess the potential for tissue damage, (a) by gingival irritation and (b) by producing excessive torque.

Intracoronal attachments can be placed so that the occlusal load is directed through the tooth axis and if the attachment is placed coronally an adequate embrasure space can be produced and pressure in the gingival margin avoided. However, adequate tooth preparation is necessary to avoid over-contouring. The extracoronal attachments present a greater problem. The more coronal they are placed the less likely they are to produce stagnation and gingival irritation, but the greater the chance of producing excessive tipping forces. This load is reduced by placing the attachment more apically but if a small space is left between attachment and gingiva stagnation is inevitable (Fig. 303). The solution depends

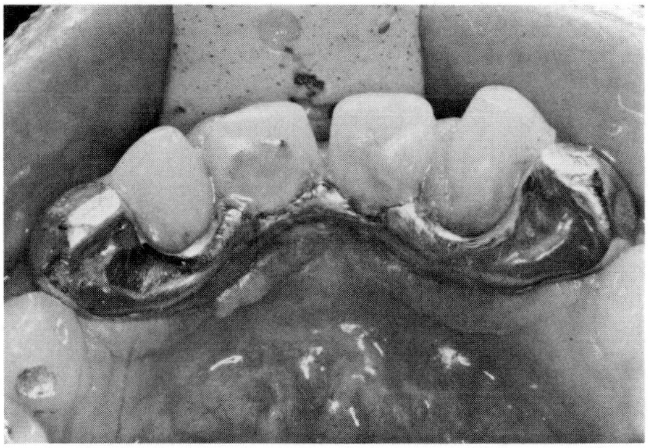

A

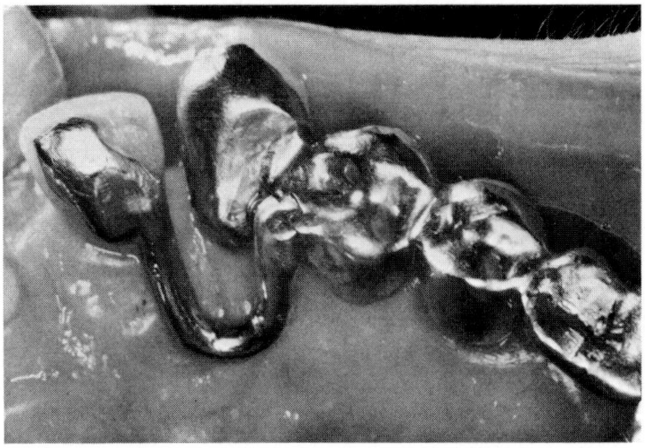

B

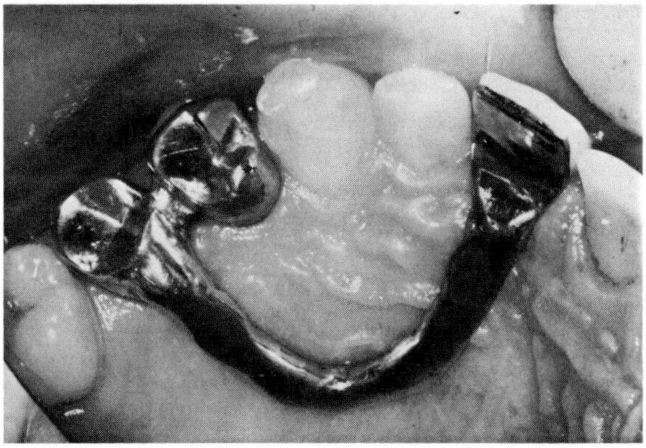

C

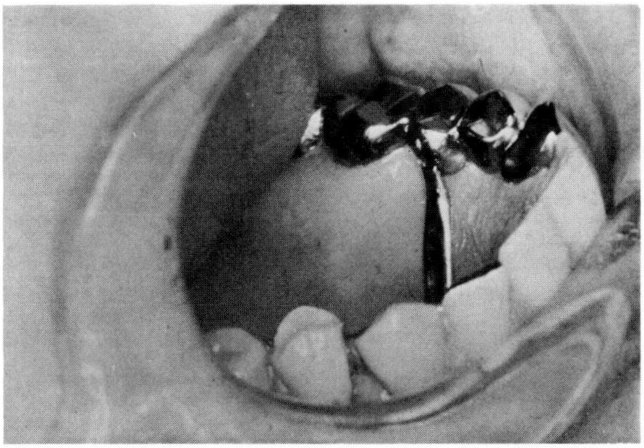

D

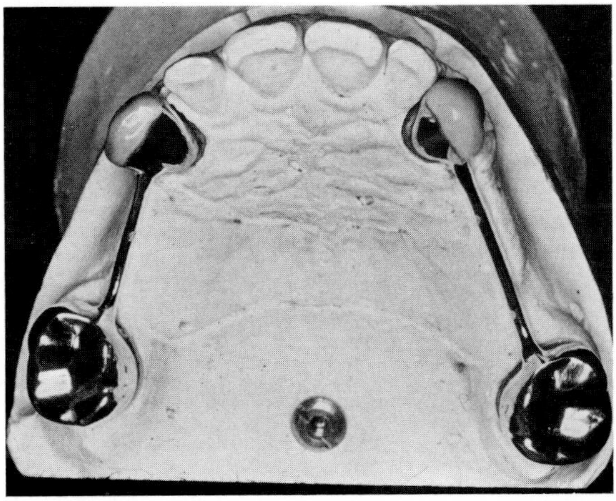

E

FIG. 301.—A variety of connector bars.

(*A*) Cantilever bridge with connector arms against gingival margin producing hyperplasia. (*B*) Connector arm minimal distance from gingival margin. (*C*) Cantilever bridge with wide clearance of gingival margin. Connector arm must be rigid to avoid springing. (*D*) Connector bar brought up to midline of abutment avoids gingival irritation. (*E*) Connector bars placed on the crests of the ridge allow cleaning.

upon crown length: if the crown is long the attachment may be placed so that the space beneath it can be cleaned: if the crown is short the attachment has to be placed touching the gingival margin without pressure and exactly at the midline of the ridge. If the situation permits placing the precision attachment on a 'fly-off' pontic rather than on the abutment tooth creates an easy to clean and non-irritant connection (Fig. 304).

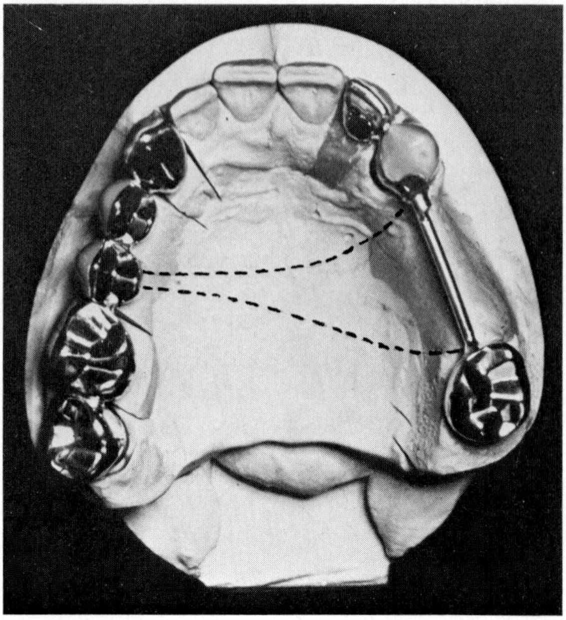

FIG. 302.—Model showing fixed and removable prosthesis in preparation. The span |456 is too long for fixed bridge and |7 is of doubtful prognosis. Provision is made in design to (*a*) give rigid mesial support to |7 without overloading, (*b*) provide easy conversion to free-end saddle if necessary. Lateral torque is counterbalanced by superstructure having palatal bar attached to fixed appliance on the right. Dolder bar is attached to |3 by Crismani attachment.

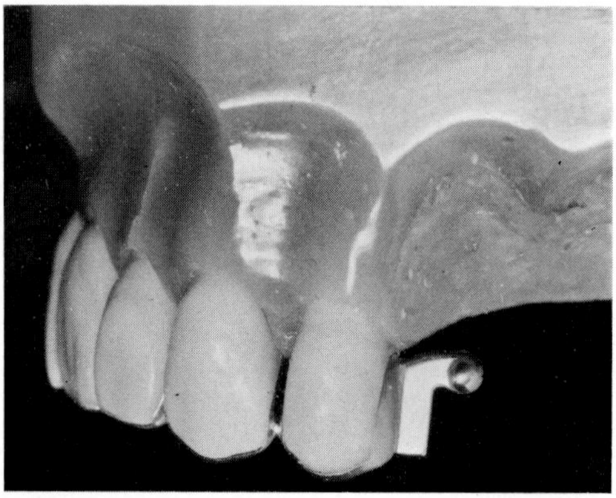

A

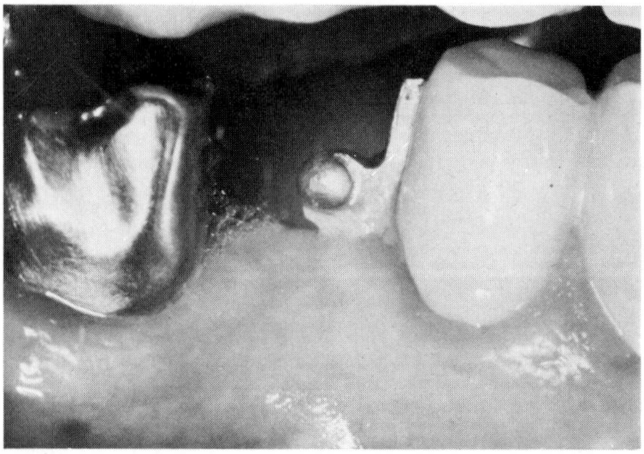

B

FIG. 303.—(*A*) Dalbo attachment on model. (*B*) Dalbo attachment close to gingival margin in mouth. If oral hygiene is not excellent stagnation is encouraged.

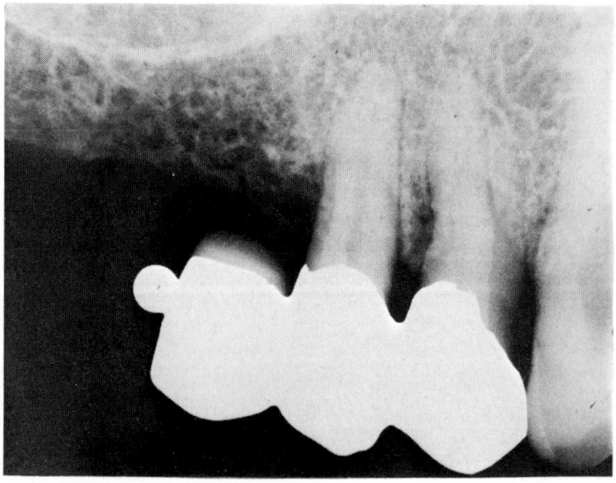

FIG. 304.—Radiograph of teeth in Fig. 297 to show fly-off pontic with precision attachment so that attachment is removed from area of gingival margin. (By courtesy of Dr L. Coppes.)

TREATMENT OF THE MUTILATED DENTITION

It is unfortunately the case that a very high proportion of all adult dentitions have suffered some mutilation, either tooth loss or loss of supporting tissue – usually both. All too frequently treatment is simply a matter of filling gaps so that more or less complete dental arches interdigitate. Then as more teeth are lost – as inevitably they must be with this kind of interference – they are replaced by additional artificial teeth until the full denture status is reached.

In the mutilated dentition teeth have drifted and tilted: haphazard contacts are made in centric occlusion and in function. With 'collapse' of the posterior segments the mandible becomes increasingly postured in a forward and elevated position so that stresses on the upper incisor teeth cause them to drift forward. It has to be kept in mind that 1 mm reduction in posterior height may bring about 3 mm increase in anterior over-bite. As supporting tissue is lost functional stresses become excessive and tooth mobility and drifting accelerate.

In attempting to conserve the mutilated dentition it is necessary to make the best use of the tissues present, *i.e.* the teeth and supporting tissues. Whatever form of appliance is employed the amount of supporting tissue cannot be increased to any significant extent unless large areas of oral mucosa are covered, and even where a partly tissue-borne appliance is used the major part of the load must be taken by the abutment teeth otherwise bone resorption under the appliance may take place.

In using the teeth present an attempt is made to create a stress-system which will allow each unit of supporting tissue to absorb its load. This is done by altering tooth form and bracing teeth against each other in such a way that the torque-producing forces are counterbalanced and the resultant load is directed through the long axes of the abutment teeth.

The management of the various problems presented by the mutilated dentition includes:

1. An improvement in jaw relationships.
   There should be:
   (a) simultaneous contact in centric occlusion.
   (b) an acceptable vertical dimension and freeway space.
   (c) multiple contacts and free movement in functional excursions: balancing contact is not desirable.

   Where forward posturing of the mandible is evident this should be corrected by restoration of the posterior segments. In doing this it is advisable to use temporary acrylic appliances, either as fixed bridgework or removable prostheses, which can be ground down or otherwise adjusted until an acceptable mandibular position is reached. This must be tested over a period of several weeks to ensure that the mandibular position and movements are commensurate with normal muscle tone.
2. Reduction in stress on incisor teeth. This is achieved by repositioning the mandible down and back and by a reduction in length of upper incisor crown and alteration of incisal edge inclination. Frequently appearance is improved by these procedures but where appearance and optimum function are not compatible some compromise has to be reached.
3. The load on the abutment teeth should be brought within the confines of the root area.
   This may be produced by:
   (a) reducing the occlusal table on abutment restorations and pontics.
   (b) orthodontic treatment to alter tooth angulation so that the occlusal load is axial.
4. Incorporate as large a number of teeth as possible within the appliance whether this is removable or fixed. Facio-lingual torque-producing forces are counterbalanced by taking appliances 'around the arch', *i.e.* across the canine tooth, or by making the appliance bilateral. This is known as cross-arch stabilization. Thus where an upper second premolar and first and second molars are missing a rigid bar between the first premolar and third molar will give mesial support to the latter tooth but will not counterbalance lateral forces. Root morphology is also inadequate for this purpose, which has therefore to be achieved by incorporating the canine and incisors in the appliance, or by taking a palatal bar across to abutments on the other side (Fig. 302).
5. Individual restorations and pontics must be designed as described to protect the gingival margin, allow effective oral hygiene measures,

and thus avoid tissue irritation and further breakdown.

In order to meet these requirements it is essential to collect all possible information from a comprehensive oral examination, reliable radiographs and study models. Frequently there is more than one way of rehabilitating a mutilated dentition: without careful consideration of the advantages and disadvantages of each approach any stability achieved may well be temporary.

REFERENCES

Johnston, J. F., Mumford, G. and Dykema, R. W. (1967). Modern Practice in Dental Ceramics. Saunders, Philadelphia, p. 171.

Johnston, J. F., Phillips, R. W. and Dykema, R. W. (1971). Modern Practice in Crown and Bridge Prosthodontics, 3rd ed. Saunders, Philadelphia, p. 393.

ADDITIONAL READING

Carlsson, G. E., Hedegard, B. and Koivumaa, K. K. (1965). Studies in partial dental prosthesis. IV. Final results of a 4-year longitudinal investigation of dentogingivally supported partial dentures. *Acta odont. scand.*, **23**, 443.

Hildebrand, G. Y. (1937). Studies in dental prosthetics, I–II. *Svensk tandläk.-T.*, **30**, Suppl.

Hirschfeld, I. (1930). Food impaction. *J. Amer. dent. Ass.*, **17**, 1504.

Hirschfeld, I. (1937). The individual missing tooth: a factor in dental and periodontal disease. *J. Amer. dent. Ass.*, **24**, 67.

Kahn, A. E. (1960). Partial versus full coverage. *J. prosth. Dent.*, **10**, 167.

Kahn, A. E. (1965). Considerations in the use of partial and full coverage in periodontal prosthesis. *J. prosth. Dent.*, **15**, 83.

Kydd, W. L., Dutton, D. A. and Smith, D. W. (1964). Lateral forces exerted on abutment teeth by partial dentures. *J. Amer. dent. Ass.*, **68**, 859.

Löe, H. and Silness, J. (1963). Tissue reaction to string packs used in fixing restorations. *J. prosth. Dent.*, **13**, 318.

Marcum, J. S. (1967). The effect of crown marginal depth upon gingival tissue. *J. prosth. Dent.*, **17**, 479.

Mosteller, J. H. (1953). The relation between operative dentistry and periodontal disease. *J. Amer. dent. Ass.*, **47**, 6.

Rosen, H. and Gitnick, P. J. (1964). Integrating restorative procedures into the treatment of periodontal disease. *J. prosth. Dent.*, **14**, 343.

Silness, J. (1970). Periodontal treatment in patients treated with dental bridges. 3. The relationship between the location of the crown margin and the periodontal condition. *J. periodont. Res.*, **5**, 225.

Stein, R. S. (1966). Pontic-residual ridge relationship: a research report. *J. prosth. Dent.*, **16**, 251.

Waerhaug, J. (1960). Histologic considerations which govern where the margins of restorations should be located in relation to the gingiva. *Dent. Clin. N. Amer.*, March, 161.

Wagman, S. S. (1965). Tissue management for full cast veneer crowns. *J. prosth. Dent.*, **15**, 106.

Wheeler, R. C. (1961). Complete crown form and the periodontium. *J. prosth. Dent.*, **11**, 722.

21. Instruments

A large variety of periodontal instruments are available. By trial and error the practitioner will come to select from these a small number which he prefers. The following description is meant as a guide to help in that selection.

POCKET MEASURING PROBES

These instruments should be slender, round-ended and highly polished with millimetre marking which is clearly visible in the mouth.

Several types are available including the Williams probe, the Fox probe, and the Ash patterns Nos. 1 and 2 (Fig. 305). The Ash pattern is rather thick and is difficult to use with accuracy where the pocket wall is fibrous and well adapted to the tooth surface. The Williams probe is slender and probably the most reliable.

The Cross Calculus Probe (Fig. 306) has been designed especially for the detection of fine particles of calculus, and is particularly useful in subgingival scaling.

Pocket Marking Forceps (Modified Crane-Kaplan type) (Fig. 307). A pair of right and left forceps is used for marking the bottom of the periodontal pocket before gingivectomy.

SCALERS AND CURETTES

Scaling instruments can be divided roughly into three basic types, the sickle, the curette and the hoe.

Cumine Scalers (Fig. 308). These are useful instruments for removing gross supragingival calculus, but their blades are large and set in line with the handle, thus limiting their application in

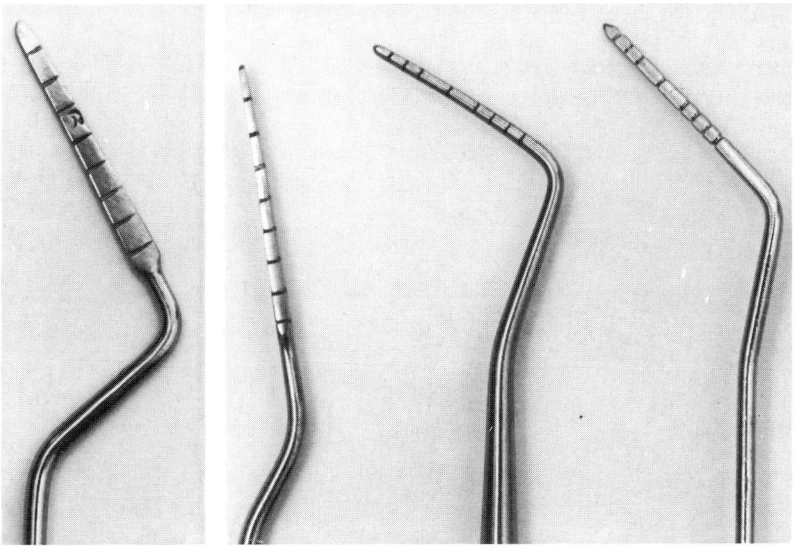

A *B* *C* *D*

FIG. 305.—Pocket measuring probes. (*A*) and (*B*) the Ash pattern Nos. 1 and 2. (*C*) the Williams probe. (*D*) the Fox probe.

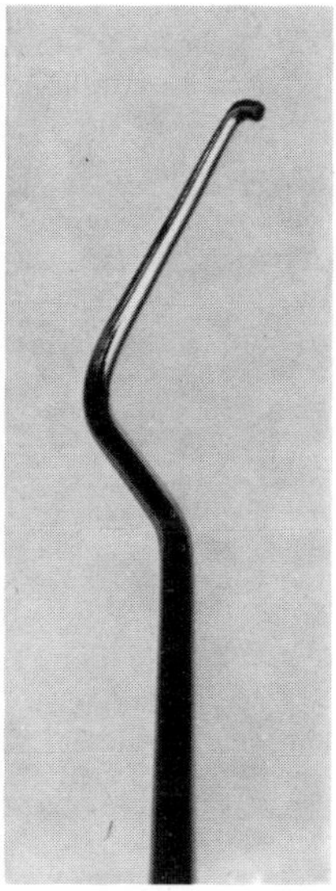

FIG. 306.—The Cross calculus probe.

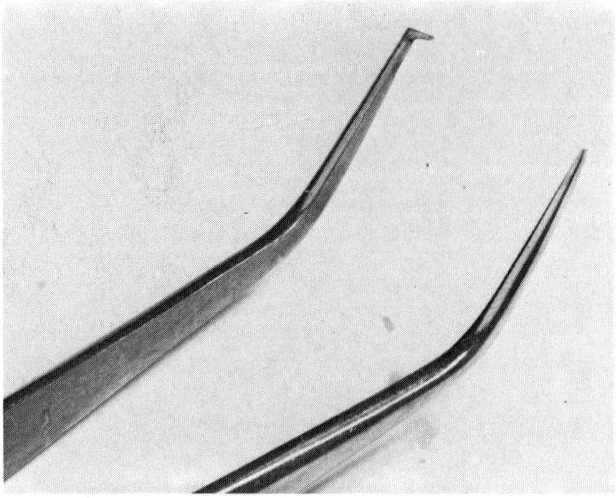

FIG. 307.—Pocket marking forceps.

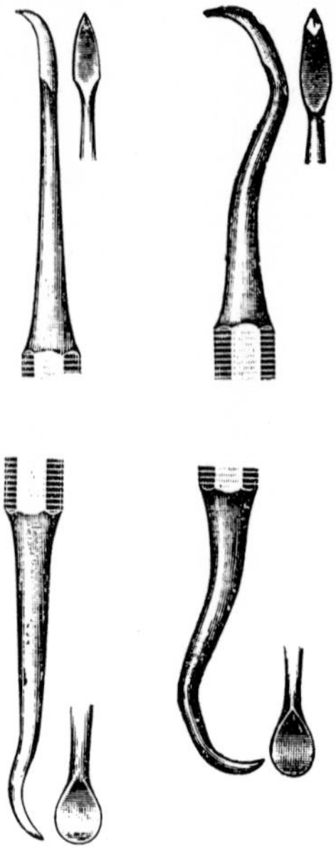

FIG. 308.—The Cumine scaler.

many parts of the mouth.

Jaquette Scalers (Fig. 309). These are sickle type scalers. The blades of these instruments are triangular in cross-section and small enough to be used for the removal of subgingival calculus. They are available in sets of three: a right and left pair with angulated shanks and an instrument with a straight shank. Access to most tooth surface is possible. They are obtainable in tungsten carbide steel in a large and miniature size. The latter is preferred by the author.

The Chisel Scaler (Watch-Spring, Push or Zerfing Scaler) (Fig. 310). This instrument, which is available in several widths, is useful for removing both supragingival and subgingival calculus from proximal tooth surfaces in the front of the mouth.

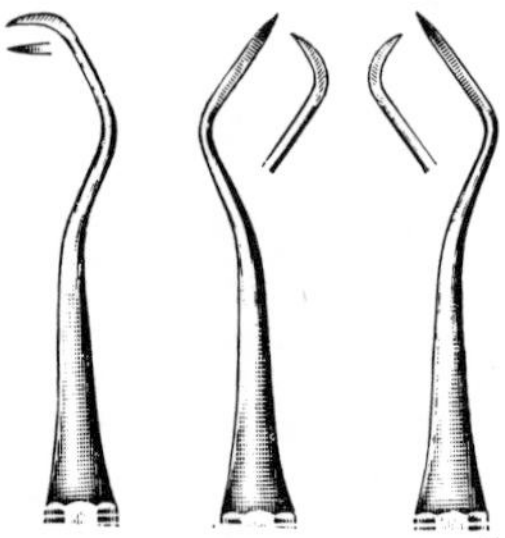

FIG. 309.—Jaquette scalers.

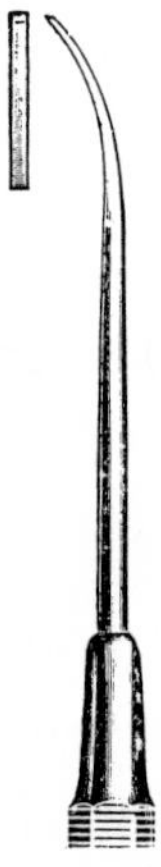

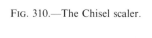

FIG. 310.—The Chisel scaler.

Periodontal Hoes (Fig. 311). These are available in sets of four instruments, each shank angulated differently so that all tooth surfaces may be reached. They are obtainable with tungsten carbide steel blades which retain their sharpness for many months. This is a considerable advantage as the standard steel hoe is a very difficult instrument to sharpen. Also the tungsten carbide blade can be made very much smaller than the blade of the standard hoe, which allows it to be inserted more deeply into the periodontal pocket.

Younger-Good Scalers (Fig. 312). These curette type instruments are very useful for both subgingival scaling and subgingival curettage. They are available in sets of five instruments: four with curette blades set at various angles on the shank; the fifth is a slim modified sickle shape. Two of these, Nos. 72 and 73, are most useful. They are obtainable in tungsten carbide steel.

McCall Curettes (Fig. 313). These are fine curettes available as two pairs of right and left instruments. They are very well designed for subgingival curettage in all regions of the mouth, and are obtainable in tungsten carbide steel.

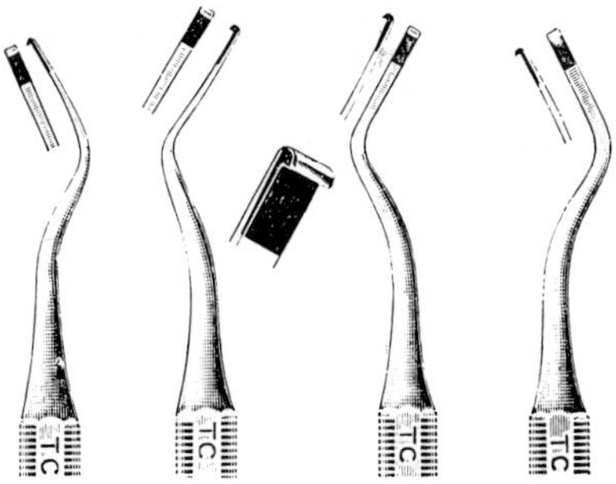

FIG. 311.—Periodontal hoes.

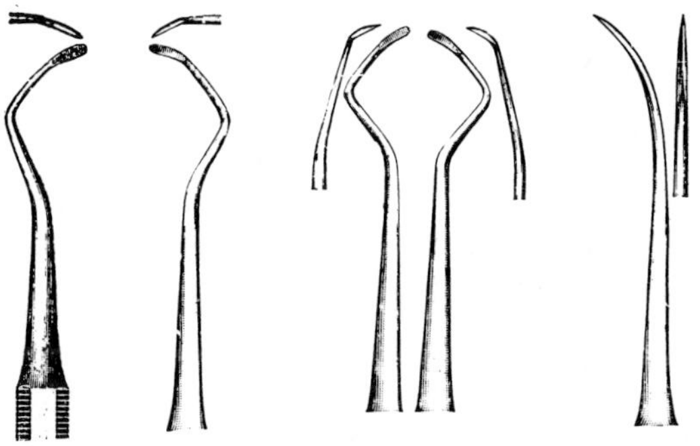

FIG. 312.—Younger-Good scalers.

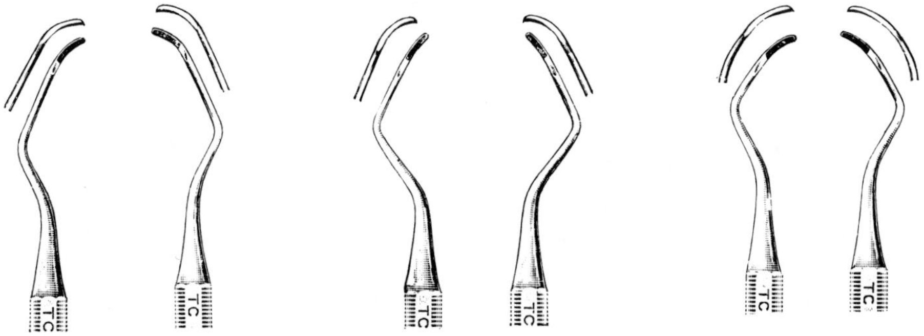

FIG. 313.—McCall curettes.

Hygienist Scalers (Fig. 314). This is a set of seven subgingival scalers of various shapes. Two are chisel scalers of different widths; three have very fine blades the same shape as the Jaquette scaler; two are very fine sickles.

The Ultrasonic Scaler (page 73). Over a decade ago ultrasonic energy was first used in the preparation of tooth cavities. More recently an ultrasonic unit (the Cavitron) has been designed primarily for scaling. The unit transmits vibra-

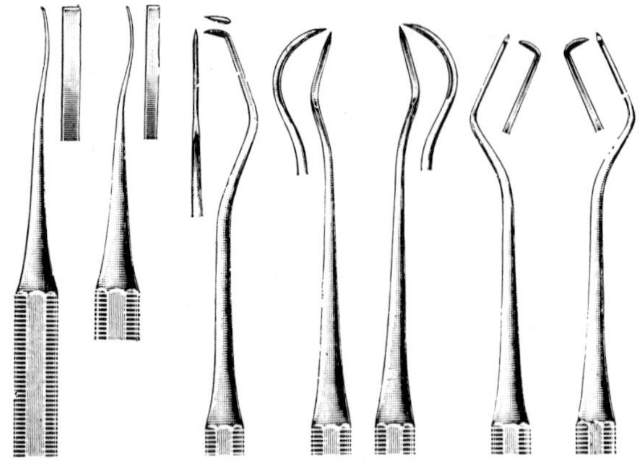

FIG. 314.—Hygienist scalers.

tions of 25,000–29,000 cycles/sec. to special stainless steel tips which are cooled by a water spray. The tips are either chisel or curette shaped, and in action are stroked lightly over the surface of the tooth. The vibration dislodges the calculus which is flushed away by the spray.

Heavy deposits of supragingival calculus and stain are rapidly removed with little fatigue to either operator or patient, and many patients prefer the ultrasonic to the conventional scaler. Copper cement remaining on teeth after the removal of a splint is also easily removed (Fig. 315) and overhanging edges of fillings are efficiently cut down and polished. The thorough removal of subgingival calculus requires all the care and time of conventional scaling, and the loss of tactile sense in using the vibrating instrument means that some deposits may be left. These have to be

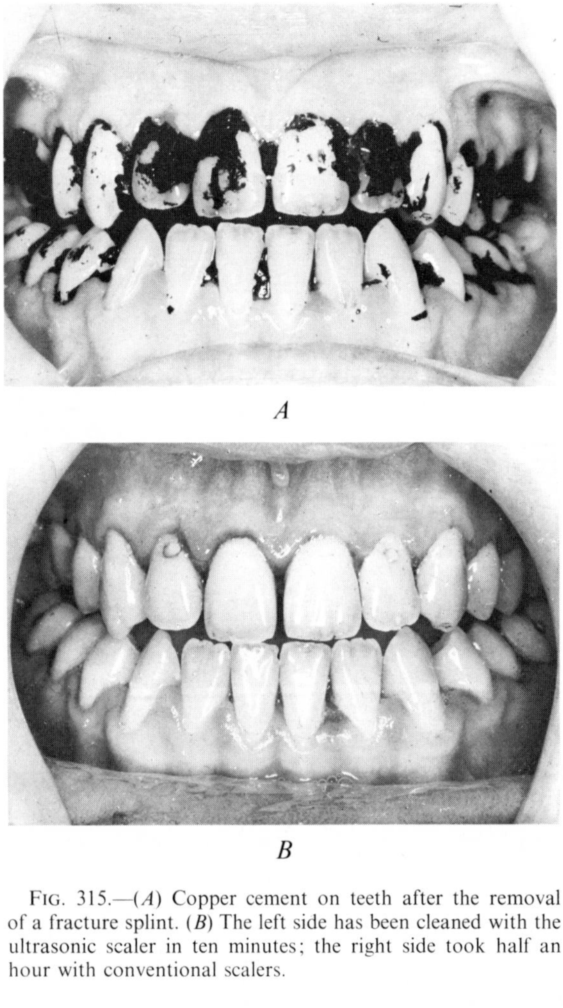

FIG. 315.—(*A*) Copper cement on teeth after the removal of a fracture splint. (*B*) The left side has been cleaned with the ultrasonic scaler in ten minutes; the right side took half an hour with conventional scalers.

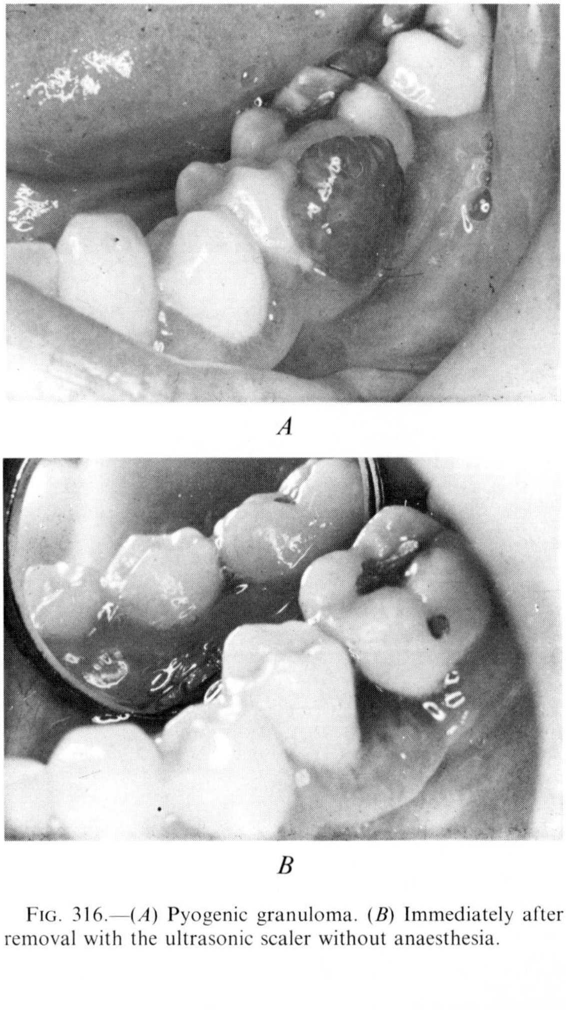

FIG. 316.—(*A*) Pyogenic granuloma. (*B*) Immediately after removal with the ultrasonic scaler without anaesthesia.

removed by the conventional scaler. Efficient suction is essential to the use of the instrument. It may also be used to advantage in the treatment of Vincent's disease, and even for the removal of soft tissue (Fig. 316).

With practice the use of the ultrasonic scaler causes no more tooth damage than conventional scaling. By relieving the operator of fatigue the ultrasonic scaler would seem to be very suitable for use by dental hygienists.

PERIODONTAL KNIVES

Making an incision with the correct bevel presents special problems in many parts of the mouth. A number of knives have been designed for this purpose, and the following list is by no means complete.

The Kirkland Knife (Fig. 317). This is a very well-designed instrument which the writer uses routinely. The blade is scalene shaped with a cutting edge all round its periphery. The shank is angulated so that the left and right pair of knives can make a correct incision in all parts of the mouth. The one disadvantage is that these instruments must be sharpened regularly.

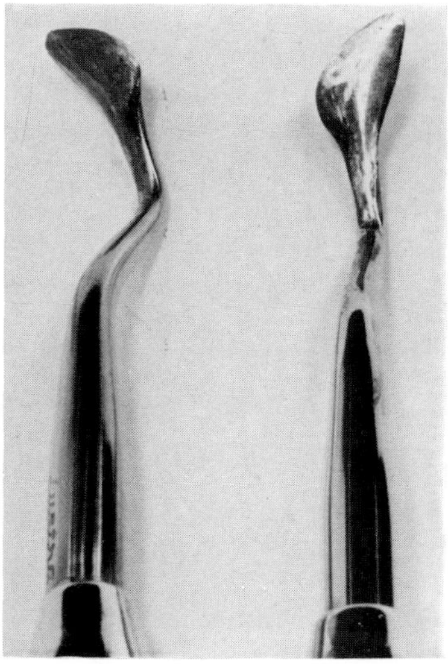

FIG. 317.—Kirkland knives.

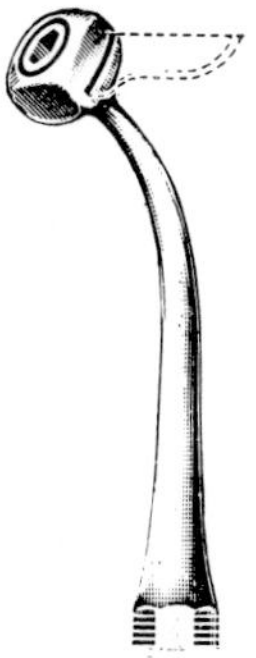

FIG. 318.—The Universal (Blake) knife.

The Universal (Blake) Knife (Fig. 318). This is an ingeniously designed instrument which makes use of standard Swann-Morton or Bard-Parker scalpel blades. Two instruments are required so that the blades may be set at opposing angles to make access possible to all parts of the mouth. They have the very real advantage of using disposable blades so that sharpening is unnecessary. Because the cutting edge of the blade is at right-angles to the handle, and therefore to the operator's arm, it takes some practice to use them efficiently and, as they are fairly broad from scalpel tip to handle back, their use at the correct angle is difficult if the vestibule is shallow.

The Swann-Morton Blades (Fig. 319). On a Swann-Morton scalpel the No. 12 blade can be

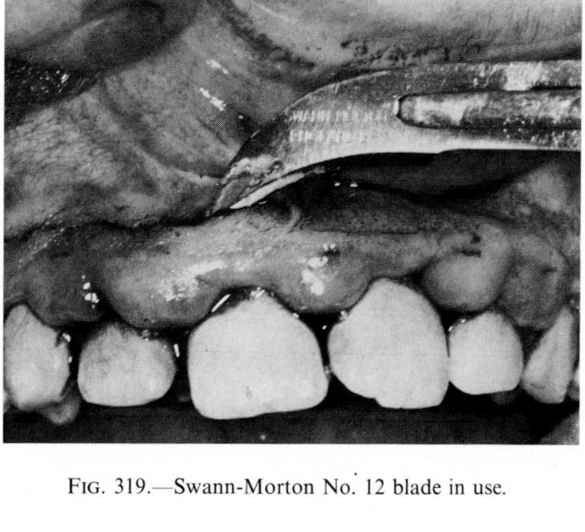

FIG. 319.—Swann-Morton No. 12 blade in use.

used to make an excellent gingivectomy incision on all labial and buccal surfaces. It is sickle-shaped with the cutting edge on the inside of the curve so that it conforms to the tooth surface. The pointed end of the blade can be inserted deep into interdental areas so that papillae are completely incised. The blade is narrow from back to front and can be used at the correct angle even where the vestibule is shallow, as it is in the lower molar region. The No. 11 blade is useful for making an inverse bevel incision in the front of the mouth. The No. 15 blade is the standard scalpel blade which with practice can be used for most incisions except those going behind the last molar. Disposable sterile handles and blades are obtainable.

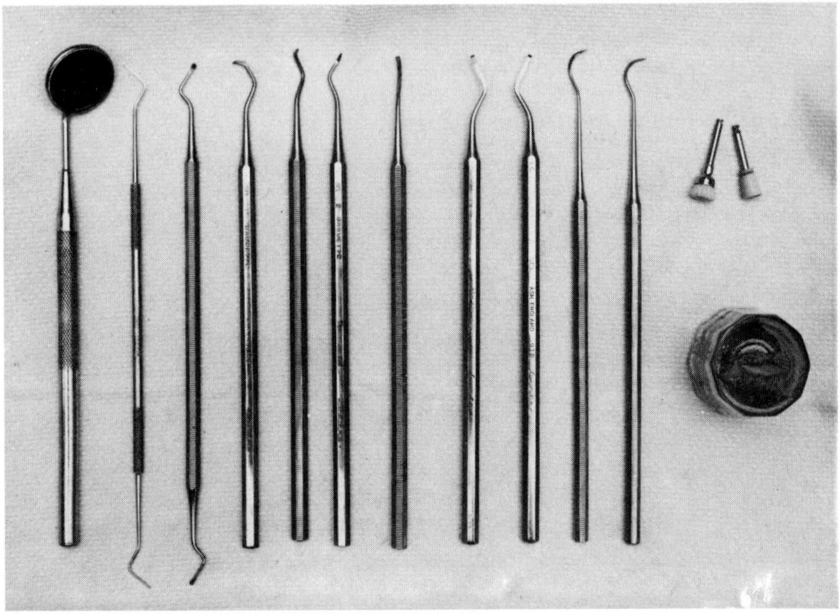

FIG. 320.—Tray of instruments for scaling.

EXAMPLE TRAYS

The following sets of instruments for use in periodontal procedures are given as a guide.

Scaling

Set A (Fig. 320)
Mirror
Probe
Small spoon excavator
Jaquette scalers 1, 2, 3
G.1 push scaler
Tungsten carbide hoes 212, 213
Hygienist sickle scalers, H6, H7
Small cup bristle brush
Rubber polishing cup
Prophylactic paste
(Curettes are added if pockets are deep.)

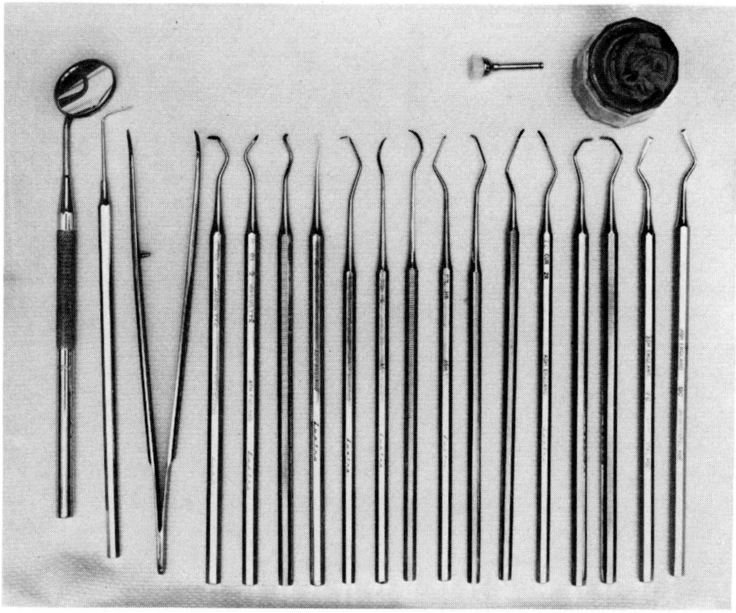

FIG. 321.—Tray of instruments for scaling.

Set B (Fig. 321)
Mirror
Probe
College tweezers
Jaquette scalers
G.1 push scaler
Hygienist scalers
McCall's tungsten carbide curettes 2R, 2L
Tungsten carbide hoes 210, 211, 212, 213
Small cup bristle brush
Prophylactic paste

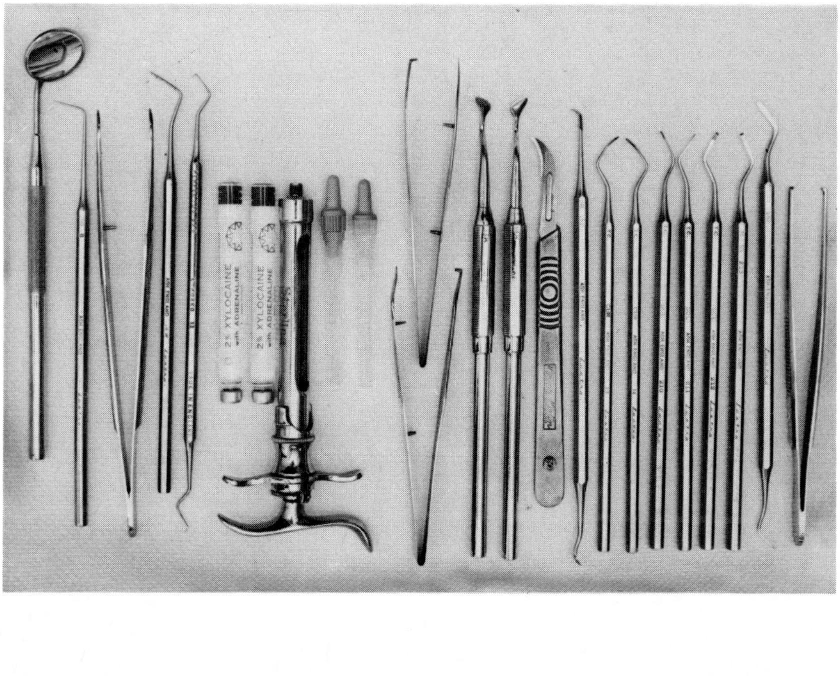

FIG. 322.—Tray of instruments for gingivectomy.

Gingivectomy (Fig. 322)
- Mirror
- Straight probe
- College tweezers
- Briault probe
- Williams pocket measuring probe
- Two 2 cc cartridges of local anaesthetic solution
- Hypodermic syringe with disposable needles
- Kirkland knives
- Swann-Morton scalpel with No. 12 blade
- Cumine scaler
- McCall's tungsten carbide curettes 13, 14
- Tungsten carbide hoes 210, 211, 212, 213
- Flat plastic instrument
- Tissue tweezers

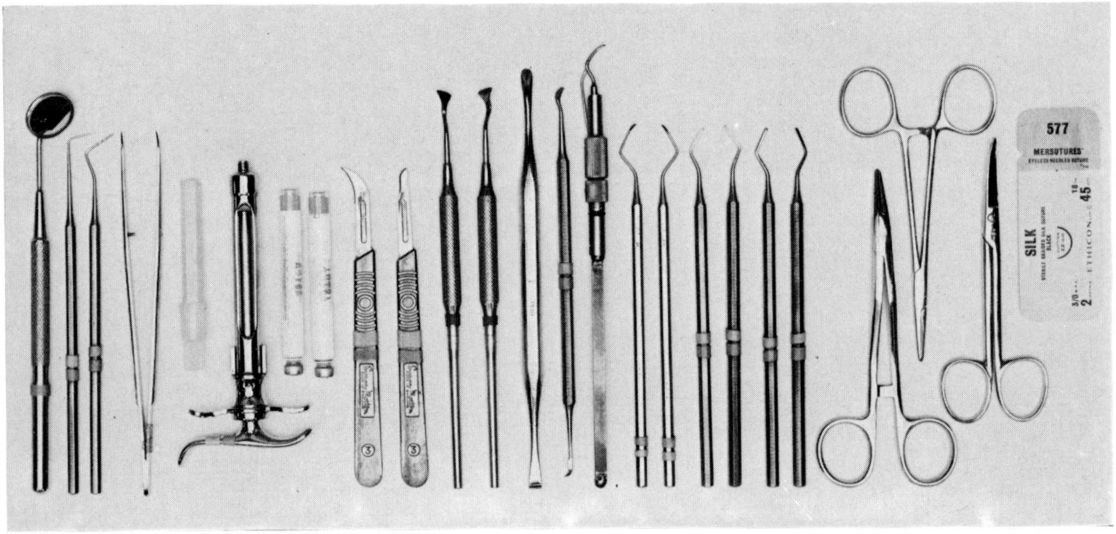

FIG. 323.—Tray of instruments for curettage at open operation (flap operation).

Flap Operation (Fig. 323)
- Mirror
- Probes
- College tweezers
- Hypodermic syringe with disposable needle
- Two 2 cc cartridges of local anaesthetic solution
- Scalpels with Nos. 15 and 12 blades
- Kirkland knives
- Periosteal elevator
- Cumine scaler
- Ultrasonic curette tip
- McCall's tungsten carbide curettes 13, 14
- Tungsten carbide hoes 210, 211, 212, 213
- Needle holder
- Mosquito artery forceps
- Pointed scissors
- Ethicon Mersuture No. 577 3/0 silk.

INSTRUMENT STERILIZATION

All instruments should be scrubbed clean before sterilization.

In the absence of an autoclave or dry heat oven, instruments should be immersed in boiling water for 20 minutes.

Instruments which might lose their cutting edge in boiling may be sterilized in solutions of Hibitane. After immersion in solution A for 20 minutes they are stored in solution B. The two solutions may be easily distinguished by making up with different colouring agents. Solutions must be renewed regularly.

Solution A

100 ml 5 per cent chlorhexidine gluconate B.P.C.
150 ml distilled water
750 ml industrial methylated spirits
} per litre

Solution B

10 ml 5 per cent chlorhexidine gluconate B.P.C.
1 gm sodium nitrite
990 ml distilled water
} per litre

INSTRUMENT SHARPENING

Cutting instruments, *i.e.* scalers, curettes and gingivectomy knives, need to be sharpened regularly. Blunt scalers and curettes are inefficient and time-wasting; blunt gingivectomy knives will tear the tissues and retard healing. The introduction of tungsten carbide steel blades for hoes and curettes has lightened this burden, but even tungsten carbide will blunt and, as a special stone is necessary for regrinding the blades, the instruments have to be returned to the manufacturer.

Instruments may be sharpened by hand using a lubricated stone which fits the surface of the instrument. Thus a sickle-shaped instrument is sharpened on a cylindrical stone by drawing the stone several times across the cutting surface of the instrument (Fig. 324). Instruments with flat cutting surfaces, *e.g.* Jaquette or Hygienist scalers, can be sharpened on a flat slip of stone, but it is easier to sharpen them with a rotating sandpaper disc.

Hoes are sharpened on a flat stone with short backward and forward strokes, the instrument being held so that the surface of the blade contacts the stone evenly.

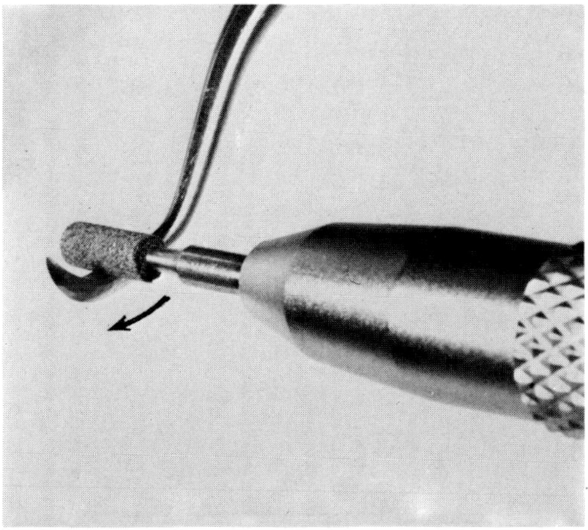

A

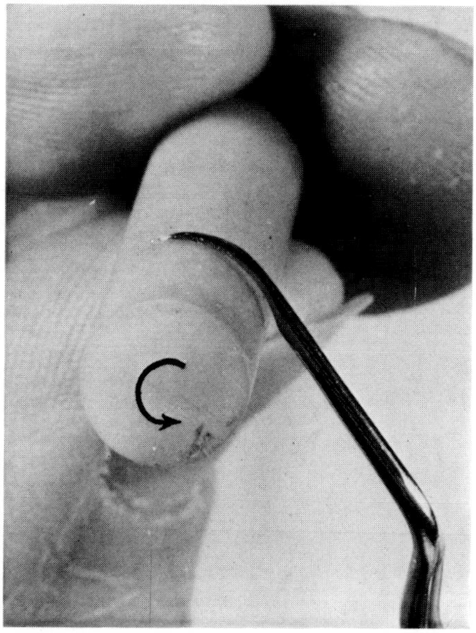

B

FIG. 324.—Sharpening curved instruments. (*A*) With a rotating stone. (*B*) With an oiled Arkansas stone.

Kirkland knives are sharpened by rotating sandpaper discs or on a flat block with small circular movements (Fig. 325). Each side of the blade is sharpened in turn. It is advisable to sharpen these instruments after every gingivectomy and with practice this can be done very quickly.

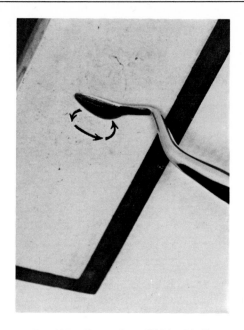

FIG. 325.—Sharpening a Kirkland knife.

Index